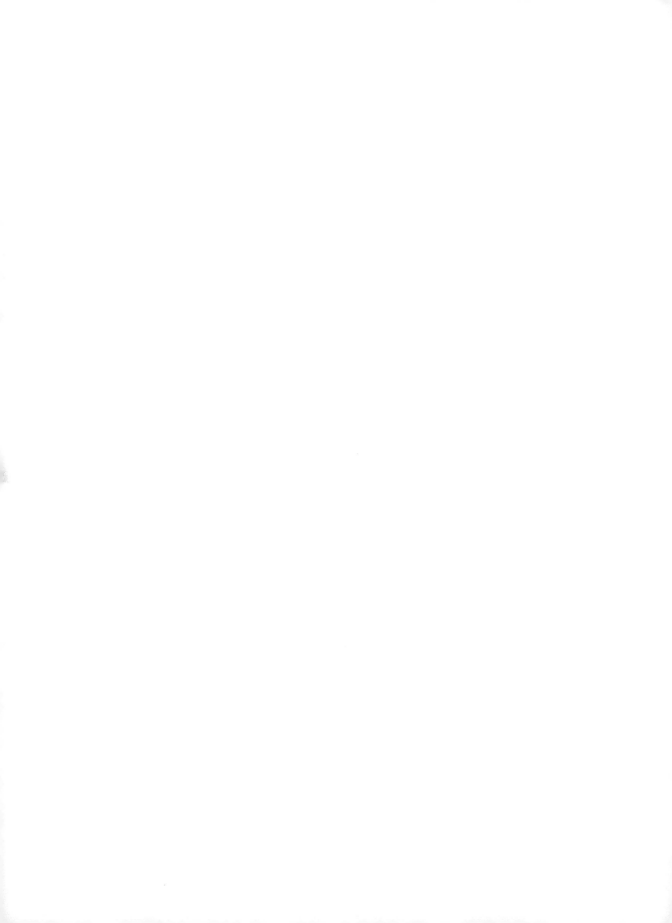

Peripheral Vascular Stenting

This textbook is dedicated to my wife Shari, the research staff at Saint Joseph's Hospital, and the staff at the Phoenix Heart Center.

Peripheral Vascular Stenting

Editors
Richard R Heuser
Giancarlo Biamino

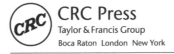

CRC Press
Taylor & Francis Group
Boca Raton London New York

CRC Press is an imprint of the
Taylor & Francis Group, an **informa** business

Contents

Contents

Contributors

J Michael Bacharach MD MPH FACC
Section Head, Vascular Medicine and
Peripheral Vascular Intervention
North Central Heart Institute
Sioux Falls, South Dakota, USA
Clinical Assistant Professor of Medicine
University of South Dakota School of Medicine

Giancarlo Biamino MD PhD
Interventional Angiologists
Division of Clinical and Interventional Angiology
Department of Angiology
University of Leipzig – Heart Center
Strümpellstrasse, Leipzig
Germany

Emmanouil S Brilakis MD MSc
Assistant Professor of Medicine
University of Texas Southwestern Medical School,
Dallas, Texas, USA

Frank J Criado MD
Director, Center for Vascular Intervention
Chief, Division of Vascular Surgery
Union Memorial Hospital/MedStar Health
Baltimore, Maryland, USA

Gregory S Domer MD
Division of Vascular Surgery and Intervention
Union Memorial Hospital/MedStar Health
Baltimore, Maryland, USA

Kathryn Dougherty CRTT RCVT
Peripheral Vascular Research
St. Luke's Episcopal Hospital and
The Texas Heart Institute
Houston, Texas, USA

Kirk N Garratt MD
Associate Professor of Medicine
Mayo Clinic College of Medicine
Mayo Clinic and Foundation
Rochester, Minnesota, USA

Brendan P Girschek BS
Research Assistant
Division of Vascular Surgery
Union Memorial Hospital–MedStar Health
Baltimore, Maryland, USA

Isabelle Henry MD
Interventional Cardiologist
Polyclinique Bois-Bernard
Bois Bernard, France

Michel Henry MD FACA FASA FAHA
Interventional Cardiologist
80 rue Raymond Poincaré
Nancy, France

Richard R Heuser MD FACC FACP
Director of Cardiovascular Research, Saint Joseph's
Hospital and Medical Center
Medical Director, Phoenix Heart Center
Clinical Professor of Medicine, University of Arizona
College of Medicine
Phoenix, Arizona, USA

Michèle Hugel RN
Interventional Cardiologist
80 rue Raymond Poincaré
Nancy, France

J Stephen Jenkins MD FACC FSCAI
Associate Section Head, Interventional Cardiology
Director, Interventional Cardiology Research
Ochsner Heart & Vascular Institute
New Orleans, Louisiana, USA

Raghunandan Kamineni MD
Interventional Cardiologist
Phoenix Heart Center
Phoenix, Arizona, USA

Lisa Kelly BSN MBA
Clinical Director of Cardiovascular Services
St. Joesph's Hospital
Phoenix, Arizona, USA

Zvonimir Krajcer MD FACC
Clinical Professor of Medicine
Baylor College of Medicine and
The University of Texas Health Science Center
Director Peripheral Vascular Intervention
St. Luke's Episcopal Hospital and
The Texas Heart Institute
Houston, Texas, USA

Philip Morales MD
Interventional Cardiologist
Legacy Heart Center,
Plano, Texas, USA

Kasja F Rabe
Student
Cardiovascular Center Frankfurt, Sankt Katharinen
and Sankt Katharinen Hospital
Frankfurt, Germany

Stephen R Ramee MD
Section Head Invasive and
Interventional Cardiology
Director
Cardiac Catheterization Laboratories
Ochsner Clinic Foundation
New Orleans
Los Angeles, USA

Dierk Scheinert MD
Interventional Angiologists
Division of Clinical and Interventional Angiology
Department of Cardiology
University of Leipzig – Heart Center
Strümpellstrasse, Leipzig
Germany

Andrej Schmidt MD
Interventional Angiologists
Division of Clinical and Interventional Angiology
Department of Cardiology
University of Leipzig – Heart Center
Strümpellstrasse, Leipzig
Germany

Horst Sievert MD
Professor of Medicine
Director of the Cardiovascular Center Frankfurt, Sankt
Katharinen
and Sankt Katharinen Hospital
Frankfurt, Germany

Ron Waksman MD FACC
Professor of Medicine
Georgetown University
Associate Chief of Cardiology
Washington Hospital Center
Washington DC, USA

Christopher J White MD
Chairman, Department of Cardiology
Ochsner Clinic Foundation
New Orleans, Louisiana, USA

Preface

The idea for the first edition of this book came from discussions I had with Alan Burgess of Martin Dunitz Ltd after I wrote a chapter entitled 'Peripheral stenting for the cardiologist' for *Frontiers in Interventional Cardiology*, a text that was published as part of the Second International Meeting of Interventional Cardiology in Jerusalem, Israel. Currently there continue to be few books describing endovascular treatment of peripheral vascular disease. *Peripheral Vascular Stenting* discusses this approach for interventional physicians, a group that includes interventional cardiologists, interventional radiologists, vascular surgeons, neuroradiologists, neurosurgeons, and angiologists.

The prevalence of peripheral vascular disease in the general population and the overall success of interventional procedures, especially those involving stents, have generated substantial interest in the endovascular approach. Stenting has revolutionized the treatment of aortoiliac disease and renal artery stenosis, two maladies that are often discovered when the cardiologist screens patients with congestive heart failure, hypertension, and/or pulmonary edema. Many interventional cardiologists, as well as radiologists, now have a great deal of experience with stenting, and it has become clear that treating the peripheral vessels is no longer the sole province of vascular surgeons. Indeed, vascular surgeons also appreciate the benefits of the endovascular approach in patients who, in the past, would only have had the option of traditional bypass surgery.

In this book we have adopted a format that first reviews anatomy and details access techniques. We also explore equipment choices and device placement and examine the numerous imaging options now available to us. In addition, we describe interventions in the renal, aortoiliac, femoral, and popliteal vessels. The book also details more specialized interventions, such as carotid stenting and abdominal aortic aneurysm repair. These procedures are not solely the domain of either interventional radiologists or interventional cardiologists – a number of specialties are now happy to claim them as their 'very own'. It is important that all clinicians be aware of the latest research regarding carotid stenting, as recent clinical trials indicate it may be the preferred therapy, particularly in those at high risk for an open surgical procedure. Similarly, the results of endoluminal grafting in patients with abdominal aortic aneurysms have shown that patients may often be discharged in less than 24 hours, making the procedure appealing even to vascular surgeons who might otherwise choose a more traditional surgical approach.

This book stands as tribute to the pioneering work of Drs Charles Dotter and Andreas Gruentzig. Their initial vision and successful demonstration of early techniques for peripheral intervention have guided the development of endovascular intervention for the last 35 years. We are indebted to them and to the many talented researchers and interventionists who came after them. We are fortunate enough to have a number of these distinguished clinicians as contributors to this textbook. My sincere thanks to them and to Alan Burgess, whose tireless efforts have helped to shape this outstanding text. *Peripheral Vascular Stenting* provides an important source of information for students and practicing cardiologists and serves as a comprehensive introduction to endovascular techniques. For further advancement of training and research in this technology, I have donated all my royalties for this textbook to two important research institutions: The American Heart Association, an organization committed to combating the nation's number one killer, whose members continue to show that we can reduce the likelihood of death and morbidity from this devastating disease, and The Osler Fund at Johns Hopkins Hospital, which is dedicated to the training of physicians in medicine. I received my housestaff and fellowship training at Johns Hopkins Hospital.

Richard R Heuser
2005

1. Introduction

Richard R Heuser

During the last three decades, percutaneous endovascular intervention has revolutionized the treatment of vascular disease. The technology was pioneered by Dotter and Judkins, who first canalized an iliac artery obstruction with coaxial catheters in 1964.[1] Although Dotter envisioned the use of stents, his initial attempts were largely unsuccessful.[2,3] In the late 1970s, Andreas Gruentzig introduced percutaneous transluminal balloon therapy, a dilation technique now known as angioplasty.[4] Nearly a decade later, the successful application of metallic stents in the human peripheral arterial circulation was described by Sigwart and colleagues.[5]

Currently, a wide variety of balloons and stents are being used to treat stenoses and total occlusions in the carotid, subclavian, coronary, aortic, renal, mesenteric, iliac, femoral, popliteal, and distal leg vessels.[6–8] Stents are also used to treat elastic recoil, arterial dissections, intimal flaps, and residual stenoses not amenable to balloon angioplasty. The benefits of stenting, in particular, have been very apparent in the coronaries,[6–7] where stent implantation has successfully reduced restenosis in vessels greater than 3.0 mm in diameter. Indeed, interventional cardiologists frequently use stents in treating triple vessel disease and even consider their use in left main disease. Recently, drug-eluting stents have been so successful in defeating restenosis – the Achilles heel of angioplasty – that the indications for coronary bypass surgery have changed dramatically, emphasizing a true paradigm shift in the treatment of cardiovascular coronary disease.[8]

A number of specialists, including radiologists and vascular surgeons, now incorporate angioplasty and stenting in the treatment of peripheral vascular disease. Indeed, the advent of percutaneous endovascular intervention has allowed the successful treatment of patients who are at high risk for classic surgical intervention. Given current demographics, this is extremely important as many of our patients are elderly and have comorbidities that limit treatment options.

As the field of endovascular intervention has advanced, the division of labor among interventional cardiologists, radiologists, and vascular surgeons has become less obvious than in the past. In fact, the cardiologist may be the first specialist to see a patient with symptoms of peripheral vascular disease, and concomitant peripheral artery disease is frequently identified and treated by cardiologists. While this approach has the potential to escalate a 'turf battle' between the cardiologist and vascular surgeon or radiologist, patient care remains the most important issue.

We must ask ourselves: Who is best equipped to offer successful treatment? The answer will surely vary, depending both upon the physicians and the facilities available in any given community. If a hospital has a skilled radiologic or vascular surgery team with vast experience and all the appropriate equipment at their disposal, a cardiologist benefits by working with them. When no such established team exists, patients may still be treated safely and effectively by a single specialist. Given the variety of specialties involved in endovascular intervention, a national accreditation program should be established to ensure quality of care – unfortunately, this idea remains controversial.

DIAGNOSING PERIPHERAL VASCULAR DISEASE

Peripheral vascular disease is frequently detected by the following symptoms: intermittent claudication or resting leg pain, acute ischemia with blue toe syndrome, impotency, severe hypertension or hypertension associated with worsening renal function, transient cerebral ischemia, recent stroke, or subclavian steal symptomatology. Atherosclerotic disease is ubiquitous, and in patients with peripheral vascular disease, nearly half will have concomitant coronary disease.

NON-INVASIVE STUDIES

The use of non-invasive studies has improved the diagnosis of peripheral vascular disease.

- Duplex studies with color flow and measurements of ankle–brachial studies can give an accurate assessment of peripheral vascular disease and define the extent of the disease in critical limb ischemia.
- Duplex scanning can also be used to establish a baseline for intervention.
- Computed tomography (CT) and magnetic resonance imaging (MRI) allow the acquisition of images for visualizing aneurysmal disease in some populations.

Although careful clinical examination and non-invasive assessment will permit an initial evaluation of a patient with peripheral vascular disease, angiography is often necessary.

ANGIOGRAPHY

The equipment available in the radiology suite or cardiac catheterization department dictates the type of angiographic images that can be obtained. Equipment that permits continuous, variable-speed, and motion imaging is now available. Digital subtraction angiography incorporates a dedicated computer to subtract real-time images and allows images to be stored electronically. Hence, these images can be electronically manipulated to integrate frames and compensate for a certain amount of motion. Some systems are sophisticated enough that there is active rotary motion of the C-arm gantry to 300 rotations per second during injection, allowing multiple projections from a single angiographic run.

Several contrast media are now available. Low-osmolality contrast media are usually better tolerated by patients during leg and carotid arteriograms and are associated with fewer adverse reactions; they may also be less nephrotoxic than ionic agents. The cost, however, is considerably more than that of conventional media.

Patient monitoring and preparation, as well as sedation and physiologic monitoring, are similar in coronary and peripheral vessel arteriography. Careful monitoring is extremely important for patients undergoing carotid stenting, as stimulation of the carotid sinus may provoke severe bradycardia and, in some cases, prolonged hypotension.

EQUIPMENT CHOICES FOR ENDOVASCULAR INTERVENTION IN THE PERIPHERAL ARTERIES

The equipment now used in peripheral balloon angioplasty incorporates design features pioneered from experience in the coronaries. Low-profile balloons and small-diameter shaft catheters allow access to the majority of lesions, including even small-caliber arteries such as those below the knee. Chronic total occlusions may be recanalized with hydrophilic guidewires and, in some cases, the procedure is aided by a 24- to 48-hour infusion of urokinase, which is a thrombolytic therapy. Aneurysms can be treated with endoluminal grafts (ELGs), and carotid disease may also be approached non-surgically.

SUCCESS WITH ENDOVASCULAR INTERVENTION IN THE PERIPHERAL ARTERIES

The success of percutaneous intervention and stenting in the peripheral arteries is determined by the physician's experience, technique, level of training, and the type of lesion being treated. Angioplasty and stenting have both demonstrated important benefits in the treatment of peripheral vascular disease. In comparison to coronary angioplasty, the success rate of angioplasty in the peripheral arteries is probably higher due to the larger size of the vessels. Success rates are as high as 95–100%

for stenoses and 85–90% for occlusions. In general, results are better in proximal stenoses as compared to those more distal. For example, intervention in the iliac artery is usually far more successful than that in the femoral artery, and the best results are probably in the aorta.

SUMMARY

Endovascular intervention allows physicians to treat patients with severe and potentially disabling peripheral vascular disease using safe and highly successful techniques that have the potential to provide lasting results. In this book, we review anatomy and access approaches and describe the use of angioplasty, stents, and endoluminal grafts in the peripheral arterial circulation.

REFERENCES

1. Dotter C, Judkins MP. Transluminal angioplasty of atherosclerotic obstructions: description of a new technique and a preliminary report of its application. Circulation 1964;30:654–70.

2. Dotter C. Transluminally placed coil-spring endoarterial tube grafts: long-term patency in canine popliteal artery. Invest Radiol 1969;4:329–32.

3. Dotter C. Transluminal angioplasty: a long view. Radiology 1980;135:561–4.

4. Gruentzig AR. Transluminal dilatation of coronary artery stenosis (letter). Lancet 1978;i:263.

5. Sigwart U, Puel J, Mirkovitch V. Intravascular stents to prevent occlusion and restenosis after transluminal angioplasty. N Engl J Med 1987;316:701–6.

6. Serruys PW, de Jaegere P, Kiemeneij F et al. A comparison of balloon-expandable stent implantation with balloon angioplasty in patients with coronary artery disease. Benestent Study Group. N Engl J Med 1994;331:489–95.

7. Fischman DL, Leon MD, Baim D et al. A randomized comparison of coronary stent placement and balloon angioplasty in the treatment of coronary artery disease. N Engl J Med 1994;331:496–501.

8. Morice MC, Serruys PW, Sousa JE, et al. A randomized comparison of a sirolimus-eluting stent with a standard stent for coronary revascularization. N Engl J Med 2002;346:1773–80.

2. Angiographic Anatomy of the Peripheral Vasculature and the Non-invasive Assessment of Peripheral Vascular Disease

Philip A Morales and Richard R Heuser

ANGIOGRAPHIC ANATOMY OF THE PERIPHERAL ARTERIAL SYSTEM

The anatomy of the peripheral vascular system can be complex. Using an angiographic rather than a surgical approach helps to simplify matters. The focus of this chapter is therefore on the more proximal anatomy of the upper and lower extremities, specifically to the level of the elbow and the knee, which are the territories that are amenable to endovascular stent procedures. The extracranial carotid and first-order branches of the abdominal aorta are also described in some detail.[1] An angiographic atlas by Uflacker[2] provides detailed descriptions of the vascular anatomy, which is beyond the scope of this chapter.

ARTERIES OF THE HEAD AND NECK

The arterial vessels of the head and neck are derived from the three main branches (the great vessels) of the aortic arch (Fig. 2.1). The brachiocephalic artery, also known as the innominate artery, is the first branch of the arch. This artery quickly divides into the right common carotid and right subclavian arteries. Shortly after the takeoff of the right common carotid artery, the right vertebral branch arises on the superior–posterior aspect of the right subclavian artery. The next branch of the aortic arch is the left common carotid artery. Following this is the left subclavian artery, which subsequently gives rise to the left vertebral artery.

In up to 30% of patients this normal relationship is not seen. The most common variation is a

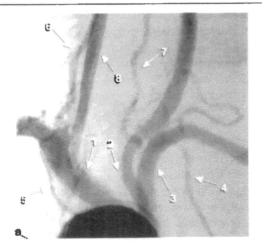 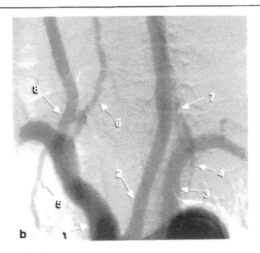

Fig. 2.1 (a) Right anterior oblique 30° and (b) left anterior oblique 60° of the aortic arch.

(1) Right innominate/brachiocephalic; (2) left common carotid, here seen sharing the takeoff with the innominate, best seen on the left anterior oblique view; (3) left subclavian; (4) left internal mammary; (5) right internal mammary; (6) right vertebral; (7) left vertebral; (8) right common carotid.

shared ostium of the brachiocephalic trunk and the left carotid artery, or the left carotid artery arising from the proximal aspect of the brachiocephalic trunk. Other common variants include the right subclavian artery arising from the arch distal to the left subclavian artery, and the left vertebral artery arising directly from the aortic arch between the left carotid and left subclavian arteries.

CAROTID ARTERIES

The common carotid arteries rarely give rise to any significant arterial branches prior to the carotid bifurcation. At the level of the third or fourth cervical vertebral body or the upper border of the thyroid cartilage, the common carotid arteries bifurcate into the external and internal carotid arteries (Fig. 2.2). In some patients, the bifurcation is significantly higher, placing it deep to the

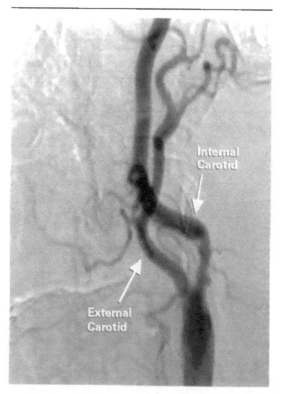

Internal
Carotid

External
Carotid

Fig. 2.2 The carotid bifurcation.

mandible. This is important in the planning of the surgical approach to carotid endarterectomy requiring dislocation of the mandible in order to gain exposure to the bifurcation, significantly increasing the morbidity of the procedure.

Proximal to the carotid bifurcation, the common carotid artery gradually dilates forming the carotid sinus, which is innervated with parasympathetic fibers from the glossopharyngeal nerve. These nerves are responsible for the baroreceptor reflexes that cause bradycardia and hypotension seen during percutaneous intervention including balloon angioplasty and stent placement in the carotid artery. The proximal portion of the internal carotid artery is also dilated (carotid bulb), and should not be used for calculating the normal reference diameter of the internal carotid artery. Rather, an uninvolved segment 3–4 cm beyond the bulb should be used as the reference diameter for the internal carotid artery. Atherosclerotic disease of the carotids usually involves the bifurcation and proximal internal carotid artery. Disease of the external carotid artery rarely causes symptoms and would not often come to the attention of the interventional cardiologist or radiologist. Some patients develop temporary jaw claudication after a carotid stent procedure in which the ostium of the external carotid is compromised. However, this is usually short lived and infrequently leads to the need for repeat intervention.

Differentiating angiographically between the internal and external carotid arteries can be done systemically. First, the external carotid artery courses more anterior on the lateral (90° left anterior oblique) projection compared to the internal carotid artery. Second, the external carotid artery gives rise to a fair number of branches, whereas the internal carotid artery usually does not give off branches in its extracranial portion. As the internal carotid artery enters the cranium, it traverses the cavernous sinus and forms a siphon-like S-curve (Fig. 2.3). Is it imperative that, during carotid interventional procedures, the distal end of the guidewire is maintained below the level of the siphon as a perforation could occur, inducing an arteriovenous malformation.

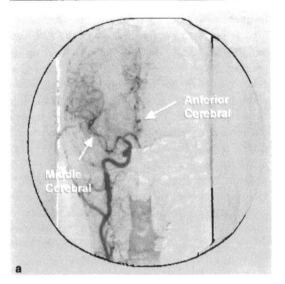
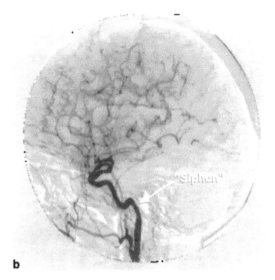

Fig. 2.3 (a) Anteroposterior and (b) lateral projections of the intracranial circulation showing the 'siphon' and the bifurcation of the carotid into the anterior and middle cerebral arteries.

It is also imperative that, when performing carotid stent procedures, the intracranial carotid be imaged both before and after stent implantation. The branches of main importance to the interventionist are the ophthalmic, anterior cerebral and middle cerebral arteries. If persistent symptoms develop in the catheterization laboratory, these branches should be scrutinized for drop-out.

ARTERIES OF THE UPPER EXTREMITIES

After the vertebral artery, the subclavian artery gives rise to four major branches: internal mammary, thyrocervical trunk, dorsal scapular artery, and suprascapular artery (Fig. 2.4). Next, the subclavian artery heads inferiorly and crosses the first rib. At this landmark, it becomes the axillary artery and gives rise to the following branches: superior thoracic artery, thoracoacromial artery, lateral thoracic artery, subscapular artery, and the circumflex humeral branches (Fig. 2.5). Next the axillary artery crosses the lower border of the tendon of the teres major where it becomes the brachial artery. The main branches of the brachial artery are the pro-

funda brachial and the superior ulnar collateral arteries, both of which form a collateralization network around the brachial artery. The brachial artery bifurcates into the ulnar and radial arteries below the elbow.

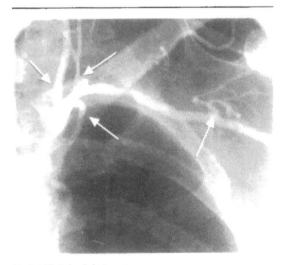

Fig. 2.4 The left subclavian artery.

Branches from proximal to distal are: vertebral, internal mammary, thyrocervical trunk, thoracoacromial.

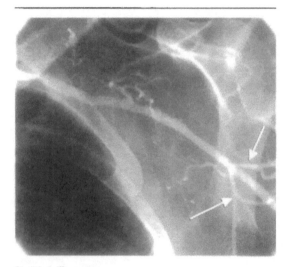

Fig. 2.5 Axillary artery.

Branches are: posterior circumflex humeral (superior arrow), subscapular artery (inferior arrow).

ABDOMINAL AORTA AND ITS BRANCHES

The descending thoracic aorta courses inferiorly to continue on as the abdominal aorta when it pierces the diaphragm through the median arcuate ligament (Fig. 2.6). Just inferior to the median arcuate ligament and at the level of the first lumbar vertebral body, the celiac axis arises from the anterior aspect of the aorta. The celiac axis gives rise to the left gastric artery. A rare cause of abdominal angina can be the median arcuate compression syndrome in which the celiac axis arises at the level of the ligament, thus impinging on the artery (Fig. 2.7). Next, the superior mesenteric arises from the anterior surface of the aorta. The superior mesenteric artery is responsible for the vascular supply of the small intestine, right colon and the transverse colon. The most distal anterior branch of the aorta is the inferior mesenteric artery, arising several centimeters above the aortic bifurcation. It is significantly smaller in caliber than either the celiac axis or the superior mesenteric artery. The inferior mesenteric artery is responsible for the vascular supply of the distal portion of the transverse colon, left colon, sigmoid, and a portion of the rectum. The origin of the major visceral branches of the aorta is best seen in the lateral projection (90° left anterior oblique).

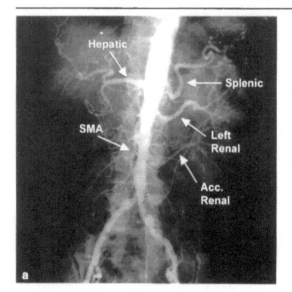
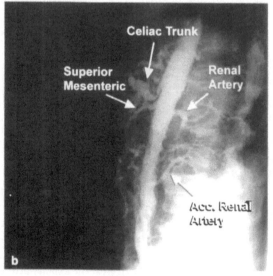

Fig. 2.6 Abdominal aorta: (a) anteroposterior, (b) lateral.

In this case the patient is status-post right nephrectomy. There are two left renal arteries. The celiac axis is compressed by the median arcuate ligament (best seen on the lateral picture, b)

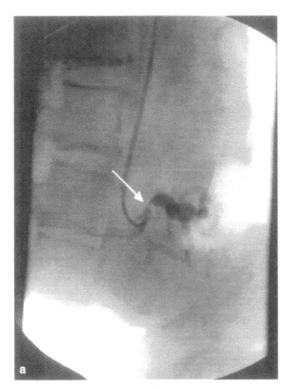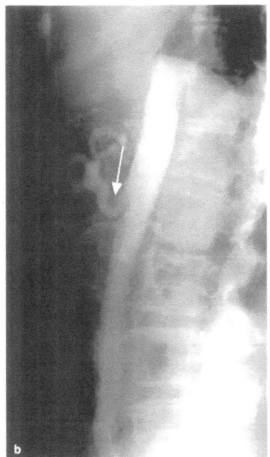

Fig. 2.7 (a) Selective arteriography of the celiac trunk in a patient with median arcuate compression syndrome and intestinal angina (arrow). (b) Celiac axis after stenting.

The renal arteries most commonly arise as single vessels from the aorta at the level of the second lumbar vertebral body (approximately 1–2 cm below the takeoff of the superior mesenteric artery), most often coursing inferiorly prior to entering the renal hilum. The left renal artery usually has a higher origin than the right renal artery. Multiple renal arteries are relatively common, occurring in up to 30% of patients. The most common abnormalities are two distinct arteries to the hilum, or one artery to the hilum and one to either the superior or the inferior pole of the kidney.

ARTERIES OF THE LOWER EXTREMITIES

The common iliac arteries form the terminal bifurcation of the abdominal aorta approximately at the level of the fourth vertebral body (i.e. L4) (Fig. 2.8). The internal iliac artery arises from the medial aspect of the bifurcation of the common iliac artery. Thus, the iliac bifurcation is best seen angiographically with a 20° right or left anterior oblique (RAO or LAO) view. The internal iliac arteries supply the reproductive organs, the distal rectum,

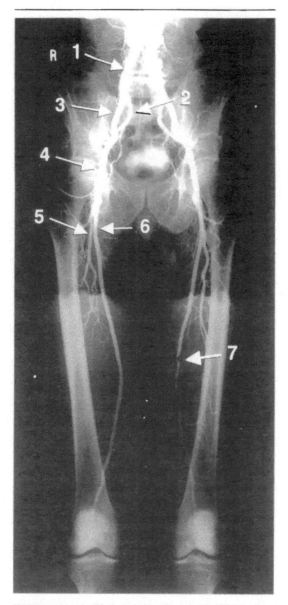

Fig. 2.8 Angiogram of the lower extremities to the level of the knee.
(1) Common iliac; (2) internal iliac (hypogastric); (3) external iliac; (4) common femoral; (5) profunda femoris; (6) superficial femoral artery (SFA). Note the near total occlusion of the left SFA (7).

and the gluteal arteries, which supply the buttocks and proximal thigh. There are dense anastomotic connections between the left and right internal iliac territories that can form collateral networks.

Therefore, unilateral internal iliac disease is unlikely to cause symptoms. Anastomotic connections also exist between the inferior gluteal and the perforating arteries of the thigh from the femoral circulation. This explains the fact that common iliac arterial disease, which affects both internal iliac and femoral circulation, can cause claudication in the buttocks and proximal thigh.

The external iliac artery forms the continuation of the common iliac artery. The external iliac artery courses inferiorly and exits the pelvis deep to the inguinal ligament. There are two main branches of the external iliac artery: the deep circumflex iliac artery and the inferior epigastric artery, which anastomoses with the superior epigastric artery, a terminal branch of the internal mammary.

The common femoral artery is the continuation of the external iliac artery after it passes through the inguinal canal. The common femoral artery gives rise to the superficial circumflex iliac artery and the pudendal branches. The common femoral artery then bifurcates into the superficial femoral artery and the arteria profunda femoris (profunda). The femoral profunda artery comes off posterolaterally, and thus the femoral bifurcation is best seen angiographically with a 30° RAO or LAO view. The superficial femoral artery courses along the medial aspect of the thigh and continues on as the popliteal artery when it exits the adductor canal via the adductor hiatus. Prior to passing through the adductor canal, it gives rise to the superior genicular artery. It provides the superior, middle, and inferior genicular arteries which have anastomoses with genicular branches from the superficial femoral and femoral profunda arteries. The popliteal artery continues below the knee until it bifurcates into the anterior tibial (lateral takeoff) and tibioperoneal trunk, which subsequently bifurcates into the peroneal artery and the posterior tibial artery, which is the medial-most artery (Fig. 2.9). The anterior tibial artery passes between the tibia and fibula to run anterior to the interosseous membrane and eventually forms the arteria dorsalis pedis.

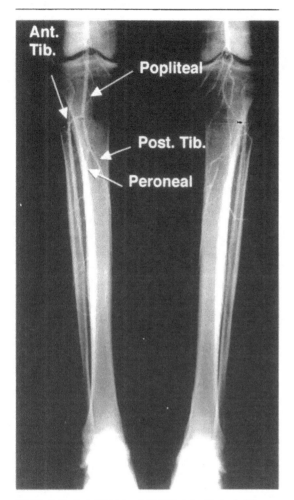

Fig. 2.9 Angiogram of the lower extremities below the level of the knee.

Ant. tib., anterior tibial; Post. tib., posterior tibial. Note the occlusion of the right popliteal, with collaterals filling the posterior tibial.

NON-INVASIVE EVALUATION OF
PERIPHERAL ARTERIAL DISEASE

ANKLE–BRACHIAL INDICES

Without question, the ankle–brachial index (ABI) is the easiest to perform and is the test most widely used to detect significant arterial insufficiency of the lower extremities. In its most simple form, a Doppler device and standard blood pressure cuff are used to obtain systolic pressures of both brachial arteries in the supine position at rest. Next, blood pressures are again obtained with the pressure cuff at the ankle, and the Doppler transducer is used to determine systolic pressures of the dorsalis pedis and posterior tibial arteries. The ratio of ankle pressure to brachial pressure (ABI) is then derived. A ratio of ≥0.9 is found in patients without claudication. Patients with intermittent claudication generally have ABIs of at least 0.5 and no more than 0.9. Patients with rest pain usually have ABIs less than 0.5 and an absolute pressure less than 50 mmHg. More accurate anatomic localization of disease can be obtained by performing segmental pressure recordings at the thigh, calf, and ankle.

Some patients with hemodynamically significant obstruction may have normal ABIs at rest. In these patients, exercise ABI may improve the sensitivity of detecting significant disease. Patients exercise on a treadmill at 1.5–2.0 mph and a 10–12% grade until they develop leg pain. Owing to vasodilation induced by exercise, a steal phenomenon causes increased shunting of blood from the stenosed arteries and the ABI will drop in patients with hemodynamically significantly vascular disease.

Patients with diabetes or end-stage renal disease may have significant calcification of their peripheral vasculature, thus making pressure measurements inaccurate or impossible. In these patients, toe pressures may be helpful. Normal toe–brachial pressure indices should be at 0.6. Those with non-healing ulcers or rest pain often have toe pressures less than 30 mmHg.

ULTRASOUND IMAGING: 2-D AND COLOR-FLOW DOPPLER WITH SPECTRAL ANALYSIS

The combination of 2-D and Doppler analysis (duplex scanning) can yield highly useful and accurate assessments of the severity and location of stenoses in the peripheral vasculature. Currently, ultrasound is most often used in the evaluation of carotid arteries, abdominal aortic aneurysms, renovascular disease, and in the monitoring of bypass grafts. Ultrasound is also highly effective at detecting venous thrombosis, and at detecting and guiding the treatment of access site pseudo-aneurysms.

In the evaluation of the native peripheral vasculature, 2-D and color-flow Doppler are displayed simultaneously as the artery of interest is surveyed for areas of stenosis. A stenosis will be detected by the appearance of plaque on 2-D and by turbulence on Doppler. This site is interrogated by placing the pulsed-wave gate at the site of maximum turbulence and stenosis and by obtaining velocity measurements. Velocity measurements are also made at an uninvolved arterial segment proximal to the stenosis. A ratio of peak systolic velocities (PSV) at the area of stenosis and at the area proximal to the stenosis can then be calculated. The PSV ratio is directly related to the severity of the stenosis and has been validated angiographically (Table 2.1).[3]

The technique can also be adapted for the follow-up and surveillance of lower extremity bypass grafts, and in fact has become the recommended non-invasive imaging modality for this purpose.[4] Gray-scale imaging is used to evaluate the anastomotic areas for stenosis and pseudoaneurysm formation. The same color-flow and pulsed-wave Doppler techniques are then used to estimate the degree of stenosis. A PSV ratio of 3 or greater is consistent with a hemodynamically significant stenosis that will probably lead to graft failure, and is felt to be an indication for intervention. Of note, a PSV ratio of 2 at the distal anastomosis is typical due to the discordance in size between the graft and the distal vessel.

Carotid arterial evaluation requires much the same technique as the rest of the peripheral vasculature. A number of different criteria have been developed to correlate Doppler findings with angiographically proven stenosis. The most often used are the Washington criteria, which grade the stenosis based on Doppler parameters as A (no disease) to E (complete occlusion) (Table 2.2).[5] In the North American Symptomatic Carotid Endarterectomy Trial (NASCET), Doppler indices were developed that showed a high sensitivity and specificity to define stenoses of at least 70% (Table 2.3).[6] Currently, symptomatic patients with 70% or greater carotid stenosis are felt to be candidates for endarterectomy due to the benefit shown in NASCET.[7]

Table 2.1 Peak Systolic Velocity Compared to Diameter Stenosis on Angiography

PSV Ratio	Diameter Stenosis (%)
<2.0	<50
2.0–3.9	50–75
4.0–6.9	75–90
>7.0	>90

PSV, peak systolic velocity.

Table 2.2 University of Washington Doppler Criteria for Carotid Stenosis Grading

Grade	Diameter Stenosis (%)	PSV (cm/s)	EDV (cm/s)	Spectral Waveform
A	None	<125	—	Normal, no broadening
B	1–15	<125	—	Minimal broadening
C	16–49	<125	—	Pansystolic broadening
D	50–79	≥125	<140	Marked broadening
D+	80–90	≥125	≥140	Marked broadening
E	100	0	—	No flow signal

EDV, end diastolic velocity; PSV, peak systolic velocity.

Table 2.3 Doppler Indices of 70% or Greater Internal Carotid Artery Stenosis

	Sensitivity	Specificity	PPV	NPV	Accuracy
PSV of ICA >210 cm/sec	94	77	68	96	83
EDV of ICA >70 cm/sec	92	60	73	86	77
PSV$_{ICA}$/PSV$_{CCA}$ >3.0	91	78	70	94	83
EDV$_{ICA}$/EDV$_{CCA}$ >3.3	100	65	65	100	79

All results as percentages. CCA, common carotid artery; EDV, end diastolic velocity; ICA, internal carotid artery; NPV, negative predictive value; PPV, positive predictive value; PSV, peak systolic velocity.
Adapted from Carpenter.

EVALUATION OF RENOVASCULAR DISEASE

Renovascular hypertension is prevalent in less than 5% of the general hypertensive population.[8] However, the prevalence of renovascular disease among hypertensive patients undergoing cardiac catheterization may be as high as 23%.[9] Therefore, widespread screening examinations of the hypertensive population are not effective. Instead, certain clinical clues should raise the suspicion of renovascular hypertension. Among the most likely findings are:

- onset of hypertension before age 30 or after age 50;
- abrupt onset of hypertension;
- azotemia induced by the institution of angiotensin-converting enzyme inhibitors;
- multidrug-resistant hypertension;
- other symptoms of atherosclerotic cardiovascular disease;
- smoking history;
- recurrent acute pulmonary edema.

Physical findings are largely unhelpful; however, an abdominal bruit may suggest renovascular disease. Laboratory findings may include azotemia, proteinuria, hyperreninemia, and hypokalemia (due to high circulating aldosterone induced by high renin levels). Younger, predominantly Caucasian females may develop fibromuscular dysplasia as the cause of their renovascular hypertension, and they do not have the typical atherosclerotic phenotype.

The non-invasive evaluation of renovascular hypertension can be quite complex and is hampered by a number of tests with low sensitivity and/or specificity. Pickering has suggested a rational approach to this evaluation.[10] After selecting a suitable patient based on the demographic criteria listed above, the first test would be an oral captopril test. The criteria for a positive test after an oral dose of captopril are a rise in renin level of 10 ng/ml per hour, with a maximum renin level greater than 12 ng/ml per hour, and an increase of 150% over baseline renin level (400% if baseline <3 ng/ml per hour). This test provides a sensitivity of 73–100% and a specificity of 72–100%.[11-15] Duplex scanning can then be used as a confirmatory test prior to the decision to proceed with arteriography. The sensitivity of duplex scanning is 84–91% with a specificity of 95–97%.[16] Duplex scanning can confirm the site of stenosis, but is technically limited in up to 40% of patients due to body habitus or excessive bowel gas, and may miss accessory renal arteries; it should therefore not be used as a stand-alone procedure.

Another and perhaps simpler method for evaluating renal artery stenosis is radionuclide angiography with technetium-99m-diethylenetriamine pentaacetic acid (DTPA). The concept is similar in that an oral dose of captopril is administered. Radionuclide angiography is performed prior to (pre-captopril imaging) and after (post-captopril imaging) the administration of oral captopril. The criteria for a positive test are based on asymmetry of renal function and the presence of captopril changes. Specifically, it is:

- a percentage uptake of DTPA by the affected kidney of less than 40% of the combined bilateral uptake;
- a delayed time to peak uptake of DTPA; and/or
- a delayed excretion of DTPA.

The sensitivity and specificity of captopril renal radionuclide angiography are not significantly different from the more conventional captopril–renin vein sampling test.[17]

Future non-invasive assessments for renal artery stenosis may include the use of electron-beam dynamic CT scanning (EBCT).[18] Although the current use of EBCT in evaluating for coronary artery disease is controversial, this may hold different for other applied uses of EBCT.

EVALUATION OF ABDOMINAL AORTIC ANEURYSMS

Over 95% of abdominal aortic aneurysms are infrarenal in origin and most extend to the level of the aortic bifurcation. As previously mentioned, ultrasound is an excellent technique to detect and follow-up aneurysms of the abdominal aorta. Accurate measurements of the size can be made, and these measurements can be followed serially to detect growth in the size of the aneurysm, and to define the timing of possible surgical intervention. Ultrasound, however, is not able to show fine detail (resolution is approximately 3 mm) clearly enough to help guide the type of intervention. Computed tomography (CT) scanning, particularly helical or spiral CT, and magnetic resonance imaging (MRI) are superior to ultrasound in precisely defining the anatomy of the aneurysm, including involvement of side branches such as the renal arteries, and involvement or extension into the iliac arteries. These factors are critical in determining whether patients are suitable for endovascular or open surgical therapies.

REFERENCES

1. Woodfield SL, Heuser RR. Angiographic anatomy of the peripheral vasculature and the noninvasive assessment of peripheral vascular disease. In: Heuser RR, ed. Peripheral Vascular Stenting for Cardiologists. London: Martin Dunitz, 1999: 5–16

2. Uflacker R. Atlas of Vascular Anatomy: An Angiographic Approach. Baltimore: Williams and Wilkins, 1997.

3. Ranke C, Creutzig A, Alexander K. Duplex scanning of the peripheral arteries: correlation of the peak systolic velocity ratio with angiographic diameter reduction. Ultrasound Med Biol 1992;18:433–40.

4. Mills JI, Harris EJ, Taylor LM Jr, et al. The importance of routine surveillance of distal bypass grafts. A study of 379 reversed vein grafts. J Vasc Surg 1990;12:379–89.

5. Roederer GO, Langlois YE, Jaeger KA, et al. A simple spectral parameter for accurate classification of severe carotid artery disease. Bruit 1989;20:174–8.

6. Carpenter JP. Determination of duplex Doppler ultrasound criteria appropriate to the North American Symptomatic Carotid Endarterectomy Trial. Stroke 1996;27:695–9.

7. North American Symptomatic Carotid Endarterectomy Trial Collaborators. Beneficial effect of carotid endarterectomy in symptomatic patients with high-grade stenosis. N Engl J Med 1991;325:445–53.

8. Gifford R. Evaluation of the hypertensive patient with emphasis on detecting curable causes. Millbank Q 1969;47:170–86.

9. Vetrovec GW, Landwehr DM, Edwards VL. Incidence of renal artery stenosis in hypertensive patients undergoing coronary angiography. J Interv Cardiol 1989;2:69–76.

10. Pickering TG. Diagnosis and evaluation of renovascular hypertension: indications for therapy. Circulation 1991;83(suppl I):I147–54.

11. Muller FB, Sealy JE, Case CB, et al. The captopril test for identifying renovascular disease in hypertensive patient. Am J Med 1986;80:633–44.

12. Thibonnier M, Sassano P, Joseph A, et al. Diagnostic value of a single dose of captopril in renin- and aldosterone-dependent, surgically curable hypertension. Cardiovasc Rev Reports 1982;3:1659–66.

13. Idrissi A, Fournier A, Renaud H, et al. The captopril challenge test as a screening test for renovascular hypertension. Kidney Int 1988;34(suppl 25):S138–41.

14. Salvetti A, Arzilli F, Nuccorini A, Mauro M, Giovanetti R. Does humoral and hemodynamic response to acute ACE inhibition identify true renovascular hypertension? In: Glorioso N, Laragh JH, Rapelli A, eds. Renovascular Hypertension. New York: Raven Press, 1987; pp 305–16.

15. Svetky LP, Himmelstein SI, Dunnick NR, et al. Prospective analysis of strategies for diagnosing renovascular hypertension. Hypertension 1989;14:247–57.

16. Lewis BD, James EM. Current applications of duplex and color Doppler ultrasound imaging: abdomen. Mayo Clinic Proc 1989;64:1158–69.

17. Mann SJ, Pickering TG, Sos TA, et al. Captopril renography in the diagnosis of renal artery stenosis: accuracy and limitations. Am J Med 1991;90:30–40.

18. Paul JF, Ugolini P, Sapoval M, et al. Unilateral renal artery stenosis: perfusion patterns with electron-beam dynamic CT – preliminary experience. Radiology 2001;221:261–5.

3. Vascular Access

J Stephen Jenkins

Multiple methods of arterial access have been described since the first documented arterial cannulation in 1733 when Reverend Stephen Hale inserted a brass rod into the surgically exposed artery of a horse and measured pressure via a manometer.[1] Since the most common procedural complications involve the initial access to the circulation, this important step deserves full study. The widely used technique of percutaneous retrograde common femoral artery access will not be described here as it is well described in the literature.[2] This chapter will describe the percutaneous techniques of antegrade femoral artery access, contralateral iliofemoral artery access and popliteal artery access.

ANTEGRADE FEMORAL ARTERY ACCESS

ANATOMY

Although the common femoral artery (CFA) is considered by many angiographers to be the safest site for arterial puncture, there is little published data relating the CFA and its bifurcation to the landmarks used to guide arterial puncture. Lechner et al showed the inguinal skin crease to be distal to the bifurcation of the CFA in 75% of limbs but did not consider other landmarks.[3] A thorough understanding of the relationship of the CFA to anatomic landmarks is necessary to ensure safe antegrade CFA puncture, the technique for which was first described by Dotter and Judkins in 1964.[4]

The regional anatomy relevant to percutaneous femoral artery puncture is demonstrated in Fig. 3.1. The femoral artery and vein are shown coursing underneath the inguinal ligament which is a band of dense fibrous tissue connecting the anterior superior iliac spine to the pubic tubercle. The

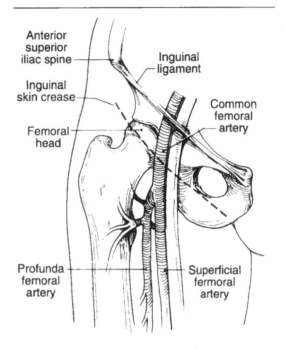

Fig. 3.1 The most important landmark is the femoral head. Puncture of the femoral artery at this level almost assures entry caudal to the inguinal ligament and cranial to the femoral artery bifurcation.

inguinal skin crease which can be highly variable in location is shown as a dotted line.[3] The most important landmark shown in this illustration is the femoral head. In a morphologic study of computed tomographic (CT) scans in 50 patients, there was not a single case in which a puncture would have passed cranial to the inguinal ligament or caudal to the femoral artery bifurcation if the CFA was entered at the level of the center of the femoral head.[5] Caudal to the femoral head, the CFA is encased in the femoral sheath and bifurcates to the superficial femoral artery laterally. With these anatomic observations in mind, the importance of osseous support and entry of the needle into the CFA at the center of the femoral head is desirable.

INDICATIONS AND CONTRAINDICATIONS

Endovascular treatment of patients with femoral–popliteal atherosclerotic disease is becoming increasingly more common. Antegrade CFA puncture may be useful or desirable for diagnostic angiography, angioplasty, thrombolytic therapy or the use of artherectomy devices. Anatomic considerations where antegrade CFA puncture may be desirable include an acute angled common iliac bifurcation and aortoiliac grafts where a contralateral femoral approach may be impossible. Contraindications to antegrade CFA puncture include extreme obesity and atherosclerotic disease involving the CFA.

EQUIPMENT AND PROCEDURE

Equipment necessary to perform antegrade CFA puncture includes a percutaneous needle, a steerable guidewire and an arterial sheath. A steerable guidewire is desirable to negotiate the CFA bifurcation. A 6F arterial sheath is the initial size chosen until successful entry is obtained. The sheath size is upgraded if necessary to accommodate larger devices once a treatment plan is formulated.

After the arterial sheath is placed in an antegrade fashion, a wire, catheter or obturator is maintained at all times within the sheath lumen to prevent sheath kinking. Braided sheaths, coiled metal sheaths or kink-resistant sheaths are also useful for antegrade punctures to prevent sheath kinking.

Anatomical landmarks are initially identified by palpation of the anterior superior iliac spine and the pubic tubercle to locate the inguinal ligament; the femoral head position is confirmed fluoroscopically. Depending on the amount of subcutaneous fat, a skin incision should be made 1.0–2.0 cm cranial to the level of the center of the femoral head. The needle is directed through an oblique downward course while palpating the CFA over the center of the femoral head. Once the CFA has been entered, a steerable guidewire is then advanced under fluoroscopic guidance to select the desired branch. The bifurcation of the CFA is best separated fluoroscopically by a 20° lateral view. Once the sheath has been placed, its lumen is always occupied with a wire or catheter to prevent sheath kinking.

COMPLICATIONS

Complications of antegrade CFA puncture are most commonly related to either too high or too low arterial entry. When the puncture is too high, a retroperitoneal hemorrhage may occur.[6-8] The presence of loose connective tissue in the retroperitoneum can cause large hematomas. The lack of osseous support and the presence of the tense inguinal ligament at the arterial puncture site render manual compression inadequate. Low punctures are complicated by formation of arteriovenous fistulas, false aneurysms and hematomas as well as inadvertent entry into the deep femoral artery or superficial femoral artery, which precludes treatment of ostial disease of either of these vessels.[9,10] These complications are avoided by proper identification of bony landmarks and entry into the CFA caudal to the inguinal ligament where the artery can be compressed against the common femoral head.

SUMMARY

The consistent relationship of the CFA to the femoral head cited in the literature makes it the landmark of choice in obtaining antegrade femoral artery access. Reluctance to perform such a high skin incision for fear of entering the abdominal cavity has to be avoided to prevent complications of needle entry too low. Antegrade femoral artery access is a safe technique for performing femoro-popliteal angioplasty when reliable landmarks are used.

CONTRALATERAL ILIOFEMORAL ARTERY ACCESS

INTRODUCTION

The acquisition and maintenance of arterial access during a procedure until sheath removal plays a major role in determining whether peripheral intervention is a success or failure.[8-12] Retrograde common femoral artery access remains by far the most commonly used site and the easiest arterial access method. Peripheral interventionists should be well familiarized with the contralateral iliofemoral approach as it may be the access of choice for many lesions and a successful technique where other approaches fail.

ANATOMY

Anatomic considerations of the femoral artery and its relationship to the common femoral head have been discussed in detail earlier (see Fig. 3.1). The needle puncture is made in a retrograde fashion through a skin incision 1.0–2.0 cm below the midline of the femoral head. The standard retrograde common femoral artery access technique is used and a sheath is placed in the common femoral artery.[8]

Evaluation of the anatomy of the aortic bifurcation and common iliac arteries is important when considering a crossover technique. The two most common reasons for failure are an acutely angled aortic bifurcation or diffusely diseased and calcified common iliac arteries (Fig. 3.2). This is evaluated with an abdominal aortogram performed by placing a pigtail catheter in the terminal aorta. Once suitable anatomy is identified, a flexible guidewire placed in the terminal aorta is directed to the contralateral iliac artery by means of a 5F or 6F diagnostic internal mammary artery or Judkins' right 4 catheter (Fig. 3.3). Once a guidewire is secured into the contralateral external iliac or common femoral artery, a guiding catheter or long sheath can be advanced to the contralateral side.

INDICATIONS AND CONTRAINDICATIONS

One approach to performing angioplasty of the superficial femoral and profunda femoral arteries is via an ipsilateral antegrade common femoral artery puncture.[13,14] A contralateral approach is desirable when antegrade access may be difficult to obtain as

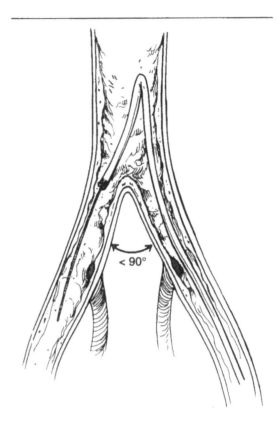

Fig. 3.2 Failure to advance this catheter is caused by the acutely angled aortic bifurcation. Heavily calcified aortic bifurcations also present difficulty in crossing with catheters.

in obese patients with large panniculus or if lesions are located within the common femoral artery or involve the ostium of the superficial femoral or profunda femoral artery. The proximity of these lesions to the arterial puncture site preclude their treatment if an antegrade ipsilateral approach is used (Fig. 3.4). Bifurcation anatomy of the common femoral artery into the superficial femoral and profunda femoral arteries may also render an ipsilateral approach technically impossible and require either a contralateral or a popliteal approach.[15,16]

A contralateral approach also allows treatment of bilateral disease with a single arterial puncture. Other anatomic considerations where a contralateral approach may be desirable include angioplasty of internal iliacs or renal transplant artery stenosis

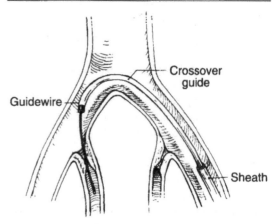

Fig. 3.5 Internal iliac stenoses are best treated from a contralateral approach. An ipsilateral approach necessitates negotiating an acute angle, which is rarely successful.

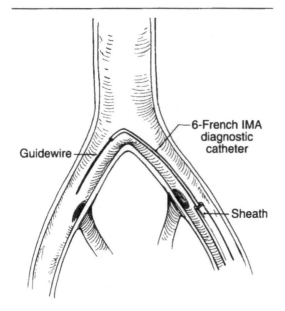

Fig. 3.3 A 6F internal mammary artery (IMA) or Judkins' right 4 catheter will direct the guidewire to the contralateral iliac artery.

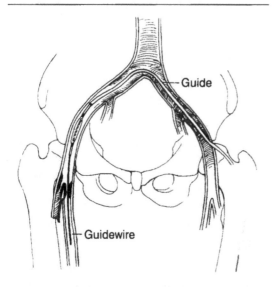

Fig. 3.4 The proximity of these lesions to the common femoral artery puncture site precludes antegrade femoral artery access.

(Fig. 3.5). Contraindications to the contralateral approach are generally related to the anatomy of the terminal aortic bifurcation and the anatomy of the lesions to be treated. Acute bends at the bifurcation of the terminal aorta make it difficult to manipulate catheters around the iliac bifurcation and maintain enough pushability in tortuous arteries to cross heavily calcified or obstructive lesions. There is a tendency for guidewires and even guide catheters to prolapse or buckle into the aorta at the bifurcation if the angle is too acute. Aortobifemoral grafts can be negotiated unless the bifurcation angle is too acute. If bulky devices such as peripheral atherocaths or non-segmented Palmaz stents longer than 30 mm are to be used, then a contralateral approach is contraindicated.[17] The currently manufactured flexible, premounted balloon expandable stents and self-expanding stents negotiate the aortoiliac bifurcation angle with ease.

EQUIPMENT AND PROCEDURE

Equipment used to gain contralateral iliofemoral access includes a percutaneous needle, guidewire and arterial sheath to obtain standard retrograde CFA access. Once arterial access is obtained, a guidewire is advanced into the abdominal aorta and a catheter is chosen to access the contralateral common iliac artery. Diagnostic catheters useful in crossing the aortic bifurcations include 5F or 6F diagnostic internal mammary artery, Judkins' right 4, pigtail and Simmons catheters (see Fig. 3.3). These catheters placed at the level of the aortic bifurcation will direct a wire into the contralateral common iliac artery. After positioning a catheter in this manner, either a steerable floppy guidewire such as a 0.035 inch Wholey or an angled glide wire with its superior lubricity is advanced far into the contralateral femoral artery. The catheter is then advanced over the guidewire into the iliac artery.

There are a number of guiding systems which may be used for contralateral iliofemoral angioplasty. They all add the ability to inject contrast during lesion dilations and provide more back-up support when crossing stubborn lesions. Guide catheters which may be used include a Mullins transseptal sheath, a 40 cm long Arrow-Flex sheath (Arrow International, Reading, PA), a 55 cm long multipurpose coronary or renal guiding catheter, or a kink-resistant crossover guide currently available from a number of manufacturers. Any long sheath chosen should be a braided one as non-braided sheaths have a tendency to kink. The guide is advanced over the aortic bifurcation using the stiff wire. If the guide is a long sheath it is inserted with a dilator, and if a guiding catheter is used then a diagnostic multipurpose catheter approximately one French size smaller is inserted through the lumen to extend approximately 1 cm distal to the end of the guide and is secured in place with a Tuohy-Borst Y connector. This minimizes the chance of dissection of the terminal aorta during advancement of the guide contralaterally. Once a guiding system is in place, selective injection of contrast allows visualization of the target lesion. The angioplasty catheter and wire can be positioned under direct visualization with contrast avoiding the need for multiple catheter exchanges over the terminal aortic bifurcation.

COMPLICATIONS

Complications of contralateral iliofemoral artery access are most commonly related to the retrograde common femoral artery puncture. They include pseudoaneurysms, arteriovenous fistulas, thrombo-embolism, infection, retroperitoneal hematomas and bleeding complications.[18-20] The most common bleeding complication is hematoma formation at the arterial access site.[21-25]

If care is not taken to protect large-bore guides when advancing them over the iliac bifurcation, terminal aortic and common iliac dissections may occur. This complication can be best avoided by protecting the tip of the guide with a diagnostic catheter placed within its lumen to provide a smooth transition from the guidewire to the guiding catheter (Fig. 3.6). Crossover sheaths with dilators that create a smooth transition minimize this complication.

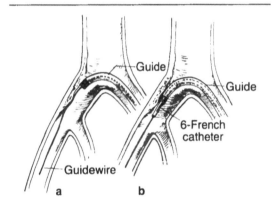

Fig. 3.6 (a) Without protection, the large-bore guide can cause complications. (b) A 6F diagnostic catheter through the guide lumen will protect against such complications.

SUMMARY

Historically the ipsilateral approach has been used for superficial femoral artery angioplasty but is limited when treating common femoral artery and proximal superficial artery lesions.[13,15,17] With the development of peripheral guiding catheter systems, the contralateral approach extends our ability to perform percutaneous transluminal angioplasty of bilateral disease with a single arterial puncture and treatment of proximal superficial femoral, proximal profunda and common femoral artery lesions which would be impossible with an ipsilateral approach.

Many devices can be used and most stents implanted through this access if the anatomy of the terminal aortic bifurcation is not excessively acute and allows passage of a guiding system. Bulky devices such as the directional atherectomy catheter and long rigid stents are difficult if not impossible to deliver using a contralateral approach. This technique can be performed safely as described and broadens the indications for endovascular treatment of peripheral vascular disease in the lower extremities.

POPLITEAL ARTERY ACCESS

INTRODUCTION

Endovascular treatment of atherosclerotic peripheral vascular disease is most commonly approached via the common femoral artery. Lesion location and anatomy in some scenarios dictate the use of an alternative approach from the brachial artery or popliteal artery which may be successful when standard approaches fail. This section will describe the popliteal anatomy, the technique of popliteal access and its indications.

ANATOMY

It is critical to understand the anatomy of the popliteal fossa when performing percutaneous popliteal artery access to prevent the creation of an arteriovenous fistula. Textbooks of anatomy describe the popliteal artery as being anterior and medial to the popliteal vein.[26] This anatomic relationship between the artery and vein predisposes percutaneous posterior access to puncture of the popliteal vein (Fig. 3.7). The popliteal artery, vein and sciatic nerve are encased in a common sheath, which courses upwards along the diagonal of the popliteal fossa as shown. These structures usually remain superficial in location well above the level of the joint space. The semitendinous muscle is seen anterior to the artery.

Anatomic variations were described by Trigaux et al by use of cadaveric specimens, CT scans and

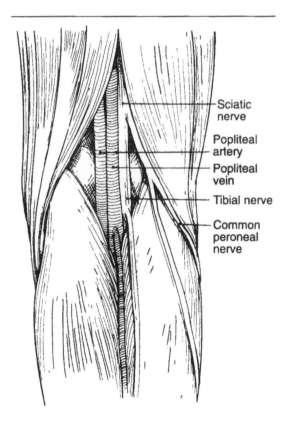

Fig. 3.7 The popliteal artery courses medial to the popliteal vein and overlaps 60% of the time at a level of 6.5 cm above the joint space.

plain radiographs of the knee in 67 patients.[27] Five levels were studied on CT scan ranging from the joint space to 6.5 cm cranially. In 92% of all levels studied on CT, the artery was anterior to the vein and in 87% of the levels, more than 25% of the arteries overlapped the vein. However, when the most cranial level was considered (6.5 cm cranial to the joint space), overlap occurred in only 60% and the artery was medial to the vein in 25%, resulting in the most desirable location for arterial puncture. The plain radiographs of the knee demonstrated the popliteal skin crease to be above the femorotibial joint space in 97% of the cases.

This study would indicate the most reliable bony landmark to be the femorotibial joint space and the most favorable puncture site to be 6.5 cm cranial to this space with the puncture needle directed from a medial to lateral course. Puncture of the popliteal artery at this level will also avoid arterial entry below an anomalous high popliteal bifurcation which occurs in 4.7% of cases.[28]

INDICATIONS AND CONTRAINDICATIONS

The popliteal approach is utilized for lesions that have failed the antegrade approach, flush occlusions of the superficial femoral artery or superficial femoral arteries that end in large collaterals which have a tendency to divert angioplasty wires into them. An antegrade approach to superficial femoral artery occlusions generally fails due to the inability to maintain an angioplasty wire within the true lumen of the vessel. Ostial superficial femoral artery and common femoral artery lesions may also be approached via the popliteal access in patients with acute angled terminal aortic bifurcations. Obese patients with large panniculus and acute angled terminal aortic bifurcations can be approached with the popliteal access to treat superficial femoral artery disease.

Strict contraindications to popliteal artery puncture include aneurysms of the popliteal artery and pathology of the popliteal fossa such as Baker's cyst.

EQUIPMENT AND PROCEDURE

The patient is first placed in a supine position and retrograde ipsilateral common femoral artery sheath or a contralateral retrograde access is placed for direct visualization of the popliteal artery with contrast medium. This access is secured in place and connected to a high frequency pressure monitoring line for contrast injections. Visualization of the site to be treated may be afforded with this access. The patient is then turned and placed in a prone position on the angiography table and the popliteal fossa is prepared and draped. The femorotibial joint is the most reliable landmark determined fluoroscopically. An area 3–4 cm above this space is then infiltrated with local anesthetic and a skin incision is made medial to the popliteal artery. Contrast is then injected into the previously

placed common femoral artery access for direct fluoroscopic visualization of the popliteal artery during puncture. The puncture needle is directed obliquely from medial to lateral so that the artery is entered 6–7 cm above the level of joint space. A 0.035 inch floppy guidewire is then advanced into the popliteal artery over which a 6F arterial sheath is placed. In addition to direct contrast visualization, ultrasound guidance can be employed to gain retrograde popliteal artery access. This technique avoids ipsilateral or contralateral CFA access.

COMPLICATIONS

As with any arterial puncture, hematomas occur at rates of 2–4% when popliteal artery access is used.[29-31] The anatomic relationship of the popliteal artery to popliteal vein increases the risk of arteriovenous fistula due to transvenous arterial puncture. The risk can be minimized with attention to the anatomic considerations previously discussed and higher punctures directed from medial to lateral.

SUMMARY

Popliteal access is a useful technique which allows endovascular treatment of peripheral arterial disease not approachable by other techniques. Still, it is probably the least used access by the peripheral interventionist. With close attention to the anatomic considerations and technique, it is a safe and reliable approach to many lesions using percutaneous methods.

REFERENCES

1. Hales S. Statistical Essays: Hemostaticas, Vol. 2, 3rd edn. London: W Innys and R Manby, 1738.
2. Seldinger SI. Catheter placement of the needle in percutaneous arteriography. A new technique. Acta Radiol 1953;39:368–76.
3. Lechner G, Jantsch H, Wanech R, Kretschmer G. The relationship between the common femoral artery, the inguinal crease, and the inguinal ligament; a guide to accurate angiographic puncture. Cardiovasc Intervent Radiol 1988;11:165–9.
4. Dotter CT, Judkins MP. Transluminal treatment of arteriosclerotic obstruction: description of a new technique and a preliminary report of its application. Circulation 1964;30:654–70.
5. Spijkerboer AM, Scholten FG, Mali WPT, van Schaik JP. Antegrade

puncture of the femoral artery: morphologic study. Cardiovasc Radiol 1990;176:57–60.

6. Bouhoutsos J, Morris T. Femoral artery complications after diagnostic procedures. BMJ 1973;3:396–9.

7. Hessel SJ, Adams DF, Abrams HL. Complications of angiography. Radiology 1981;138:273–81.

8. Greenfield AJ. Femoral, popliteal and tibial arteries: percutaneous transluminal angioplasty. AJR Am J Roentgenol 1980;135:927–35.

9. Altin RS, Flicker S, Nadiech HJ. Pseudoaneurysm and arteriovenous fistula after femoral artery catheterization: association with low femoral puncture. AJR Am J Roentgenol 1989;152:629–31.

10. Rapoport S, Sniderman KW, Morse SS, et al. Pseudoaneurysm: a complication of faulty technique in femoral arterial puncture. Radiology 1985;154:529–30.

11. Grossman M. How to miss the profunda femoris. Radiology 1974;111:482.

12. Keller FS. Percutaneous angioplasty of the femoral, popliteal and tibial arteries. In: Jang GD, ed. Angioplasty. New York: McGraw-Hill, 1986: 61–82.

13. Schwarten DE. Aortic, iliac and peripheral artery angioplasty. In: Castaneda-Zuniga WR, Tadavarthy SM, eds. Interventional Radiology. Baltimore: Williams and Wilkins, 1988: 268–97.

14. Bachman DM, Casarella WJ, Sos TA. Percutaneous iliofemoral angioplasty via the contralateral femoral artery. Radiology 1979;130:617–21.

15. Kaufman SL. Angioplasty from the contralateral approach: use of a guiding catheter and coaxial angioplasty balloons. Radiology 1990;177:577–8.

16. White CJ, Nguyen M, Ramee SR. Use of a guiding catheter for contralateral femoral artery angioplasty. Cathet Cardiovasc Diagn 1990;21:15–17.

17. Henry M, Armor M. Stenting of femoral and popliteal arteries. In: Sigward U, ed. Endoluminal Stenting. London: WB Saunders, 1996: 476–86.

18. Ricci MA, Trevisani GT, Pilcher DB. Vascular complications of cardiac catheterization. Am J Surg 1994;167:375–8.

19. Clevland KO, Gelfand MS. Invasive staphylococcal infections complicating percutaneous transluminal coronary angioplasty: three cases and review. Clin Infect Dis 1995;21:93–6.

20. Trerotola SO, Kuhlman JE, Fishman EK. Bleeding complications of femoral catheterization: CT evaluation. Radiology 1990;174:37–40.

21. Fraedrich G, Beck A, Bonzel T, Schlosser V. Acute surgical intervention for complications of percutaneous transluminal angioplasty. Eur J Vasc Surg 1987;1:197–203.

22. Garti I, Salinger H. Complications in brachial countercurrent arteriography and in retrograde femoral arteriography. Israel J Med Sci 1969;5:1192–7.

23. Lang EK. A survey of the complications of percutaneous retrograde arteriography: Seldinger technique. Radiology 1963;81:257–63.

24. Redman HC, Reuter SR. Percutaneous transarterial arteriography: complications and their avoidance. Angiology 1970;21:575–9.

25. Sigstedt B, Lunderquist A. Complications of angiographic examinations. AJR Am J Roentgenol 1978;130:455–60.

26. Paturet G. Traité d'Anatomie Humaine, tome II: Members Superieur et Inferieur. Paris: Masson, 1951: 933–89.

27. Trigaux JP, Van Berrs B, De Wispelaere JF. Anatomic relationship between the popliteal artery and vein: a guide to accurate angiographic puncture. AJR Am J Roentgenol 1991;157:1259–62.

28. Ducksoo K, Orron DE, Skillman JJ. Surgical significance of popliteal arterial variants: a unified angiographic classification. Ann Surg 1989;210:776–81.

29. Zaitoun R, Iyer SS, Lewin RF, Dorros G. Percutaneous popliteal approach for angioplasty of superficial femoral artery occlusions. Cathet Cardiovasc Diagn 1990;21:154–8.

30. Tonnesen KH, Sager P, Karle A, et al. Percutaneous transluminal angioplasty of the superficial femoral artery by retrograde catheterization via the popliteal artery. Cardiovasc Intervent Radiol 1998;11:127–31.

31. Henry M, Armor M, Henry I, et al. Percutaneous transluminal angioplasty of peripheral arteries with retrograde catheterization through the popliteal artery: series of 63 cases. Radiology 1994;193:192.

4. Endovascular Equipment and Interventional Tools

Zvonimir Krajcer and Kathryn Dougherty

INTRODUCTION

Since first described in 1964 by Charles Dotter,[1] angioplasty and the management of peripheral vascular disease has undergone tremendous changes. It has not only proven effective and durable, it has paved the way for a technological revolution that has applied percutaneous catheter techniques to progressively more complex clinical situations. This chapter will review the basic equipment and current adjunctive endovascular therapies used to manage peripheral vascular disease.

Although coronary angioplasty and peripheral angioplasty procedures are similar, there are significant differences in interventional tools and treatment of the two disease states. The success of the intervention is determined by the physician's experience, level of training, type of lesion, and technique. However, before treatment decisions can be made, an accurate diagnosis needs to be confirmed with a detailed history, physical and non-invasive studies (ankle–brachial index, duplex ultrasound, etc.). Non-invasive imaging techniques such as magnetic resonance angiography can supply detailed peripheral vascular anatomic information. The use of multidetector computed tomography has recently revolutionalized the management of cardiovascular disease, offering additional information about arterial calcification. With the use of 16 detectors imaging is easier, quicker and more readily available than magnetic resonance. Imaging from the carotid circulation through the toes in 3.2 mm sections takes less than 30 seconds. The whole-body scan can be used to assess the patency of the carotid arteries or look for the source of atheroembolism.

VASCULAR ACCESS

After obtaining the appropriate angiographic images, choosing the right vascular access ensures a successful procedure. Most peripheral vascular interventions can be performed from different access sites (e.g. brachial artery, common femoral artery). There are some interventions, however, that require a specific access to achieve a successful result. Knowledge and proficiency with the various access sites is one of the most important basic skills in peripheral vascular intervention.

OVERVIEW OF BASIC ENDOVASCULAR EQUIPMENT

The disposable products required for peripheral vascular interventions, while similar to those used for coronary interventions, incorporate technological design features adapted to the anatomic variances of the arterial site being treated. Low-profile balloons and small-diameter shaft catheters allow access to the majority of lesions, even small-caliber arteries such as those below the knee.

INTRODUCER SHEATH

Hemostatic introducer sheaths are generally used for all endovascular procedures. They establish a secure path from the skin to the vascular lumen. In addition to providing a safe port of access to the vascular system, they allow catheter instrumentation without ongoing blood loss or damage to the vessel. Sheath size is dependent upon the type of procedure, the outer diameter of the catheters or equipment used during the intervention. Sheaths are generally 10–11 cm in length, although shorter and longer (7.5–100 cm) sheaths are used for a variety of purposes, for example to straighten out the tortuous iliofemoral vessels, to improve torque control and to facilitate guide catheter, stent and stent graft advancement. The Super Arrow-Flex™ introducer sheath (Arrow International, Reading, PA) is popular for peripheral intervention because of its flexibility, and numerous sizes and lengths. It can provide all of the features of a guide catheter, with the added advantages of a built-in hemostatic valve and side-port. It incorporates a highly radiopaque coil-wire design which allows it to flex at any point, in any direction, without kinking. A hydrophilic coating added to the tip allows successful negotiation through the tortuous peripheral anatomy.

Many introducer sheaths can be used in place of guiding catheters for selective catheterization and visceral/branch artery intervention. Cook Incorporated (Bloomington, IN) has a variety of peripheral introducer sheath sizes, lengths and configurations to accommodate radial, brachial or femoral access. The Cook Flexor™ (Cook, Bloomington, IN) introducer systems are thin walled, with large lumens. The Flexor™ is equipped with a Tuohy-Borst side-arm that allows contrast injections, prevents blood reflux and permits unimpeded catheter and guidewire introduction. It

is kink resistant with a hydrophilic coating and easily accommodates contralateral access. The Balkin Contralateral™ sheath (Cook, Bloomington, IN) is frequently used for the contralateral iliofemoral approach. The Shuttle™ (Cook, Bloomington, IN) has a radiopaque marker band in the distal tip that allows accurate positioning and facilitates endoluminal maneuvers in the supra-aortic vessels.

Cook also makes the Extra Large (14F–24F) introducer. The 24F Keller-Timmerman is used to introduce large devices such as endovascular stent grafts for abdominal aortic aneurysm exclusion. These sheaths range from 25 to 50 cm in length. They are also available with a special hemostasis valve or CheckFlow™ valve that prevents blood reflux and allows flushing around the larger devices while they are positioned inside the sheath (Fig. 4.1).

The Pinnacle™ Destination™ (Boston Scientific, Natick, MA) was also developed as a guide sheath. These sheaths come in various lengths and are either straight or shaped for renal, visceral or contralateral iliofemoral access. They have two detachable valve types and are available in 6F and 7F sizes. Like the Shuttle™, the Destination™ has coil reinforcement and is kink resistant. The Destination™ also incorporates the hydrophilic coating that helps decrease resistance when it is passed through tortuous and/or calcified vessels.

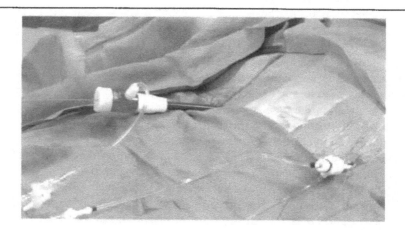

Fig. 4.1 A 22F Keller-Timmerman sheath with the CheckFlow™ valve is in the right femoral artery and a 16F Extra Large introducer is in the left femoral artery.

GUIDEWIRES

Guidewires permit safe transluminal navigation of catheters and devices. Guidewire design variables include tip configuration, length, diameter, stiffness, antifriction coatings, and radiopaque markers. The fundamental attributes of a guidewire include the ability to transmit torque, minimize friction, tip flexibility, and steerability. All guidewires should only be advanced under fluoroscopic guidance and never advanced against resistance. This will eliminate the risk of subintimal guidewire passage, vessel dissection, and perforation.

Guidewire diameters are measured in inches. The standard range is 0.014–0.038 inches. The diameter of the guidewire should match the required diameter of the catheter. This provides better support of the catheter during manipulation and decreases the amount of blood leakage around the wire.

Guidewires are straight, angled, or have a J-shaped tip. Flexible tip lengths range from 3 to 20 cm. The J-tipped wire is the most commonly used guidewire for initial passage into the vessel because of its low risk of subintimal dissection. The main components of the traditional guidewire are:

- the central core, which provides body, steerability and torque control;
- a tightly wound outer spring coil containing a forming ribbon for tip shaping;
- a Teflon outer coating to decrease friction.

Hydrophilic guidewires were developed to satisfy a wide variety of procedural requirements. Terumo Glidewire™ (Boston Scientific, Natick, MA) uses a unique design of a nitinol inner core and a tapered distal tip that has a polyurethane outer surface instead of a spring coil and a hydrophilic polymer coating. The hydrophilic coating is chemically bonded to the polyurethane jacket to reduce friction and thrombogenicity. The Magic Torque™ hydrophilic guidewire (Boston Scientific, Natick, MA) has enhanced radio-opacity with distal platinum markers to facilitate accurate vessel measurements and accurate placement.

The length of the guidewire is determined by its intended use. Most guidewires are 145–180 cm long. Exchange length guidewires are 260–450 cm long and allow catheters, balloon and other device exchanges while the guidewire is maintained in the distal position. The length of the guidewire will generally depend on the distance of the lesion from the access site and on the length of the catheter or the device that is being used.

For diagnostic procedures it is not necessary to use guidewires that are longer than 180 cm. However, during the interventional procedure it is generally recommended that exchange length (260 cm) guidewires be used. This length is necessary so as to have an adequate length of guidewire to be able to remove the device without losing the guidewire position across the lesion. It is occasionally necessary to use a 450 cm wire when brachial access is used for an intervention of femoral, popliteal or tibioperoneal arteries. In this circumstance a 450 cm long, 0.035 inch Geenan™ (Meditech, Boston Scientific, Natick, MA) guidewire is very useful.

When attempting to traverse severely stenotic lesions or occlusions of vessels it is essential to select a guidewire that is flexible and can be easily steered, yet has sufficient body stiffness. There are several products that are commonly used for this purpose. A 0.035 inch super-stiff angled Glidewire™, because of good steerability and sufficient support, is the wire of choice when crossing occluded vessels. The 0.018 inch angled Goldwire™ (Boston Scientific, Natick, MA) is another guidewire that has a hydrophilic coating and can be of great advantage for crossing severely stenotic or occluded femoral and tibioperoneal arteries. One of the disadvantages of wires with a hydrophilic coating is their propensity to cause perforations of the vessels when not used with caution. It is therefore not advisable to use these wires for renal or visceral interventions, for which shorter guidewires are more suitable. The 0.018 inch Steel Core or the 0.014 inch HI-TORQUE SPARTACORE™ 14 (Guidant, Santa Clara, CA) with a 3 and a 5 cm floppy tip, respectively, are currently used for renal and visceral interventions.

For endoluminal repair of abdominal aortic aneurysm (AAA) it is essential to have sufficient support to advance a large profile stent graft device across the iliac arteries. In this type of procedure a 0.035 inch, 260 cm long, Amplatz Super Stiff™ (Meditech, Boston Scientific, Natick, MA) guidewire or an even stiffer 0.035 inch, 260 cm long, Lunderquist™ (Cook, Bloomington, IN) guidewire should be used.

The Bentson™ (Cook, Bloomington, IN) wire is a 0.035 inch guidewire with a very soft body that allows easy tracking in a tortuous vessel. This wire is frequently used for advancing the catheter in the renal and other visceral vessels when other wires are not able to achieve this goal. It is also routinely used for advancing the vascular coils through the catheter for coil embolization.

Guidewires are available with different lengths of the flexible segments at their distal ends. Some products are available with 1, 3, 6, and 10 cm flexible tip segments. The purpose of the flexible segment of the wire is to conform itself to the vessel anatomy and avoid vessel trauma and spasm. The choice of length of the flexible segment will depend on the location of the vessel and the amount of support that is needed to advance the device. For carotid and renal interventions a 3 cm flexible segment length is commonly used; for endovascular AAA repair a 10 cm flexible tip length is usually selected.

Other specialty guidewires include infusion wires such as the ProStream™ (Micro Therapeutics, San Clemente, CA), the Katzen™ wire, the Cragg™ FX™ wire, and the Cragg™ Convertible™ wire (Meditech, Boston Scientific, Natick, MA) (Fig. 4.2). They have an outside diameter of either 0.035 or 0.038 inches and range from 145 to 180 cm in length. Multiple side-holes with various infusion port lengths from 3 to 50 cm and/or an open end-hole allow pharmacologic agents to be delivered to the occluded vessels. This wire configuration also permits the use of infusion catheters in a coaxial fashion. Some of the commonly used infusion catheters include the Meiwissen™, the Cragg™ McNamara™ valved infusion catheter (Meditech, Boston Scientific, Natick, MA), the MicroMewi™ (Micro Therapeutics, Irvine, CA) and the Tracker™ (Target Therapeutics, Freemont, CA). The infusion catheters are 0.018 inch guidewire compatible and also permit multiple lengths of coaxial infusion. The Meiwissen™ and the Cragg™ McNamara™ catheters are 4F and 5F and 135–150 cm long with infusion lengths of 5–30 cm.

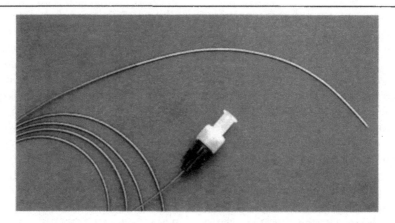

Fig. 4.2 The Cragg Convertible™ wire has an outer diameter of 0.038 inches and inside diameter of 0.027 inches.

For occluded vessels the Safe-Steer™ (IntraLuminal Therapeutics, Carlsbad, CA) guidewire system incorporates guidance technology (optical coherence reflectometry) to help safely negotiate and prevent vessel perforation. The Safe-Steer™ is available in several diameters ranging from 0.014 to 0.035 inches and has straight or angled tip configurations. It has been used in conjunction with the excimer laser to safely redirect the laser catheter using real-time feedback and recanalize a totally occluded superficial femoral artery.[2]

DISTAL PROTECTION GUIDEWIRE DEVICES

There are several guidewires systems that are designed to provide distal protection from embolization during coronary, cerebral, and peripheral intervention. Protective guidewire systems were developed in an effort to reduce the incidence of embolization during coronary and saphenous vein bypass graft intervention. More recently these devices have been tested and used during carotid and renal artery stenting. The devices used for cerebral protection during carotid artery stenting include the NeuroShield™ (MedNova, USA, Topsfield, MA), the GuardWire™ (PercuSurge™, Sunnyvale, CA) (Fig. 4.3), AngioGuard™ (Cordis/Johnson & Johnson, Warren, NJ) (Fig. 4.4), and the FilterWire EX™ embolic protection system (Boston Scientific, Natick, MA) (Fig. 4.5). Protective wires basically consist of a 0.014 inch wire with a filter basket or occluding balloon incorporated into the distal wire segment that captures any thromboembolic debris. So far these protective wires appear to be beneficial in reducing ischemic complications associated with coronary, renal and carotid interventions.[3-5]

DIAGNOSTIC CATHETERS

Diagnostic angiography is always performed prior to endovascular therapy since it determines the complexity of the procedure, the access site, and the equipment that may be needed to successfully complete the intervention.

Diagnostic catheters, like guidewires, are available in multiple shapes, sizes, and materials and serve many purposes. Diagnostic catheters are usually introduced into the vasculature over a J-shaped wire that has a soft distal tip. Diagnostic catheters can be divided into two basic categories: selective and non-selective. Non-selective catheters are usually designed with multiple side-holes – for example the 'pigtail' and the Omniflush™ (AngioDynamics, Queensbury, NY) – and are placed within a large vessel, such as the aorta or vena cava. These non-selective shapes provide high flow and rapid dispersion of a contrast agent. Angiography of high-flow vessels requires contrast injection by a power injector to obtain adequate opacification. The pigtail catheter is designed to protect the vessel walls from the whipping effect during power-injected boluses of contrast. Calibrated marker pigtail catheters are used to determine accurate sizing of vessel lumen. This is

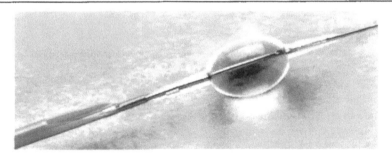

Fig. 4.3 The GuardWire™ distal protection wire.

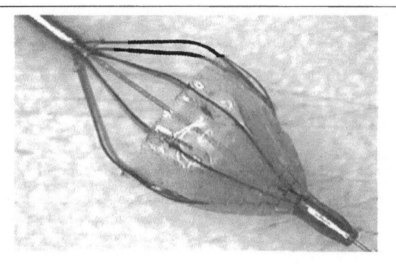

Fig. 4.4 The AngioGuard™ cerebral protection wire.

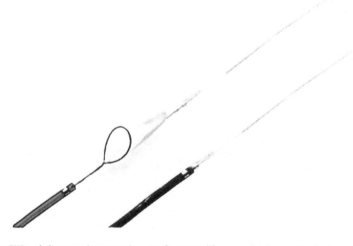

Fig. 4.5 The FilterWire EX™ embolic protection system is currently approved for use as distal protection during saphenous vein bypass graft intervention.

particularly important during endoluminal AAA repair. Radiopaque marker bands delineate a 20 cm segment, at 1 cm intervals, for precise measuring.

Catheter types and shapes are infinitely variable and choice is based on the type and location of the lesion. Selective catheters are pre-shaped to allow direct branch vessel engagement, pressure measurements, and contrast angiography. Specific catheters are recommended for specific anatomic locations and are designed to facilitate selective manipulation into branch vessels. Favorite pre-shaped catheter configurations are listed in Table 4.1. It is best to

Table 4.1 Pre-shaped Catheter Configurations

Area For Visualization	Size	Suggested Diagnostic Catheter
Aortic arch and branches (vertebral, subclavian, carotid)	4–6F	H1, H2, SIM1, SIM2, SIM3, JB1, JB2, JB3, MANI, VITEK, HINCK, MPA, Angled, Vertebral (100–125 cm length)
Visceral (renal, celiac, superior mesenteric)	4–6F	C1, C2, RDC, RDC2, HS, MPA, SIM1, SIM2 (65 cm length)
Abdominal aorta and iliac run-off	5–6F	PT, Tennis Racket
Contralateral iliac	5–6F	MPA, Hook, RIM, IM, SIM1, SIM2 (50 cm length)

have a variety of catheter shapes available for challenging anatomic situations. Precise knowledge of the type of catheter is very important for angiography so that appropriate and accurate information can be obtained prior to the intervention (Fig. 4.6). Each manufacturer provides detailed product information on the catheters and their use. Hydrophilic catheters are useful for a selective approach of the carotid arteries and to study the intracranial branches. Shorter length catheters (50 cm) are used for visceral, renal or contralateral iliac artery injections.

Selective catheters generally have a single hole, located at the tip, through which all injected contrast exits. Because of the single end-hole, flow rates are much lower than non-selective catheters and therefore power injectors should not be used. Furthermore, high-flow power injection through

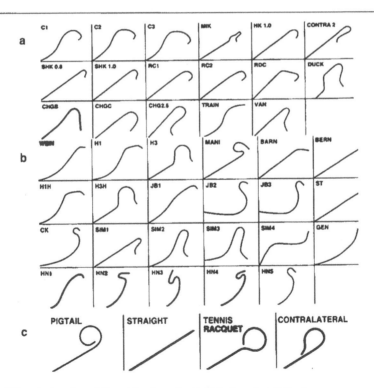

Fig. 4.6 (a) Visceral and (b) cerebral pre-formed diagnostic catheter shapes. (c) Angiography catheter shapes.

an end-hole catheter carries a considerable risk of vessel injury due to the end-hole jet effect.

Catheter size or outer diameter is measured in 'French' (1 mm = 3F), whereas catheter inner lumen diameter is measured in inches. Common inner lumen diameters range from 0.018 to 0.038 inches. This inner diameter measurement denotes the acceptable guidewire size for the catheter. A mismatch in size can cause problems, such as the guidewire not fitting inside the catheter or blood leakage around the guidewire. Diagnostic catheter sizes range from 4F to 6F, and lengths from 50 to 125 cm, respectively. Most of these catheters are braided, with a soft tip. Different catheter materials have specific functional characteristics such as stiffness or rigidity and kink-free torque control. Some catheters have inner and outer hydrophilic coatings to reduce friction for ease of passage and manipulation.

GUIDE CATHETERS

Like diagnostic catheters, guide catheters come in a variety of lengths and shapes designed to facilitate their manipulation into branch vessels. However, they differ from diagnostic catheters by having a substantially larger luminal diameter. Guide catheters are sized in the same fashion as diagnostic catheters with the outer diameter in French and the inner diameter in inches. To allow passage of the endovascular device, guide catheters must have a lumen diameter at least twice that of a typical diagnostic catheter. Guide catheters are similar to sheaths in that they provide protection to the vasculature when passing multiple devices into the same vessel. Important guide catheter characteristics include the ability to provide stable coaxial alignment between catheter tip and ostium of the vessel and kink-free torque control.

A properly selected guide catheter should also provide back-up support for balloon catheter advancement, reliable pressure monitoring, and adequate contrast delivery during injections. In comparison to diagnostic catheters, guide catheters have reinforced construction and a much stiffer shaft to provide back-up support for the advancement of guidewires, balloons and stents. Peripheral guide catheters are generally 6F, 7F or 8F and range from 65 to 100 cm in length with internal diameters ranging between 0.064 and 0.091 inches.

BALLOON DILATION CATHETERS

Balloon catheters are available in a wide variety of sizes, shapes, lengths, and compositions and are designed for different functions. They are the universal tool of endovascular intervention. The most important characteristic of a balloon dilation catheter is its ability to inflate to a precisely defined diameter at a known pressure. Factors that determine balloon characteristics are dependent on balloon composition. All of the percutaneous transluminal angioplasty (PTA) balloons are made of plastic polymers, which are then altered to enhance the physical properties of the balloon. The balloon's composition dictates its performance and is the primary determinant of compliance, burst pressure, and scratch or puncture resistance. A balloon's compliance is a measure of how much it continues to grow beyond its predetermined size when pressure is applied. Compliant balloons will stretch and expand in the direction of least resistance. The more it expands beyond its predetermined size, the greater the reduction of dilating force on the stenosis and the greater the chance of transmitting that force and causing trauma to the healthy, non-diseased vessel.

Non-compliant balloons, such as those made of polyethylene terephthalate (PET) or nylon reinforced polyurethane, have minimal expansion and have a high rated burst pressure. Manufacturers use proprietary additives to strengthen the balloon material and improve puncture resistance. Non-compliant balloons are more desirable because they provide a high dilating force up to the stated diameter and length, which may be necessary for highly calcified lesions.

Balloon dilation catheters are available in two basic designs: over-the-wire and on-the-wire. The over-the-wire system is when the wire and balloon move independently of each other; on-the-wire (fixed) systems consist of a balloon mounted directly on a steerable wire core. Because of advances in balloon and catheter technology, over-the-wire systems have as low a profile and perform competitively with on-the-wire systems. Unfortunately, although lower profile and smaller diameter shafts may allow access to smaller vessels, they may not be stiff enough to push through tight, heavily calcified lesions. Therefore, stiffer catheter shafts and lubricous coatings such as silicone have been applied to the outside of balloon catheters to help prevent kinking and ease the passage through tortuous and tight lesions. The best results achieved with a balloon catheter are on short, concentric, and non-calcified lesions.

Balloons are available in several shapes that vary by manufacturer and balloon type. Other very important considerations when selecting a balloon is the length of the catheter tip, the length of taper to the shoulders of the balloon, and the length of the balloon. The use of short tip, short taper balloons minimizes the trauma to the adjacent non-diseased vessel wall and is especially useful at vessel branch points or at sites of acute angulation, which is commonly seen in the extracranial vasculature. Balloon lengths range from 1.5 to 10 cm and the shortest balloon that completely straddles the lesion should be used. Longer balloons may be necessary in the iliac, femoral or popliteal area. The carotid, renal, celiac, and mesenteric vessels generally require shorter balloons. The 'kissing' balloons are advisable when treating bifurcation vessels such as those in the aortoiliac region.

Balloon size is selected after measuring the diameter of the reference artery distal to the target lesion using digital subtraction angiography. Depending on the anatomy, balloon sizes can vary (Table 4.2) from 2 to 40 mm in diameter. The smaller balloons are generally used for dilating vessels below the knee. In many instances, such as in carotid intervention, a smaller coronary balloon (3–4 mm) is used to pre-dilate the stenosis prior to stent implantation and a larger balloon (5–6 mm) is used after stent implantation. Balloon dilation after endoluminal exclusion of AAA is performed with larger balloons such as the XXL™ (12–18 mm) (Meditech, Boston Scientific, Natick, MA) and the

Table 4.2 Balloon Sizes

Target Vessel	Balloon Diameter (mm)	Balloon Length (cm)
Internal carotid	4–6	2
Common carotid	5–7	2–4
Subclavian	5–8	2–4
Vertebral	3–5	2
Abdominal aorta	10–26	2–4
Renal	4–8	2
Celiac and mesenteric	4–6	2
Common and external iliac	6–10	2–4
Common or superficial femoral	4–6	2–10
Popliteal	3–5	2–4
Tibial or peroneal	<4	2–4

Impact™ (20–35 mm) (B Braun Medical, Bethlehem, PA).

Contrary to dilating balloons, occlusion balloons are used to temporarily occlude arterial blood flow. Occlusion balloons such as the Equalizer™ (Boston Scientific, Natick, MA) are made of latex rubber and have a large liquid capacity. They range from 20 to 40 mm in diameter and are indicated during applications of temporary vessel occlusion during angiographic visualization, accurate stent graft deployment or emergency control of hemorrhage. Finally, placement or positioning of balloons should be accomplished under fluoroscopic guidance using road-mapping techniques and anatomic landmarks.

ADJUNCTIVE ENDOVASCULAR TOOLS

STENTS

In spite of significant improvements in technology, balloon angioplasty remains plagued with unacceptable restenosis rates for complex lesions, requiring reintervention. Vascular stents were developed to deal with residual stenosis after angioplasty, dissection, recoil, and late failure due to restenosis. Some of these problems, however, have not been completely resolved by using stents.

The concept of vascular stenting originated with Charles Dotter in 1969, but it did not become a clinical reality until the 1980s. Endovascular coils were first described in 1983 using a nitinol coil to support the arteries in an animal model.[6,7] These initial experiments were the catalyst for further development in stents to treat vascular disease non-surgically. Since that time, many stents have been designed and evaluated in both the animal laboratory and clinically. Stents have become the most important mechanical innovation for percutaneous revascularization.

In 1985, Palmaz and colleagues[8] described preliminary results of balloon expandable stainless steel stents in canine arteries. Of the 18 arteries stented, 22% developed thrombotic occlusion. It was in this small series that the need for adequate antithrombotic and antiplatelet therapy at the time of stent deployment became well recognized.[9] Since that time, an antiplatelet regimen has been included as a standard clinical practice for all stent procedures, which has had a pivotal effect in reducing the incidence of stent thrombosis. Although the rates today are low compared to early results, stent thrombosis can be a disastrous complication with a high risk of ischemic sequelae. Those who receive stents for high-risk indications should be considered for an even more intense antithrombotic regimen.

All stents share a common function of enlarging and supporting the vascular lumen and decreasing the incidence of complications and restenosis. They do, however, differ in their fundamental designs. There are two basic types of stent that differ considerably: balloon expandable and self-expanding. Balloon expandable stents are generally pre-mounted on a balloon and can be placed accurately and offer greater radial strength. They initially resist deformation, but can eventually yield under stress (compression) and become irreversibly deformed. Because of a risk of deformation or 'crush', balloon expandable stents are not recommended for use in extracranial carotid or femoropopliteal locations. Balloon expandable stents are best suited for accurate placement at the site of ostial lesions such as in the renal, celiac, and mesenteric arteries and are ideal for ostial aortic arch lesions.

Conversely, self-expanding stents behave elastically and do not become deformed. However, they have less radial strength than balloon expandable stents. In addition, their placement is less accurate than balloon expandable stents and they have sharp strut ends.

BIOCOMPATIBILITY

Other stent characteristics include biocompatibility, which refers to the stent's ability to resist thrombosis. The stent surface is an important determinant of its thrombogenic potential. All currently available stents are made of metal. The composition and characteristics of the stent itself have been shown to initiate a complex interaction between the blood components and the metallic surface of the stent. The nature of the flow in the vessel also determines the degree to which blood elements interact with the structures on the vessel wall.[10] Special coatings have been added to metallic stents to provide a biological inert barrier between the stent surface and the circulating blood to improve the hemodynamic compatibility as well as the biocompatibility of the stent.[11-14]

FLEXIBILITY

Flexibility is another very important stent characteristic because of the tortuosity and angulation that is encountered in the periphery. The flexibility of a stent is the amount of force required to flex it a given amount, or the force with which it resists bending. A flexible stent can be deployed in a tortuous artery without altering its normal course, whereas an inflexible stent when deployed can straighten the vessel, forcing it to conform to its shape rather than vice versa. Most balloon expandable stents are less flexible than self-expanding stents. The least flexible stent is the non-articulated stent – for example the Palmaz™ (Cordis/Johnson & Johnson, Warren, NJ) (Fig. 4.7) – and therefore the majority of the newer stent designs have articulations.

ANATOMIC APPLICATIONS

Different types of stent are used for specific anatomic applications. The newer pre-mounted,

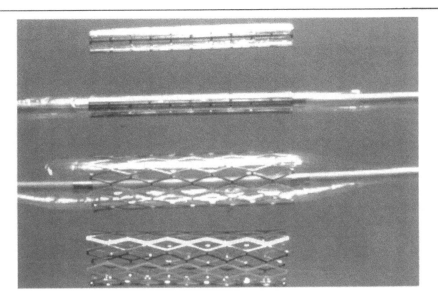

Fig. 4.7 The non-articulated Palmaz™ stent.

low profile, balloon expandable stents such as the HERCULINK™ PLUS (Guidant, Santa Clara, CA), NIRROYAL™ (Meditech, Boston Scientific, Natick, MA), the Express™ (Boston Scientific, Natick, MA), the Genesis™ (Cordis/Johnson & Johnson, Warren, NJ) and the Bridge™ Assurant™ (Medtronic AVE, Santa Rosa, CA) are well suited for iliac, renal, celiac, and mesenteric arteries. The lower profile self-expanding nitinol stents such as the Luminexx™ and Conformexx™ stents (CR Bard, Temple, AZ), PROTEGE™ GPS™ (IntraTherapeutics, St Paul, MN), the 0.018 inch S.M.A.R.T.™ or 0.014 inch PRECISE™ (Cordis/Johnson & Johnson, Warren, NJ) and the Absolute™ (Guidant, Menlo Park, CA) provide minimal shortening for accurate placement and are useful in subclavian, iliac, and extracranial carotid intervention. As far as femoral and popliteal stenting is concerned, the IntraCoil™ (IntraTherapeutics, St Paul, MN) (Fig. 4.8) has shown encouraging results.

Renal artery stenting has shown superior results to balloon angioplasty by avoiding recoil and dissection. In the early stages of renal artery stenting

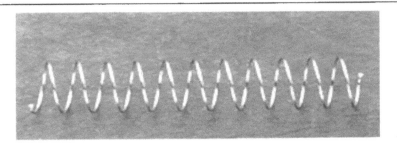

Fig. 4.8 The IntraCoil™ stent.

the Palmaz™ 15, 20 or 29 mm stent was mounted on a peripheral balloon that was from 5 to 8 mm in diameter and 20 mm in length. The majority of current generation stents are pre-mounted on a balloon that is lower in profile and specifically designed for visceral and renal artery stenting. They are available in over-the-wire or monorail design. The HERCULINK™ PLUS (Guidant, Santa Clara, CA) comes pre-mounted on a ViaTrax 90 or 135 cm monorail balloon system that is 0.014 inch guidewire compatible. Deployed stent diameters range from 4.5 to 7.0 mm. The Bridge™ Assurant™ stent and the Palmaz™ Genesis™ stent (Cordis/Johnson & Johnson, Warren, NJ) are pre-mounted. They are available on 0.018 inch over-the-wire systems that are either 80 or 135 cm in length. Deployed stent diameters range from 5.0 to 9.0 mm and are between 12 and 39 mm in length.

FUTURE STRATEGIES

Stent coatings are also being investigated as a way of decreasing neointimal hyperplasia. For reasons that remain unclear, some patients develop an aggressive neointimal hyperplasia, leaving restenosis as the main clinical obstacle of stent technology. In an attempt to deal with the shortcomings of stents, future strategies include:

* stents made of biological materials and stent grafts;
* polymer-coated stents that are thromboresistant;
* biodegradable stents that absorb, avoiding a permanent prosthetic implant;
* drug-eluting stents;
* radioactive stents or using adjunctive radiotherapy.

CRYOPLASTY

Despite extensive research, restenosis remains the major limitation to the long-term success of angioplasty. While stents have addressed the problems of recoil and intimal dissection, an ideal solution for neointimal proliferation has been elusive. Endovascular radiation therapy has shown results

for the prevention of restenosis; however, it may be associated with a higher risk of late thrombotic complications and long-term tissue effects are not well characterized.

Cryotherapy has been used as a surgical modality to reduce scar formation.[15] PolarCath™ (Boston Scientific, Natick, MA) has been developed as a cryoplasty system that delivers a precisely controlled temperature and pressure to the arterial wall using a liquid nitrous oxide-filled balloon (Fig. 4.9). The PolarCath™ peripheral dilation system incorporates conventional balloon angioplasty with cryotherapy to reduce post-dilation elastic recoil by triggering freezing-induced apoptosis. The PolarCath™ is available in a broad range of balloon diameters and lengths and is capable of multiple inflations for treating long lesions.

ENDOGRAFTS

The rapid evolution of transcatheter devices for the delivery of vascular endoprostheses has given non-surgical interventional radiologists and cardiologists the opportunity to get involved in the vascular surgical arena. Endoluminal stent grafts are now being used to treat aneurysmal and occlusive arterial disease.[16–21] The vascular endoprosthesis represents a joining of stent and surgical bypass graft technology. A variety of graft materials are used to line or cover the stent. Although it is yet to be proven, the covered stent may limit the intimal hyperplasia and improve long-term patency compared with balloon angioplasty and stenting.

Indications for using a covered stents include:

* arterial rupture;
* arteriovenous fistulas;
* arterial trauma;
* aneurysms.

Possible indications for using covered stents include:

* long occlusions or stenosis;
* long dissections.

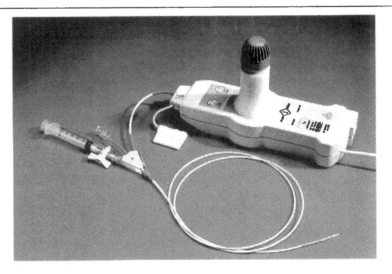

Fig. 4.9 The PolarCath™ combines traditional balloon angioplasty with cryotherapy by cooling the inflation balloon to –10°C during dilation.

There are several covered stents that have been approved for non-vascular use or are used in clinical investigation, including:

- the Viabahn™ (WL Gore, Flagstaff, AZ);
- the Wallgraft™ (Boston Scientific, Natick, MA);
- the JOSTENT™ (JOMED International AB, Helsingborg, Sweden);
- the Fluency™ (Bard Peripheral Vascular, Temple, AZ).

All but one of the currently available endoluminal grafts are made of self-expanding nitinol. The JOSTENT™ stent graft is a balloon expandable system (Fig. 4.10). This system uses a double thin, stainless steel stent with expandable polytetrafluoroethylene (PTFE) material sandwiched between the two stents. It ranges from 5 to 10 mm in diameter and is from 28 to 58 cm long. It has been implanted successfully in renal, iliac, femoral, and tibioperoneal arteries.

The Wallgraft™, which is still in clinical trials in the United States, has been used to successfully treat iliac, femoral, and popliteal aneurysms and iliac artery occlusive disease.[22,23] It is composed of PET graft material covering a Wallstent™ (Fig.

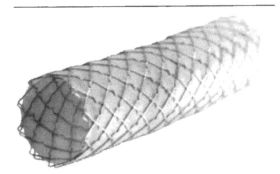

Fig. 4.10 The JOSTENT™ graft is stainless steel, balloon expandable and covered with an expandable PTFE coating.

4.11). The UNISTEP™PLUS delivery system has a working length of 90 cm and is supplied with the Wallgraft™. This stent graft is available in diameters from 6 to 14 mm and lengths of 20, 30, 50, and 70 mm. The system accommodates a 0.035 inch guidewire.

In an international trial,[24] the Viabahn™ endoprosthesis showed promising patency rates at 1 year for treatment of iliac and femoral artery occlusive disease. This device is composed of a

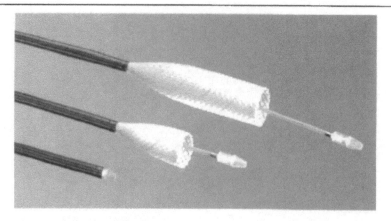

Fig. 4.11 The Wallgraft™ is a self-expanding stent graft.

self-expanding nitinol stent, which is incorporated in an ultrathin PTFE cover (Fig. 4.12).

The Fluency™ is made of nitinol and PTFE similar to the Viabahn™ although it incorporates radiopaque tantalum markers which enhance visualization during deployment. This device is loaded in a kink-resistant delivery system. Expanded stent diameters range from 6 to 10 mm, and lengths from 40 to 80 mm.

ENDOLUMINAL GRAFTS FOR TREATMENT OF ABDOMINAL AORTIC ANEURYSMS

Endoluminal grafts are gaining acceptance in the treatment of thoracic and abdominal aortic aneurysms (AAA). Initial experience with endovascular AAA exclusion was performed with straight, non-bifurcated devices.[25,26] The early prostheses

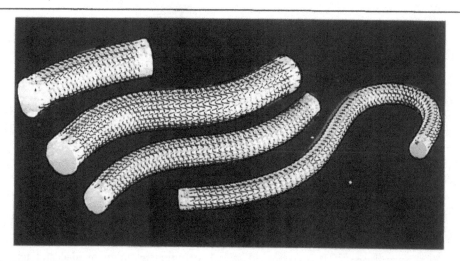

Fig. 4.12 The Viabahn endoprosthesis.

were relatively inflexible and required a 24F internal diameter introducer sheath. Few patients, however, were candidates for the tubular endo-prosthesis. Nowadays, bifurcated grafts are available and are smaller in diameter and more flexible than the first generation devices. Most of the stent grafts used today are fully supported by a self-expanding stent.

There are multiple systems used around the world; however, only four are commercially available in the United States. The first two such systems were the Ancure™ (Guidant, Menlo Park, CA) and the AneuRx™ (Medtronic AVE, Santa Rosa, CA). Both devices are over-the-wire systems that require bilateral femoral artery access; however, fundamental differences exist between these two systems.

ANCURE™

The Ancure™ was an unsupported single piece of woven Dacron fabric. The graft was bifurcated with no intragraft junctions. The device was delivered through a 24F introducer sheath; a 12F sheath was required to facilitate the deployment of the contralateral limb. The graft was attached by a series of hooks located at the proximal aortic end and at both the distal iliac limbs. The hooks are seated transmurally in the aorta and the iliac arteries and affixed by low-pressure balloon dilation. Radiopaque markers are located on the body of the graft for positioning and alignment. The use of the unibody design eliminated the endoleaks that can originate in the 'overlaps' between various components of modular endografts. Tortuous anatomy and narrowed, calcified iliac arteries, however, can make the deployment of this stiff, one-piece system very difficult. Several investigators have reported that less than 30% of patients that were referred to their institutions for endoluminal AAA repair were candidates for Ancure™ device.[24-28]

This adds to the complexity and the duration of the procedure. Because of the increasing number of clinical complications with Ancure™, in April 2001 the manufacturer of this device announced a voluntary recall of the endograft and halted the production until these problems were resolved. This device was again released for clinical use in August 2001 but in July 2003 Guidant voluntarily halted production of the stent graft system and withdrew it from the market because of increased competition after the release of two new endograft systems.

ANEURX™

The AneuRx™ device (Medtronic AVE, Santa Rosa, CA) is a modular two-piece system (Fig. 4.13) composed of a main bifurcation segment and a contralateral iliac limb. The graft is made of

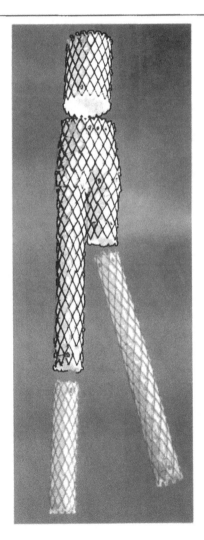

Fig. 4.13 The AneuRx™ modular stent graft system.

thin-walled woven polyester that is fully supported by a self-expanding nitinol exoskeleton. The main bifurcated body is delivered through a 21F or 22F sheath; the contralateral limb requires a 16F sheath. The body of the graft has radiopaque markers for alignment and positioning; attachment is accomplished by radial force.

In September 2002, a new version of AneuRx Expedient™ Delivery was released. This innovation offers a tapered tip, which is more flexible and allows introduction of the device via a percutaneous approach (without a sheath). Another improvement in the delivery device includes the use of a lubricous coating that allows easier stent graft deployment. This stent graft is easily deployed by retracting a protective sleeve.

EXCLUDER™

The Excluder™ endograft (WL Gore, Flagstaff, AZ) was approved for use in November 2002. It is a fully supported, self-expanding modular device. The Excluder™ consists of expanded PTFE on the luminal surface and a nitinol-supporting frame on the outer surface (Fig. 4.14). The two modular components are pre-mounted on separate delivery catheters and constrained using a lacing suture, which courses the length of the catheter and is attached to a deployment knob at the operator end. When the knob is loosened and pulled back it releases the suture and the stent-graft component expands immediately. An 18F sheath is used to advance the bifurcated aortic component and a 12F sheath is used for the contralateral iliac limb.

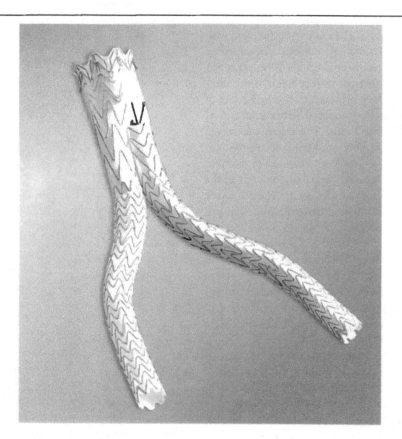

Fig. 4.14 The Excluder™ endoprosthesis is an 18F stent graft system.

ZENITH™

The Zenith™ stent graft (Cook, Bloomington, IN) is the most recent stent graft system to be approved for clinical use. It is a fully supported modular bifurcated system that incorporates a polyester fabric on a network of Z-stents (Fig. 4.15). This device utilizes uncovered stents and a series of suprarenal barbs which, when released, are designed to mimic a surgical anastomosis.[17] A 20F sheath is used to advance the bifurcated aortic component and a 12F sheath is used for the contralateral iliac limb deployment. Positioning and deployment of this stent graft system is more complex than for the AneuRx™ and the Excluder™.

OTHER STENT GRAFT SYSTEMS

Other systems being investigated include the Talent™ (Medtronic AVE, Santa Rosa, CA) (Fig. 4.16), the PowerLink™ (Endologix, Irvine, CA), Lifepath™ (Edwards Lifesciences LLC, Irvine, CA), EndoFit™ (Endomed, Phoenix, AZ), Fortron™ (Cordis, Miami, FL) and Enovus™ (TriVascular, Santa Rosa, CA). Some of these systems incorporate a design feature that affixes the graft in a healthy segment in the suprarenal aorta with the proximal end of the graft left uncovered to accommodate patients with more complex anatomy.[27,28]

There are several devices available in clinical trials for endovascular treatment of descending thoracic aortic aneurysms.[29-31] Clinical trials are slow in the United States and have been limited to the use of the thoracic Excluder™ endoprosthesis and the Talent™. The Excluder™ stent graft is composed of a self-expanding nitinol stent exoskeleton lined with an ultrathin-walled PTFE. Graft diameter ranges from 26 to 40 mm and length from 7.5 to 20 cm. The grafts can be implanted singly or in multiples according to the length of the diseased segment. In the initial feasibility trial,[30] there were no instances of deployment failure, conversion to open surgery, graft occlusion or paralysis. Later follow-up has unfortunately revealed evidence of stent fractures, primarily affecting the dorsal (spine) wire that traverses the length of the device. Upon removal of this wire the manufacturer has not reported any further problems.

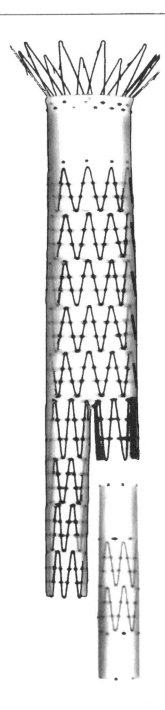

Fig. 4.15 The Zenith™ AAA endovascular graft bifurcated three-component system.

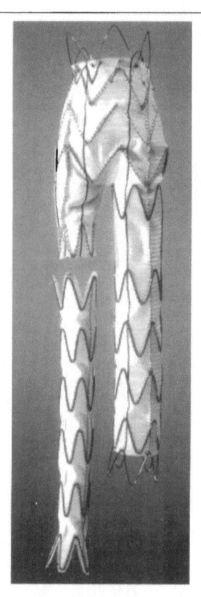

Fig. 4.16 The Talent™ bifurcated stent graft allows suprarenal fixation.

The Talent™ thoracic stent graft consists of a self-expandable stent that is sutured to a PET material. The stent graft segments range from 26 to 46 mm in diameter and from 76 to 131 mm in length. The delivery device ranges from 22F to 25F.

MECHANICAL THROMBECTOMY DEVICES

Mechanical thrombectomy has been developed to address a number of significant problems associated with chemical thrombolysis. These problems include frequent bleeding complications, prolonged procedure times, the cost and the risk of the thrombolytic agent, and residual clot. A number of mechanical devices have been developed to disrupt and remove freshly formed thrombus from the circulation. There are three hydrodynamic devices currently in use: the AngioJet™ Rheolytic™ thrombectomy system, the Hydrolyser™ thrombectomy catheter, and the Oasis™ Amplatz thrombectomy system

ANGIOJET™

The AngioJet™ Rheolytic™ thrombectomy system (Possis Medical, Minneapolis, MN) is approved for use in the arterial circulation and is an over-the-wire system that uses high-velocity saline jets (Fig. 4.17). Pulverized clot is then aspirated by the Bernoulli effect induced vacuum at the tip of the catheter. Microfragments are discharged through the outflow lumen into the collecting bag.[32] Wagner et al reported a success rate of 90% and low incidence of amputation and mortality using rheolytic thrombectomy for treatment of limb ischemia.[33] AngioJet™ catheters were first designed for coronary vessels, 5F in size and requiring a 0.018 inch guidewire. A second generation AngioJet™ device (Xpeedior™) is 6F in size and 0.035 inch guidewire compatible, offering greater effectiveness in thrombus removal and better suited for treating larger peripheral vessels. There is now a 4F thrombectomy device (XPI™) available from the same manufacturer (Possis Medical, Minneapolis, MN).

HYDROLYSER™

The Hydrolyser™ thrombectomy catheter (Cordis Europa NV, Roden, The Netherlands) is another over-the-wire hydrodynamic thrombectomy system. This system uses the Venturi principle for aspiration and removal of intravascular thrombus. Negative pressure pulls the thrombus into the

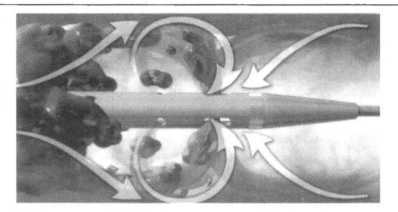

Fig. 4.17 The AngioJet™ Rheolytic™ thrombectomy system.

heparinized saline stream, resulting in microfragments that are discharged through the outflow lumen into the collection bag. In reports from the European trials,[34,35] this device may be of benefit in thrombus-containing lesions and in degenerated vein grafts.

OASIS™

The Oasis™ Amplatz thrombectomy system (Meditech, Boston Scientific, Natick, MA) is the third hydrodynamic system that has been used in the United States for obstructed renal dialysis grafts. It is also an over-the-wire system that works on the same Venturi principle as the Hydrolyser™.

There are several other systems that do not work on the hydrodynamic principle (Table 4.3). They include impeller devices, therapeutic ultrasound, suction and clot-macerating devices, all of which all are designed to remove thrombus.

DEBULKING DEVICES

There are a variety of debulking devices, including directional atherectomy, plaque excision, rotational atherectomy, and laser ablation that have been investigated as potential means of improving long-term patency and reducing restenosis. None thus far has clearly demonstrated clear advantage

Table 4.3 Commercially Available Thrombectomy Devices

Hydrodynamic Devices (thrombus is broken up by a high-velocity saline stream):
- Oasis™ Amplatz thrombectomy system (Meditech, Boston Scientific, Natick, MA)
- AngioJet™ Rheolytic™ thrombectomy catheter (Possis Medical, Minneapolis, MN)
- Hydrolyser™ thrombectomy catheter (Cordis Europa NV, Roden, The Netherlands)

Impeller Devices (thrombus is cleared by a rotating internal impeller):
- Clotbuster™ Amplatz thrombectomy catheter (Microvena, White Bear Lake, MN)
- Straub Rotarex™ (Straub Medical AG, Straubstrasse, CH-7323 Wangs)

Ultrasonic Devices (thrombus is dissolved with therapeutic ultrasound):
- Sonicath (Guidant, St Paul, MN)
- Acolysis System™ (Angiosonics, Morrisville, NC)

Suction Devices (thrombus is extracted by manual aspiration):
- GuardWire™ (PercuSurge™, Sunnyvale, CA)

Clot-Macerating Devices (thrombus is macerated):
- Arrow-Trotola™ thrombectomy device (Arrow International, Reading, PA)
- Cragg Thrombolytic Brush™ (Micro Therapeutics, Irvine, CA)
- Gelbfish EndoVac (NeoVascular Technologies, New York, NY)
- PMT (Baxter, Irvine, CA)

over other devices for peripheral revascularization.[36-40] The technique of debulking (EVI™ remote endarterectomy catheter; EndoVascular

Instruments, Vancouver, WA) prior to endoluminal femoropopliteal bypass is now being tested as a means of increasing long-term patency rates after lower extremity bypass. In addition, atherectomy devices such as the REDHA-CUT™ (SherineMed, Irvine, CA), designed specifically to treat in-stent restenosis, are under investigation.

DIRECTIONAL ATHERECTOMY

Directional atherectomy has the unique capability of resecting and retrieving intact atherosclerotic plaque. The atherectomy catheter (Atherotrack™, Mallinckrodt, St Louis, MO) is a coaxial multi-lumen catheter designed for percutaneous resection of atheromatous material. It consists of a catheter shaft equipped distally with a balloon mounted opposite a housing unit and proximally with a central adapter and a battery-operated motor drive unit. The distal housing contains a rigid cutter within an open window. The balloon is used to support the rigid cutter housing and push the plaque into the housing window. A lever on the motor drive unit allows the operator to activate and slowly advance the cutter through the lesion as it rotates at 2000 rpm. Excised atheroma is stored in a distal nose cone collection chamber. Peripheral catheters are 7F to 11F with working diameters of 5.3–9.7 mm. Directional atherectomy may be useful to debulk focal or eccentric stenosis, but there is no clear-cut, long-term improvement over balloon angioplasty alone.

PLAQUE EXCISION

Similar to directional atherectomy, the Silverhawk™ (Foxhollow Technologies, Redwood City, CA) mechanically excises large volumes of plaque while minimizing vessel barotrauma. The Silverhawk™ is a monorail system (Fig. 4.18) and has clinical approval in both the coronary and peripheral circulation and excises vessels between 2 and 6 mm in diameter. Unlike directional atherectomy, the Silverhawk™ cutter is apposed to the plaque wall mechanically without any balloon dilation and the length of excision is not limited by the device design but rather by the operator passing the device through the lesion.

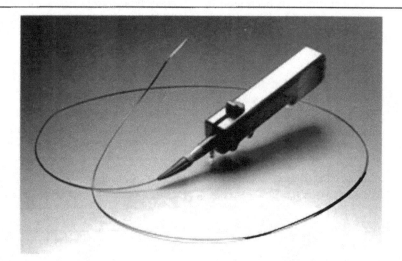

Fig. 4.18 The Silverhawk™ plaque excision system.

The Silverhawk™ consists of a 0.014 inch monorail catheter with a rotating inner blade that is contained within a tubular housing. The device is powered by the battery-driven cutter driver. Excised tissue is captured and stored in the tip of the catheter.

ROTATIONAL ATHERECTOMY

The Rotablator™ system (Boston Scientific Northwest, Redmond, WA) consists of a reusable console that controls the rotational speed of an olive-shaped, nickel-plated, brass burr, which is coated on its leading edge with 20–30 micron diamond chips and is bonded to a flexible drive shaft. The rotating burr is regulated by a compressed air or nitrogen-driven turbine. The rotating burr (160,000–170,000 rpm) is cooled by a saline flush as it is slowly advanced through a stenosis. Rotational atherectomy can achieve a lumen that is 90% of the selected burr size. It has not, however, been demonstrated to have an advantage for iliac and superficial femoral artery lesions but may be useful to debulk short calcified lesions and branch stenosis in the smaller popliteal and tibioperoneal arteries. This device today is rarely used in the periphery.

EXCIMER LASER ABLATION

The excimer laser energy (Spectranetics, Colorado Springs, CO) emits a pulsed, ultraviolet light at 308 nanometers. Ablation of inorganic material is achieved by photochemical mechanisms that involve the breakdown of molecular bonds without generating heat.[41] The role of laser angioplasty in peripheral revascularization is still investigational in the United States. Preliminary results of a phase I clinical trial (Laser Angioplasty for Critical Ischemia) indicate that excimer laser angioplasty is safe and feasible in popliteal occlusive disease with a 3-month patency rate of 88%.[42] Laser angioplasty may also be useful in total occlusions that are refractory to other techniques. Several clinical trials, however, have not shown any advantage of this device over balloon angioplasty for treatment of superficial femoral and popliteal artery lesions.

RADIATION THERAPY

Low dose radiation has been suggested to inhibit intimal hyperplasia. Recent clinical data indicate that peripheral vascular brachytherapy may be effective in the prevention of restenosis.[43] The double lumen PARIS centering catheter (Guidant, Santa Clara, CA) with multiple segmented centering balloons is used to deliver gamma ^{192}Ir to the target site. Radioactive stents with low-activity beta emitters (^{32}P) have been suggested as a method of treatment for the larger peripheral vessels. Balloons filled with different isotopes (^{188}RE or ^{186}RE) have also been suggested as a way of delivering radiation to the vessel. All of these methods, however, are still under investigation. Future studies will focus on isotope selection, dosing strategies, and optimal stent designs for delivery of radiation. Brachytherapy so far has not shown significant benefit over balloon angioplasty for treatment of superficial femoral and popliteal artery lesions.

Frontrunner™ X39 CTO (LuMend, Redwood City, CA) is designed to treat chronic total occlusions. The system facilitates guidewire placement by utilizing the controlled blunt microdissection technique with the Frontrunner™ X39 CTO catheter which separates the plaque, creating a microchannel as it moves through the total occlusion. The Frontrunner™ X39 CTO is supported by a microguide catheter that serves as the conduit for guidewire exchange once the total occlusion is crossed.

PERCUTANEOUS CLOSURE DEVICES

A variety of devices are available for arterial hemostasis after sheath removal. They include mechanical clamp (Compressar; Instrumedix, Hillsboro, OR), inflatable pressure device (FemoStop™; USCI, Billerica, MA), extravascular collagen plug (VasoSeal™; Datascope, Montvale, NJ), intravascular anchor and collagen plug (St Jude Medical, Daig Division, Minnetonka, MN), bioabsorbable pledgets (Duet™ Thrombin; Vascular Solutions, Minneapolis, MN) and vessel suturing device (Perclose™; Abbott, Redwood City, CA) deployed through specifically designed catheters.

Perclose devices (Perclose™; Abbott, Redwood City, CA) are available in 6-, 8- or 10F catheter systems. They are designed for percutaneous deployment of surgical sutures to common femoral artery puncture sites. The 10F Perclose™ has been used to repair large bore sheath sites (16F) after endoluminal repair of abdominal aortic aneurysms.[44-47] The 10F device is advanced into the femoral artery over a 0.035 inch guidewire until adequate blood marking is achieved through the dedicated marker lumen, indicating the sutures and needles are within the vessel lumen (Fig. 4.19a). Four needles are then deployed and sutures are removed from the hub (Fig. 4.19b). The upper and lower sets of sutures are identified but remain untied. The device is then partially backed out of the femoral artery and a 0.035 inch guidewire is reinserted through the guidewire port. The device is then removed and an 11F sheath is reintroduced over the guidewire. The sheath is then upsized to 16F. After completion of the procedure, the sutures are tied with a sliding knot and the knot pusher is used to assure approximation of the knot to the vessel wall for adequate hemostasis (Fig. 4.19c). The subcutaneous tissues are then infiltrated with 1% lidocaine (lignocaine) with adrenaline (epinephrine) and the incision edges are approximated with adhesive steristrips. An arterial tamper device may or may not be required to achieve adequate hemostasis.

In addition, new hemostatic pads are now available for use as topical aids to accelerate clot formation at the vascular access site. Syvek™ NT (Marine Polymer Technologies, Danvers, MA) and Chito-Seal™ (Abbott Vascular, Redwood City, CA) are

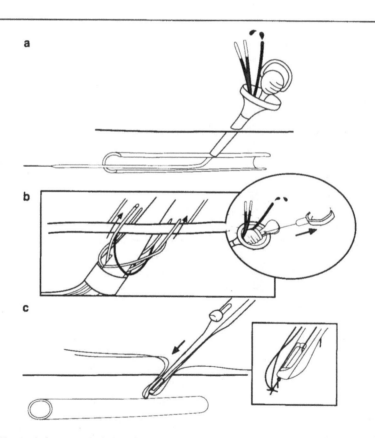

Fig. 4.19 Perclose™ is a surgical suture method of arteriotomy closure.

topical hemostasis pads that contain a potent marine biopolymer called chitin that has been positively charged, making it a potent hemostatic agent. Use of the pads can reduce compression time and accelerate hemostasis.[48,49]

VASCULAR OCCLUSION DEVICES

There are several types of vascular occlusion coil (Tornado™ Embolization Coils and Microcoils™, Gianturco-Grifka Vascular Occlusion Device; Cook, Bloomington, IN) that are used to occlude selective vessel supply to arteriovenous malformations, intrasaccular pseudoaneurysms[50] or collateral vessel branch flow feeding an aneurysmal sac. Coil embolization has been successfully used to treat pulmonary artery branch rupture after Swan-Ganz catheterization.[51] Coil embolization has become a common procedure performed to occlude internal iliac artery branches in patients with aneurysmal

common iliac arteries prior to or after endoluminal AAA repair to remedy collateral branch flow.[52] Coils (Fig. 4.20) or embolization particles are deployed percutaneously through diagnostic catheters that are coated to prevent friction. Coils range from 2 to 14 cm in length with diameters from 0.018 to 0.038 inches. Platinum coils with synthetic fibers incorporated help to maximize thrombogenicity. The microcoil design permits delivery into the target vessel by saline flush or by push technique.

VASCULAR SNARES

Vascular snares are designed specifically for foreign body retrieval and device manipulation in the cardiovascular and peripheral vascular systems. This includes fractured catheters, guidewires, balloons, embolic coils, undeployed stents or other foreign bodies. They are also used to manipulate or

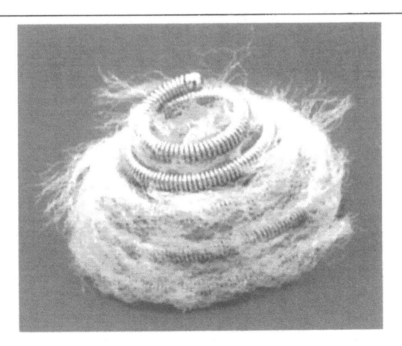

Fig. 4.20 Fibered platinum embolization coil.

reposition catheters or to facilitate contralateral guidewire pull-through during endoluminal AAA repair. Snare loops come in various sizes (2–35 mm) (Fig. 4.21) and sizing the snare loop to the vessel is extremely important for successful retrieval and manipulation. The snare loop and the vessel lumen should be coaxial for proper insertion.

FUTURE DEVELOPMENTS

Future developments remain focused on the issue of restenosis and neointimal hyperplasia. The field of 'Smart' stents, which refers to drug-eluting and thromboresistent stents, and stent grafts will have an important role in defining the future course of endovascular therapy. New opportunities being explored are those that would influence local vascular biology, for example cell-seeding, genes, and non-reactive polymer carriers that elicit optimal biologic effects.

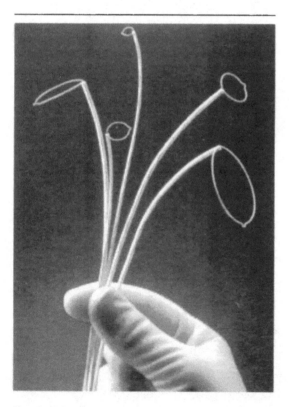

Fig. 4.21 Snares come in various loop sizes for retrieval of foreign bodies from the circulation.

REFERENCES

1. Dotter CT, Judkins MP. Transluminal treatment of arteriosclerotic obstruction: description of a new technique and preliminary results of its application. Circulation 1964;30:654–70.
2. Biamino G, Schofer J, Tübler T, Schulter M. A new vascular approach to chronic total occlusions of the superficial femoral artery [abstract]. International Congress on Endovascular Interventions 2000.
3. Al-Mubarak N, Colombo A, Gaines PA, et al. Multicenter evaluation of carotid artery stenting with a filter protection system. J Am Coll Cardiol 2002;39:841–6.
4. Diethrich EB, Rodriguez-Lopez J, Ramaiah V, Olsen D. Comparison of carotid stenting with and without cerebral protection versus carotid endarterectomy in a single center experience. J Am Coll Cardiol 2001;37(suppl A):829–32.
5. Henry M, Henry I, Klonaris C, et al. Renal angioplasty and stenting under protection: the way for the future? Catheter Cardiovasc Interv 2003;60:299–312.
6. Dotter CT, Buschmann PAC, Mckinney MK, Rösch J. Transluminal expandable nitinol coils stent grafting: preliminary report. Radiology 1983;147:259–60.
7. Cragg A, Lund G, Rysavy J, Casteneda-Zuniga W, Amplatz K. Non-surgical placement of arterial endoprosthesis: a new technique using nitinol wire. Radiology 1983;147:261–3.
8. Palmaz JC, Sibbit RR, Reuter SR, Tio FO, Rice WJ. Expandable intraluminal graft: a preliminary study. Radiology 1985;156:73–7.
9. Palmaz JC, Sibbit RR, Tio FO, Reuter SR, Peters JE, Garcia F. Expandable intraluminal graft: a feasibility study. Surgery 1986;99:199–205.
10. Williams DF. Surface interactions. In: Sigwart U, ed. Endoluminal Stenting. London: WB Saunders, 1996: 45–51.
11. Lu L, Jones MW. Diamond-like carbon as biological compatible material for cell culture and medical applications. Biomed Mater Eng 1993;3:223–8.
12. Amon M, Bolz A, Schaldach M. Improvement in stenting therapy with a silicon carbide coated tantalum stent. J Mater Sci Mater Med 1996;7:273–8.
13. Beythien C, Gutensohn K, Kühnl P, et al. Influence of 'diamond-like' and gold coating on platelet activation: a flow cytometry analysis in a pulsed floating model [abstract]. J Am Coll Cardiol 1998;31(suppl):413A.
14. Aggarwal RK, Ireland DC, Ragheb A, de Bono DO, Gershlick AH. Reduction in thrombogenicity of polymer-coated stents by immobilization of platelet targeted urokinase [abstract]. Eur J Cardiol 1996;17(suppl):177.
15. Cragg AH, Dake MD. Percutaneous femoropopliteal graft placement. J Vasc Interv Radiol 1993;4:445–63.
16. Gage AA. Cryosurgery in the treatment of cancer. Surg Gynecol Obstet 1992;174:73–92.
17. Parodi JC. Endovascular repair of abdominal aortic aneurysms and other arterial lesions. J Vasc Surg 1995;21:549–57.
18. Diethrich EB, Papazoglou CO. Endoluminal grafting for aneurysmal and occlusive disease in the superficial femoral artery: early experience. J Endovasc Surg 1995;2:225–39.

19. Marin ML, Veith FJ, Cynamon J, et al. Transfemoral endovascular stent graft treatment of aortoiliac and femoropopliteal occlusive disease for limb salvage. Am J Surg 1994;168:156–62.

20. Bergeron P. Stenting and endoluminal grafting of femoral and popliteal arteries. J Endovasc Surg 1995;2:197–8.

21. Henry M, Amor M, Cragg A, et al. Occlusive and aneurysmal peripheral arterial disease: assessment of a stent graft system. Radiology 1996;201:717–24.

22. Howell MH, Krajcer ZK, Diethrich E, et al. Percutaneous treatment of traumatic arterial injuries with the Wallgraft endoprosthesis. J Am Coll Cardiol 2001;37(suppl A):1257–33.

23. Krajcer Z, Sioco G, Reynolds T. Comparison of Wallgraft™ and Wallstent for treatment of complex iliac artery stenosis and occlusion. Tex Heart Inst J 1997;24:193–9.

24. Lammer J, Becker GJ, Cejna M, et al. A prospective study of a transluminally placed self-expanding endoprosthesis (Hemobahn Endoprosthesis) for the treatment of peripheral arterial obstructions. Cardiovasc Interv Radiol 1999;22(suppl 2):S134.

25. Parodi JC, Palmaz JC, Barone HD. Transfemoral intraluminal graft implantation for abdominal aortic aneurysms. Ann Vasc Surg 1991;5:491–9.

26. Lazarus HM. Endovascular grafting technique in the treatment of infrarenal abdominal aortic aneurysm. Surg Clin North Am 1992;72:959–68.

27. Beebe HG, Blum U. Experience with the Meadox Vanguard endovascular graft. In: Yao JST, Pierce WH, eds. Techniques in Vascular and Endovascular Surgery. Norwalk, CT: Appleton and Lange, 1998: 421–32.

28. Taheri SA, Leonhardt HJ, Greenan T. The Talent™ endoluminal graft placement system. In: Yao JST, Pierce WH, eds. Techniques in Vascular and Endovascular Surgery. Norwalk, CT: Appleton and Lange, 1998: 433–45.

29. Dake M, Semba C, Kee S, et al. Endografts for the treatment of descending thoracic aortic aneurysm: results of the first 150 procedures. J Endovasc Surg 1999;6:189.

30. Shim WH, Lee B-K, Yoon Y-S, Lee DY, Chang BC. Endovascular stent graft implantation for descending thoracic aortic dissection and aneurysm. J Am Coll Cardiol 2001;37(suppl):1230.

31. Dake MD. Thoracic excluder: initial results of a feasibility study for stent-graft treatment of descending thoracic aortic aneurysms. Oral presentation 1999 Current Issues and New Techniques in Interventional Radiology.

32. Silva TA, Ramee SR, Collins TJ, et al. Rheolytic thrombectomy in the treatment of acute limb-threatening ischemia: immediate results and six-month follow-up of the multi-center AngioJet registry. Possis Peripheral AngioJet Study Investigators. Cathet Cardiovasc Diag 1998;45:386–92.

33. Wagner HY, Muller-Hulsbeck S, Pitton MB, et al. Rapid thrombectomy with hydrodynamic catheter: results from a prospective multi-center trial. Radiology 1997;205:675–81.

34. Henry M, Amor M, Henry I, Tricoche O, Allaoui M. The Hydrolyser thrombectomy catheter: a single-center experience. J Endovasc Surg 1998;5:24–31.

35. van Ommen VG, van den Bos AA, Pieper M, et al. Removal of thrombus from aortocoronary bypass grafts and coronary arteries using the 6F Hydrolyser. Am J Cardiol 1997;79:1012–16.

36. Simpson JB, Selmon MR, Robertson GC, et al. Transluminal atherectomy for occlusive peripheral vascular disease. Am J Cardiol 1988;61:96G–101G.

37. Graor RA, Whitlow PL. Transluminal atherectomy for occlusive peripheral vascular disease. J Am Coll Cardiol 1990;15:1551–8.

38. Zacca NM, Raizner AE, Noon GP. Treatment of symptomatic peripheral atherosclerotic disease with a rotational atherectomy device. Am J Cardiol 1989;63:77–80.

39. Isner JM, Rosenfield K. Redefining the treatment of peripheral artery disease. Circulation 1993;88:1534–57.

40. Isner JM, Pieczek A, Rosenfield K. Untreated gangrene in patients with peripheral artery disease. Circulation 1994;89:482–3.

41. Grundfest WS, Segalowitz J, Laudenslager J, et al. The physical and biological basis for laser angioplasty. In: Litvack F, ed. Coronary Laser Angioplasty. Oxford: Blackwell Scientific Publications, 1992.

42. Biamino G. Laser recanalization and debulking technique in popliteal and tibial occlusive disease [abstract]. International Congress on Endovascular Interventions 1999.

43. Waksman R, Crocker IA, Kikeri D, et al. Long-term results of endovascular radiation therapy for prevention of restenosis in the peripheral vascular system. Circulation 1996;94:8,I-300:1745.

44. Haas P, Krajcer Z, Diethrich E. Closure of large percutaneous access sites using the Prostar XL percutaneous vascular surgery device. J Endovasc Surg 1999;6:168–70.

45. Krajcer Z, Howell M. A novel technique using the percutaneous vascular surgery device to close the 22 French femoral artery entry site used for percutaneous abdominal aortic aneurysm exclusion. Catheter Cardiovasc Interv 2000;50:356–60.

46. Krajcer Z, Howell M, Villareal R. Percutaneous access and closure of femoral artery access sites associated with endoluminal repair of abdominal aortic aneurysms. J Endovasc Therapy 2001;8:68–74.

47. Howell M, Dougherty K, Strickman N, Krajcer Z. Percutaneous repair of abdominal aortic aneurysms using the AneuRx stent graft and the percutaneous vascular surgery device. Cathet Cardiovasc Interv 2002;55:281–7.

48. Dangas G, Mehran R, Kokolis S, et al. Vascular complications after percutaneous coronary interventions following hemostasis with manual compression versus arteriotomy closure devices. J Am Coll Cardiol 2001;38:638–41.

49. Eidt J, Habibipour S, Saucedo J, et al. Complications from hemostatic closure puncture devices. Am J Surg 1999;178:511–6.

50. Gottwalles Y, Wunschel-Joseph, Janssen M. Coil embolization treatment in pulmonary artery branch rupture during Swan Ganz catheterization. Cardiovasc Intervent Radiol 2000;23(6):477–9.

51. Bush RL, Lin PH, Dodson TF, Dion JE, Lumsden AB. Endoluminal stent placement and coil embolization for the management of carotid artery pseudoaneurysms. J Endovasc Ther 2001;8:53–61.

52. Halloul Z, Büger T, Grote R, Fahlke J, Meyer F. Sequential coil embolization of bilateral internal iliac aneurysms prior to endovascular abdominal aortic aneurysm repair. J Endovasc Ther 2001;8:87–92.

5. The Endovascular Interventional Suite

Zvonimir Krajcer and Kathryn Dougherty

INTRODUCTION

Endovascular interventions have enjoyed an explosive growth in the last two decades. It is likely that the impact of reimbursement for medical care will stimulate even more interest: adding new endovascular procedures that involve stents and stent grafts will supplant an additional 40–70% of traditional vascular surgeries.[1] All these treatments involve the use of catheters, balloons, wires, and imaging modalities, including digital subtraction angiography, road mapping and three-dimensional reconstruction. A variety of factors must therefore be considered when designing an endovascular surgical suite.

The endovascular suite should offer full operative sterile conditions, particularly for procedures such as endoluminal grafting that incorporate prosthetic materials. Procedures involving stents or stent grafts can potentially result in catastrophic infections.[2-4] Additionally, if an endovascular intervention should require conversion to a surgical intervention, complete sterility is imperative to ensure patient safety and avoid contamination. Furthermore, the interventional suite must be large enough to accommodate the equipment and staff needed if it were necessary to convert from an endovascular to a surgical procedure (Fig. 5.1).[5-7]

DESIGN OF THE PROCEDURE ROOM

In order to accommodate the core equipment comfortably, the size of the suite should be at least 1000 square feet,[6] with at least two-thirds of that devoted to procedure area and 350 square feet to the control/observation area (Fig. 5.2). The ceiling height

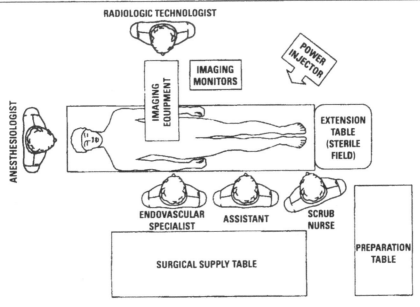

Fig. 5.1 The endovascular suite set-up.

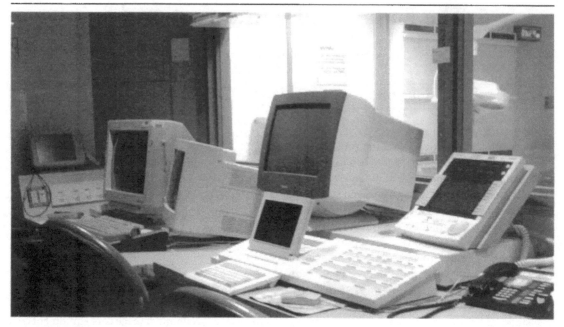

Fig. 5.2 A separate control room/observation area protected by lead shielding allows staff members to process and record procedural data without interrupting the intervention.

should be at least 10 feet,[3] and the walls should be shielded with 1 mm of lead to provide radiation protection for personnel in surrounding work areas. Observation windows and doors should also be lead treated.

The suite should be equipped with emergency power outlets located on the operating table and all four walls of the suite. The endovascular suite should have compressed air, oxygen and suction outlets at both ends of the operating table. The operating table should be radiolucent to minimize radiation exposure and provide exceptional visualization. Communication capabilities should include in-room intercoms, video input and output links to a high band width image routing network, and video/audio recording.

Most of the typical angiography suites and cardiac catheterization suites are primarily designed for catheter-based procedures and do not meet operating room requirements. The endovascular suite should have laminar or negative airflow, and seamless floors, ceilings and walls that can be washed. An electronic imaging station should also be available in the room so that digital computed tomography (CT), magnetic resonance (MR) and ultrasound images can be reviewed during the procedure (Fig. 5.3a). Multiple in-wall x-ray view boxes are also needed for viewing outside studies (Fig. 5.3b). The suite should be equipped with limited in-room storage using stainless steel cabinets with glass doors. In addition, the suite should have certified operating room, shatterproof lighting that has low, medium, and ultra-bright capabilities. Individual xenon headlamps are also necessary for surgical procedures. Vascular instrumentation should be readily available in the room, as well as adequate space for the anesthesiologists, anesthesia equipment, circulators, and instrument tables (see Fig. 5.1). The room should have controlled access and outside indicators to specify activation of the fluoroscopic equipment so that inadvertent radiation exposure is prevented.

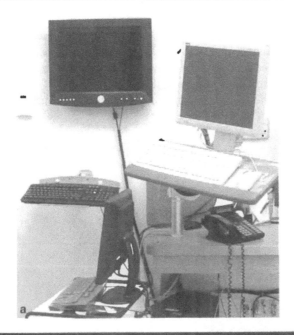

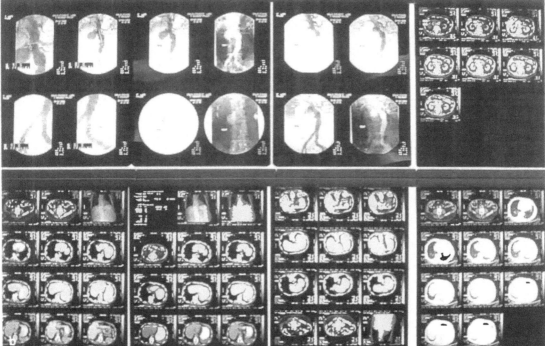

Fig. 5.3 (a) An electronic imaging workstation should be located within the endovascular suite so that angiograms, CT scans, MRIs, and ultrasound images can be reviewed during the procedure. (b) Multiple in-wall view box displays are necessary for reviewing outside diagnostic studies.

REQUIREMENTS FOR ANESTHESIA

The anesthesiologist is consulted for a variety of procedures that are performed in an endovascular suite. The spectrum of anesthesia needed in the endovascular suite ranges from local to general, depending on the needs of the patient and the interventional team. The organization of the procedural area, therefore, is case specific, and identifying the location of the high-pressure lines is important in determining where to place the anesthetic machine and accompanying equipment. Use of compact machines specifically designed for remote or ambulatory applications such as Draeger (Draeger Medical, Telford, PA) and Ohmeda (Datex-Ohmeda, Madison, WI) allow anesthetic flexibility and improve the efficiency in smaller spaces (Fig. 5.4). Additional portable lead glass shields should be available to protect the anesthesiologist during long procedures that require general anesthesia.

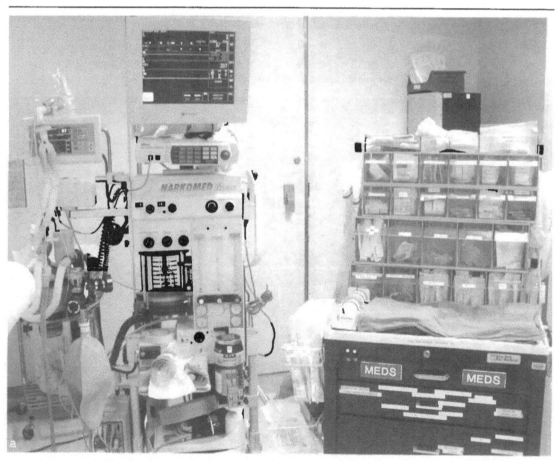

Fig. 5.4 (a) The necessary equipment that the anesthesiologist might need should be compact and portable.

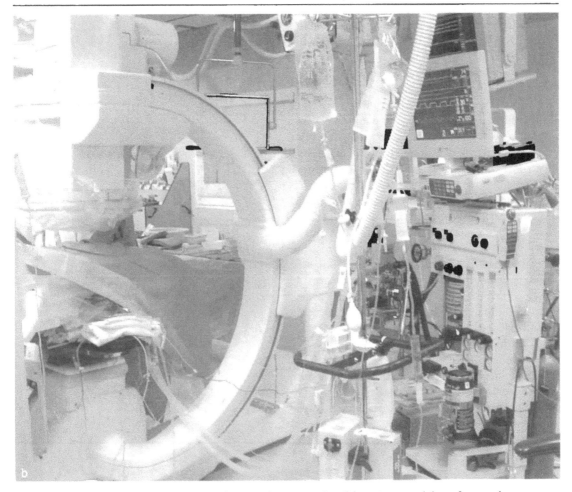

Fig. 5.3 *Continued* (b) The endovascular suite must be large enough to accommodate all the equipment needed to perform complex interventions.

FLUOROSCOPY EQUIPMENT

The key components and success of endovascular procedures are dependent on high-quality imaging equipment: 'Image-intensifier technology has been the gold standard'.[5] However, digital flat panel detector technology has since evolved and it is clear that the advantages of improved image capture, field of view, dynamic range, and dose management have improved minimally invasive techniques. Additional high-resolution monitors are essential and should be positioned for viewing on both sides of the operating table. This allows visualization from multiple angles and/or access sites either by surgical cut-down or percutaneously in the right or left femoral or right or left brachial vessels. In addition, many systems are also equipped with an integrated optional ultrasound solution to improve patient diagnosis and treatment.

The operating table should be able to rotate on its center axis 180° to allow antegrade, as well as retrograde, panning. In addition, the table should be motor driven to allow remote high-speed bolus-chase digital peripheral studies, as well as digital stepping angiography. This allows the use of automated head to toe angiographic coverage with minimal contrast usage and optimal vessel opacification. The bolus-chase technique prevents dense contrast visualization in the proximal vessels with poor contrast visualization in the distal vessels. Digital unsubtracted and subtracted angiography is a very useful modality when evaluating intracranial vascular problems. In addition, this digital feature is extremely valuable when using other contrast agents such as CO_2 or gadolinium in patients who might be at increased risk for 'traditional' iodinated contrast angiography. CO_2 and gadolinium provide less contrast than iodinated (nephrotoxic) agents but are indicated for patients with chronic renal insufficiency or congestive heart failure.

The fluoroscopy system can be single or bi-plane. Most currently used systems for peripheral vascular interventions are single plane. They are either fixed or mobile. Unless a large number of pediatric procedures are to be performed, single plane systems are adequate. A fixed flat panel detector system (Fig. 5.5) uses less radiation and provides approximately 40% more coverage with a larger field of view than image-intensifier systems. The dynamic range of a flat panel detector system is 5–10 times greater than the conventional image-intensifier, which allows improved visualization of the vasculature and views the placement of endovascular stents and stent grafts with greater precision. With improved visualization, contrast agent use can be reduced by approximately 30%.[7] This is particularly important when imaging patients with existing renal dysfunction.

Other system features include orbital and rotational C-arm movements as fast as 60° per second for three-dimensional imaging, collimator adjustments, extended dynamic range filtering, and injection triggering during rapid panning. An adjustable source to intensifier distance and processing offers results in immediate image availability. Fixed

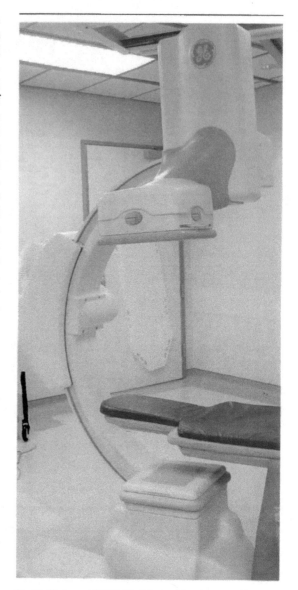

Fig. 5.5 The Innova™ 4100 digital flat panel imaging system has a much larger field of view than conventional image-intensifiers, providing approximately 40% more coverage.

systems also allow image-review functions to be directly accessible from handheld, in-room remote controls. This option can streamline procedures and minimize delays while archiving angiographic information. Post-processing, laser filming, and digital image archiving are usually performed at the system console in the control/observation bay area.

IMAGING TECHNIQUES

Proper positioning of the equipment and good radiographic imaging technique are crucial to the safety and success of endovascular procedures. Angiography using calibrated marker catheters and a graduated marker tape are useful safety measures when deploying stents and stent grafts. The flat panel detector imaging system provides constant resolution over the entire field of view up to 10 times greater than the standard 7 or 9 inch image intensifiers that are used in the cardiac catheterization laboratory (Fig. 5.6).[7] The square surface configuration of the flat panel eliminates the need for panning or multiple runs. During endovascular thoracic or abdominal aortic aneurysm repair, it is important that the entire field of endograft deployment can be seen on a single view.

'Road mapping' is an imaging technique that allows superimposition of a real life fluoroscopy on a previously recorded angiographic image. These images are retained as a road map and used to facilitate the positioning of interventional devices. They are also helpful to compare anatomy before and after intervention, and to perform on-line measurement of severity of stenosis. This technique is extremely beneficial when negotiating wires and catheters through tortuous vessels and when there is concern of contrast-induced renal dysfunction.

High-speed rotation is another useful imaging technique. This is especially helpful when evaluating the degree of stenosis and eccentricity of the vasculature such as in the extracranial carotid arteries. It can also be used effectively to evaluate the thoracic and abdominal aorta, iliac and femoral arteries. Like all digital images, however, the drawback of road mapping and high-speed rotation is that any motion of the vascular structures detracts from the quality of the image. Primary sources of movement include cardiac, diaphragmatic,

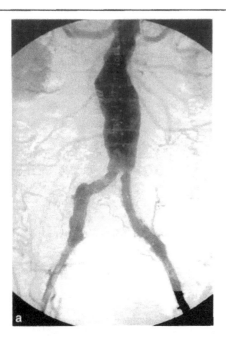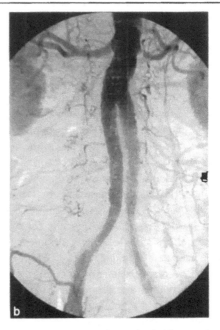

Fig. 5.6 (a, b) Using flat panel detector technology the entire infrarenal abdominal aorta and iliac arteries can be visualized without panning or using extra contrast media.

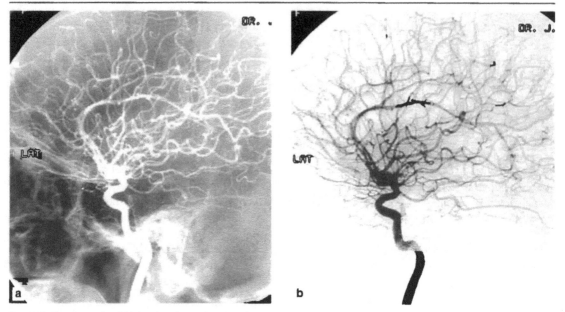

Fig. 5.7 (a) Unsubtracted and (b) digitally subtracted angiography of the intracranial anatomy from the left common carotid artery in the lateral projection.

ureteric, and interstitial. Pain is also a primary cause of patient movement and is commonly seen with high osmolality contrast agents. Adequate sedation of patients and the use of lower osmolality radiographic dyes can help reduce the motion artifact.

Another type of artifact is parallax, which is also exaggerated by movement. Because the x-ray beam is shaped like a cone, radial elongation or distortion of the structures occurs at the edges of the field: this is called parallax. There is no distortion in the center of the field, but if the position changes from the road map, relative distances change, dramatically increasing parallax artifact. To avoid image artifact caused by parallax, it is important for both the patient and the table to remain stationary during the crucial part of the intervention. Therefore, for precise placement of stents or stent grafts, no movement should occur once the road map has been obtained and no measurements attempted in the outer 20% of the field of view.[8]

There are a variety of post-processing features employed to clean images that have been degraded by patient movement and include pixel shifting, landmarking, on-screen measurements, annotation, and image zooming. The advent of digital subtraction techniques has greatly enhanced visualization (Fig. 5.7). Digital subtraction is a feature that eliminates static elements (bones and other structures) from the initial image contrast injection, allowing a clear image of the vessels.

Finally, angiography performed in multiple orthogonal views is paramount to the procedure, particularly in regions of vascular bifurcation or when bone edges overlie the area of interest. A thorough understanding of the principles of parallax, positioning and projections is instrumental when determining the precise placement of endovascular devices.

RECORD MANAGEMENT AND ARCHIVING

There continues to be a proliferation of digital technologies within the cardiovascular field. Despite continued efforts to move from cine film to all-digital approaches, to date there have been no adequate means for exchanging images between institutions in digital formats.

The American College of Cardiology, the American College of Radiology, and the National Electrical Manufacturers' Association have combined efforts to implement standards for storing and retrieving digital images on recordable compact discs, as the replacement for cine-angiographic film as the dominant archival medium.[9,10] A refined standard – Digital Imaging and Communications in Medicine (DICOM) – was developed and uses industry standard networking protocols, specifying mechanisms for image storage on removable media and added additional imaging modalities. DICOM is the key component addressed within the broader concept of computerized patient records. Industries must develop software based on user-friendly operating systems (MacOS, Windows 95, and Windows NT) that are compatible with all major vendors so that images can be stored, manipulated, and shared.

Digital images require a large hard disk for storage, while post-processing information is outputted to a compact disc and/or laser printer. This technology eliminates the need for wet processing. In fact, digital systems have largely replaced the need for videotape recorders and 'frame grabbers' (single frame images).

RADIATION SAFETY AND TRAINING

With the advent of stents and endoluminal grafts and other endovascular procedures the time needed for fluoroscopy has become much lengthier. High-quality, fixed imaging systems need high heat-capacity tubes to minimize the need for heat-cooling delays that often occur with long imaging times. Furthermore, there is an even greater need for significant lead shielding to ensure the safety of patients and health care personnel. Mechanisms to reduce radiation exposure can be divided into those directed at reducing the output of the x-ray unit and those designed to limit the amount of radiation absorbed by the interventionist and the staff. Staff

members should be properly trained in radiation safety principles, equipment, potential complications, and troubleshooting. Staff members should be able to demonstrate their understanding of the basic concepts of medical imaging and the use of newer imaging systems.

The most important method to reduce scatter radiation is to minimize patient dose and the ultimate source of scatter to the operator.[11-13] Staff members should monitor judicious use of fluoroscopy and terminate imaging runs as soon as relevant information has been obtained. Other key elements to reduce radiation exposure include collimation, pulsed fluoroscopy, imaging acquisition, frame rates, and last image hold. During long procedures the operator and staff members should stand as far back from the unit as possible to take advantage of the fact that radiation exposure decreases exponentially with increased distance from the source.

Lead shielding requirements are dictated by stringent radiation safety regulations. Protective lead aprons, thyroid shields, leaded glass screens, and leaded eye glasses with side shields are the most effective way to reduce radiation exposure. The suite itself must be lead lined, including the doors, glass, and walls,[11-13] and all personnel in the room should wear film badges that detect radiation exposure.

CONCLUSION

Endovascular procedures have already changed the way arterial and venous diseases are managed. It is likely that these techniques will have an even greater influence in the future. Transluminal angioplasty has already proven to be a helpful adjunct to arterial reconstructive surgery rather than a competitive modality. It can be used to treat lesions that produce symptoms insufficient to justify open surgery and to simplify or help manage complicated or difficult cases.[14-16]

Endovascular intervention is the fastest growing area of vascular medicine and requires dedication on the part of practitioners. Endovascular techniques require specialized skills and training in peripheral vascular diseases, diagnostic angiography, interventional techniques, and therapeutic alternatives. The challenge to the practitioner is intensified by the continual introduction of new products and methods. The establishment of a modern endovascular suite arranged in an ergonomically devised fashion is crucial to remaining on the forefront of developments in the treatment of patients with arterial and venous disorders.

REFERENCES

1. Veith FJ, Ohki T. Endovascular intervention and its impact on vascular practice: current and future perspectives. In: Criado FJ, ed. Endovascular Intervention: Basic Concepts and Techniques, Armonk, NY: Futura Publishing, 1999: 181–6.

2. Heikkinen L, Valtonen M, Lepantalo M, et al. Infrarenal endoluminal bifurcated stent graft infected with *Listeria monocytogenes*. J Vasc Surg 1999;29:554–6.

3. Deitch JS, Hansen KJ, Regan JD, et al. Infected renal artery pseudo-aneurysm and mycotic aortic aneurysm after percutaneous transluminal renal angioplasty and stent placement in a patient with a solitary kidney. J Vasc Surg 1998;28:340–4.

4. Weinberg DJ, Cronin DW, Baker AG Jr. Infected iliac pseudo-aneurysms after uncomplicated percutaneous balloon angioplasty and (Palmaz) stent insertion: a case report and literature review. J Vasc Surg 1996;23:162–6.

5. Hodgson KJ, Mattos MA, Summer DS. Angiography in the operating room: equipment, catheter skills, and safety issues. In: Yao JS, Pearce WH, eds. Techniques in Vascular and Endovascular Surgery. Connecticut: Appleton and Lange, 1998: 25–45.

6. Queral LA. Operating room design for the future. In: Yao JS, Pearce WH, eds. Techniques in Vascular and Endovascular Surgery. Connecticut: Appleton and Lange; 1998: 1–5.

7. Folander H, Martino R. Flat panel technology. Endovasc Today 2003;Dec:34–6.

8. Diethrich EB. Endovascular suite design: an integrated approach for optimal interventional performance. In: Criado FJ, ed. Endovascular Intervention: Basic Concepts and Techniques. Armonk, NY: Futura Publishing, 1999: 5–16.

9. Fillinger MF, Weaver JB. Imaging equipment and techniques for optimal intraoperative imaging during endovascular interventions. Semin Vasc Surg 1999;12:315–26.

10. ACC/ACR/NEMA Ad Hoc Group. American College of Cardiology, American College of Radiology, and industry develop standards for digital transfer of angiographic images. J Am Coll Cardiol 1995;25:800.

11. DICOM Media Interchange Standards for Cardiology. Initial interoperability demonstration by Jonathan L. Elion, Brown University Institute for Medical Computing, Providence, RI, USA. Proc Annu Symp Comput Appl Med Care 1995;591–5.

12. Implementation of the principle of as low as reasonable achievable (ALARA) for medical and dental personnel. NCRP Report No. 107. Bethesda, MD: National Council on Radiation Protection and Measurements, 1990.

13. Lowe FC, Auster M, Beck TJ, et al. Monitoring radiation exposure to medical personnel during percutaneous nephrolithotomy. Urology 1986;28:221–6.

14. Bush WH, Jones D, Brannen GE. Radiation dose to personnel during percutaneous renal calculus removal. Am J Radiol 1985;145:1261–4.

15. Veith FJ, Gupta SK, Samson RH, et al. Progress in limb salvage by reconstructive arterial surgery combined with new or improved adjunctive procedure. Ann Surg 1981;212:386.

16. Brewster DC, Cambria RP, Darling RC, et al. Long-term results after combined iliac balloon angioplasty and distal surgical revascularization. Ann Surg 1989;210:324.

6. Certification and Training in Peripheral Vascular Intervention

Raghunandan Kamineni and Richard R Heuser

INTRODUCTION

Percutaneous peripheral vascular interventions and endovascular techniques have been in widespread clinical use for more than two decades. It is estimated that approximately 100,000 of these procedures are performed annually in the United States. A variety of specialists such as interventional cardiologists, vascular surgeons, and interventional radiologists are now performing these procedures within their scope of practice. All the aforementioned specialists possess specialized training that makes them experts in one or more aspects of endovascular therapy. The interventional cardiologist is skilled in working with catheters, sheaths, balloons, wires, and stents, while the vascular surgeon has considerable experience in performing vascular cut-downs and managing complications that arise from these procedures. The radiologist brings another kind of experience – that of imaging procedures such as angiography, and duplex and intravascular ultrasound.

As new devices and techniques are developed, considerable controversy has developed among these medical disciplines about who is qualified to perform these procedures, and what training standards should be established for physicians entering this field. While it is certainly clear that each of these clinicians brings important knowledge and capabilities to the operating table, the endovascular interventionist needs to combine experience from each discipline to provide optimal care in treating peripheral vascular disease.

To address some of these concerns, in 1989 the American College of Cardiology (ACC), the American Heart Association (AHA), the Society for Cardiac Angiography and Intervention (SCAI), the Society of Cardiovascular and Interventional Radiology (SCVIR), and the Society for Vascular Surgery/International Society for Cardiovascular Surgery (SVS/ISCVS) established subcommittees on peripheral vascular disease. These organizations have explored the standardization of training and have made recommendations. The majority of the individuals that are currently performing these procedures have learned the techniques by observing experts and participating in workshops. However, the complexity of the procedures and the need for hands-on experience dictates the necessity for formal training in peripheral angioplasty and other endovascular techniques. A number of fellowship programs are now offering structured training in various aspects of endovascular techniques for the new trainees. In this chapter, a review of training and certification options is provided, and the minimum standards for endovascular facilities are reviewed.

QUALIFICATIONS

The majority of the governing organizations in endovascular interventions have outlined educational requirements for certification in endovascular therapies. The general ideal is:

Physicians who perform angioplasty of the peripheral and renal vessels or other endovascular procedures should have a thorough understanding of the clinical manifestations and natural history of peripheral and renovascular disease. They should be competent to interpret diagnostic peripheral and renal angiographic examinations and to perform arteriographic procedures via femoral (retrograde and antegrade), auxiliary and translumbar approaches.

Specific procedural training and experience may be obtained through qualification by training and qualification by experience.

QUALIFICATION BY TRAINING

An applicant may qualify to perform peripheral interventional procedures by completing a training program that provides the trainee with extensive experience in diagnostic angiography as well as percutaneous transluminal angioplasty (PTA) of peripheral vessels. This experience, at a minimum, must include performance of 100 diagnostic peripheral angiograms and 50 renal and/or peripheral PTA procedures under the direct supervision of an experienced peripheral interventionist (the applicant must be the primary operator in at least half of these procedures). In addition, the applicant should also have training and experience in at least 10 cases with the use of thrombolytic therapy in peripheral arteries. The SCVIR guidelines[1] recommend that the applicant meets these requirements during a formal 1- or 2-year subspecialty training program following completion of an approved residency program. The ACC Peripheral Vascular Disease Committee recommendations[2] are somewhat more specific, stating that:

Training in vascular medicine should be offered to physicians with training in internal medicine. The physician should have taken or be eligible to take the internal medicine examination of the American Board of Internal Medicine or its equivalent.

QUALIFICATION BY EXPERIENCE

An applicant may qualify by having previous experience in peripheral angiographic diagnosis and PTA with acceptable complication and success rates. This experience, at a minimum, must include performance of 100 diagnostic peripheral angiograms and 50 renal and/or peripheral PTA procedures under the direct supervision of an experienced peripheral interventionist (the applicant

must be the primary operator in at least half of these procedures). In addition, the applicant should also have training and experience in at least 10 cases with the use of thrombolytic therapy in peripheral arteries. The applicant should be able to present documentation of results and complications, and confirmation of these data may be requested from the institution where the experience was gained.

TRAINING

The ACC Peripheral Vascular Disease Committee[2] recommends that a basic training requirement must be met by each physician applicant and should include at least one of the following:

1. American Board of Internal Medicine eligibility or certification with additional completion of a minimum of 12-month fellowship in vascular medicine or American Board of Internal Medicine certification with additional eligibility or certification in cardiovascular medicine.
2. American Board of Radiology eligibility or certification.
3. American Board of Surgery eligibility or certification with additional completion of a general vascular surgery residency.

In some cases, recommendations recognize the importance of instruction from more than one clinician or expert in the field. There is no doubt that the trainee benefits from a variety of experiences. To this end, the ACC suggests that the trainee receive instruction from two different faculty members.

The ACC guidelines[2] suggest cognitive training and clinical exposure that includes patient care management, and experience in invasive and noninvasive imaging techniques. Didactic lectures are to include information on etiology, pathophysiology, signs and symptoms, diagnostic techniques, and treatment. Clinical rotations should constitute:

1. 3 months of hospital service, where the trainees are directly involved in patient care;

2. 3 months spent in an outpatient facility;
3. 3 months of imaging rotations spent in the non-invasive vascular laboratory;
4. at least 1 month spent in an area where angiography and catheter revascularization techniques are performed (while 1 month does not provide sufficient experience for ACC certification, it is intended to provide a basic background in arteriography, angioplasty, atherectomy, stenting, and other percutaneous procedures).[2]

Credentialing guidelines for vascular surgeons, as outlined by White et al,[3] describe the need for competence in lesion access techniques, image acquisition and interpretation, guidewire use, and experience with specific devices, such as balloons, atherectomy equipment, stents, and other devices being utilized in endovascular application. There is no doubt that the skill with various percutaneous access techniques is important to the endovascular surgeon as almost all of the transluminal peripheral vascular interventions are performed percutaneously. Establishing skill and dexterity with the equipment requires considerable practice; coordinating fluoroscopic imaging and guidance is extremely important in ensuring the success of balloon angioplasty and stenting, the primary techniques used to treat vascular lesions. The SCVIR guidelines[1] also stress the importance of formal instruction in radiation physics, radiation effects, and protection, which are clearly a vital part of understanding imaging principles and safety.

dency or fellowship, and other specialized training.[3] According to ACC guidelines,[4] in order to ensure that physicians performing PTA of the peripheral, renal, and other visceral vessels are qualified, a minimum level of training and/or experience must be documented before the privileges are granted. Physicians who have completed a formal fellowship program should provide the hospital with a list of patients that includes the total number of cases performed, the sites treated, and the complications encountered. If the physician has not completed at least 100 diagnostic peripheral angiograms, 50 peripheral angioplasty procedures, and 10 cases of peripheral thrombolytic therapy (50% of these as the primary operator), he or she should complete the requirements for postgraduate physicians.

Recommendations for postgraduate physicians state that the physician should attend at least two peripheral angioplasty seminars and learn the nature and anatomy of peripheral vascular disease, as well as the indications for and risks of alternative therapies. The physician should perform non-invasive evaluation, visit a laboratory in which peripheral angioplasty is being performed by experienced personnel, and observe at least 10 peripheral procedures. Postgraduate physicians are then required to demonstrate that they have completed at least 100 diagnostic peripheral angiograms, 50 peripheral angioplasty procedures, and 10 cases of peripheral thrombolytic therapy (50% of these as the primary operator) under supervision of an experienced interventionist.[4]

OBTAINING PRIVILEGES

The Joint Commission on Accreditation of Health Care Organizations (JACHO) mandates that specific standards be outlined to grant privileges for physicians requesting privileges to perform procedures. The training standards are intended to help medical institutions determine whether to grant initial privileges for peripheral angioplasty procedures and should be used when reviewing applications from physicians regardless of their specialty. Staff qualifications are based on training in resi-

MAINTAINING PRIVILEGES

Maintenance of peripheral angioplasty privileges requires ongoing experience in performing these procedures with acceptable success and complication rates. Maintenance of privileges should also be dependent on the physician's active participation in a JACHO mandated quality assurance program.[4] This includes the establishment of a registry that enrolls all patients who undergo peripheral interventions and the compilation of data on clinical characteristics, pertinent medical and surgical history, and examination findings. Angioplasty data are to be recorded and coded with information on the site, acute success, procedural complications and clinical follow-up in a manner that allows only the director of the registry to know the identity of the physician being reviewed. 'Blinded' review is then performed on an annual or biannual basis by a peer-review panel, and observations are forwarded to the hospital committee. When the results are deemed acceptable, privileges may be renewed for 1- or 2-year periods.

Physicians who were granted privileges before the implementation of this standard should not necessarily have their status altered if they do not meet the qualifications as outlined in the previous section. However, if they do not meet those qualifications, they should acquire necessary training or experience to do so within 3 years. They must also participate in the institution's quality improvement program and will be evaluated using the same standard for indications, success rates, and complications.[5]

Permission to study new investigational devices in the hospital setting is dependent upon review of protocols by Institutional Review Boards and the US Food and Drug Administration (FDA).[3]

FACILITIES

The design of the facility that houses the endovascular laboratory must provide for adequate space, electrical capacity, and lead shielding. Minimal requirements for angiographic facilities were outlined by the SCVIR in 1989.[1] According to these early guidelines, the angiographic facility should have the following:

- a film changer capable of obtaining rapid serial film at least 14 inches in diameter with digital subtraction angiography capability;
- a high-resolution image intensifier and television chain;
- physiologic monitoring devices;
- facilities to manage and resuscitate unstable patients;

- personnel trained to provide proper patient care and operate the equipment.

More recently, the ACC guidelines have made additional recommendations regarding peripheral angioplasty laboratories.[4] These guidelines state that the laboratory should be equipped with the following:

- An ample inventory of balloon dilation catheters, calibrated balloon inflation devices and a complete range of current guidewires allowing for differences in flexibility and steerability.
- A high-resolution fluoroscopic system and an optimal television chain that allows ready visualization of a 0.014 inch guidewire and in which still frames (road map images) can be displayed simultaneously with the real-time fluoroscopic image.
- An angulating x-ray tube image intensifier arm that allows ready determination of the anatomic position of a guidewire or balloon catheter.
- A physiologic recording system, high-resolution fluoroscope, cine-angiographic and/or digital subtraction or acquisition angiographic and/or cut film angiographic equipment, a complete set of emergency resuscitation instruments, and a full complement of drugs.
- Radiation exposure control systems, including such items as an x-ray beam with automatic collimation, a carbon fiber scattered radiation grid, a carbon fiber tabletop, and a correct tube filter. Further reduction of radiation exposure can be achieved by gap filling and using a reference monitor. Lead aprons, eyeglasses, thyroid protection and additional shielding of the x-ray tube are also recommended.
- Peripheral angiography should include contrast material and should image the entire vascular distribution; the use of video fluoroscopy alone is not sufficient.
- The surgical operating suite should be equipped to provide general anesthesia and a full complement of instruments, as well as drugs for the management of the cardiovascular patient.

Although there are no published guidelines on the use of intravascular ultrasound (IVUS), it is certainly a valuable tool in the cardiac catheterization laboratory. Intravascular ultrasound allows both pre-procedural evaluation and post-interventional assessment, providing baseline luminal dimensions and accurate determination of arterial architecture and lesion pathology. In most cases, the IVUS data help determine the need for stenting and then evaluate the adequacy of device deployment. Proper training in IVUS techniques should be a requisite part of any training program for endovascular interventionists.

CONCLUSION

A variety of recommendations from various organizations are now available and are intended to standardize training in peripheral vascular intervention. While each governing body has produced different guidelines, it is clear that all favor supervised training and subsequent demonstration of skills in imaging, angioplasty, and management of complications. There are also standards governing the choice of equipment in endovascular facilities, and adequate attention to radiation safety is clearly a priority. With ongoing advancements in endovascular technology and continued addition of new devices to treat peripheral vascular disease, it is essential that the endovascular interventionist be prepared to acquire additional training as needed. Physicians must provide evidence of competence to maintain hospital privileges and uphold the highest ethics and standards of patient care in the emerging discipline of endovascular intervention.

REFERENCES

1. Society of Cardiovascular and Interventional Radiology (SCVIR). Credentialing criteria number I: peripheral, renal, and visceral percutaneous transluminal angioplasty. SCVIR Criteria 1989.
2. Spittell JA Jr, Nanda NC, Creager MA, et al. Recommendations for training in vascular medicine. American College of Cardiology Peripheral Vascular Disease Committee. J Am Coll Cardiol 1993;22:626–8.
3. White RA, Fogarty TJ, Baker WH, Ahn SS, String ST. Endovascular surgery credentialing and training for vascular surgeons. J Vasc Surg 1993;17:1095–1102.
4. Spittell JA Jr, Nanda NC, Creager MA, et al. Recommendations for peripheral transluminal angioplasty: training and facilities. American College of Cardiology Peripheral Vascular Disease Committee. J Am Coll Cardiol 1993;21:546–8.
5. Levin DC, Becker GJ, Dorros G, et al. Training standards for physicians performing peripheral angioplasty and other percutaneous peripheral vascular interventions. J Vasc Intervent Radiol 2003;14:S359–61.

7. Stent Retrieval: Devices and Technique

Kirk N Garratt, Emmanouil S Brilakis and J Michael Bacharach

INTRODUCTION

The development of endovascular techniques for the reconstruction of peripheral arteries has been dramatic. Of all the various techniques and devices, the endovascular stent has had the single most important impact in allowing improved technical results and longer term patencies, as well as the option to treat total occlusions that were habitually unsuccessful with angioplasty techniques alone.

With the development of endovascular stents, a whole new set of technical problems and potential complications arose. Early on in the application of endovascular stents, there was a specific lack of integrated systems for balloon expandable stents and the experience in use of sheaths to protect the stents prior to deployment was quite limited. Additionally, the use of biliary stents for the treatment of vascular occlusive disease presented a number of unique challenges.

In that early period, problems with loss of stent from the balloon and deployment failures, along with inadequate or incompletely placed stents, were quite commonplace. A number of novel, as well as desperate techniques were used to retrieve or resecure a stent that had errantly come off the balloon wire or had been placed in such a position that it was insecure or unsafe to leave it there.

It was from this early experience that techniques and equipment were developed primarily to prevent the situation in which a stent had to be retrieved. There are now better guiding, as well as sheath systems that provide improved protection for the stent. Balloons have undergone significant change and modification to allow for improved stent adherence to the balloon, as well as materials that are resistant to scoring, pin-holing, or mechanical failure that would result in inability or incomplete deployment of the stent.

TECHNICAL CONSIDERATIONS

Prior to a specific discussion on technique, an evaluation and assessment of why problems occur is needed. As in most things, an ounce of prevention is worth a pound of cure. Specifically, why does stent loss occur? The most frequently encountered problem is failure to secure the stent adequately on the balloon. The development of premounted stents with sheath coverings has significantly changed the need to secure a stent to a balloon by hand. This is most typical in coronary systems. For peripheral arterial reconstruction, however, it remains quite commonplace to select a balloon and then place the stents by hand. Adequate attachment of a stent onto a balloon involves proper balloon selection, as well as proper attachment.

Several techniques have been used for crimping stents onto balloons. These include crimping devices for crimping the stent in place by hand. We prefer to crimp the balloons by hand to secure them on the balloon. By gradually turning the balloon in a circumferential pattern and crimping down, it is possible to crimp the stent on the balloon adequately and safely and to test whether the balloon is secure by ensuring that it does not slide either proximally or distally beyond the usual balloon markers.

Once the stent is secure on the balloon, there are several techniques to avoid mechanical disruption or pressure on the stent to force it off the balloon. Most commonly, sheaths or guiding systems are used and placed beyond the stenotic lesion that is to be treated. This allows for appropriate placement of the balloon and stent and the sheath has been pulled back, thereby significantly reducing the chance of mechanically disrupting the stent or causing it to come off the balloon.

Another stage commonly associated with stent loss is the time of placement at the lesion. Sometimes the stent is bare or uncovered by a sheath or guiding catheter making it susceptible to stent migration. A typical example of this is during renal artery angioplasty and stent placement, when the balloon and stent are advanced through a guiding catheter across a lesion. The guide catheter is retracted to expose the stent once it is in position. However, if the stent is not placed accurately (either too distally or too proximally) then it must be repositioned without the protection of the guide catheter. If the stent is not tightly crimped onto the balloon, then migration of the stent is possible. For this reason, the proper position of the stent should be confirmed using contrast injections and radiologic landmarks before the protective guide catheter is retracted.

At the time of placement it is also paramount to avoid forcing a balloon and stent across a tight stenosis. If a small portion of the stent is left covered with a sheath or guiding catheter and cannot move across the lesion, the stent can be safely pulled back into the sheath and the entire device removed, thereby allowing for alternative positioning or perhaps predilation with a larger balloon.

A less commonly observed cause of stent loss is during the period of balloon inflation. This is more common when the stent has migrated slightly (either forward or aft on the balloon) and during inflation the force of the balloon expanding pushes the stent either in a proximal or a distal location – the so-called watermelon seeding phenomenon. In the worst case scenario this can lead to complete loss of the stent; in other situations it may lead to incomplete or inappropriate deployment of the stent. An example of this might be a stent placed at the ostium of a renal artery that then slides back into the aorta. If this occurs, it is often best to leave the balloon in place, advance it so that the portion of the balloon is distal beyond the stent, inflate it, and gently pull the stent back out of the ostium. The entire device can then be brought down and the stent can often be placed successfully in the iliac artery without significant problem or complication.

Perhaps the most important technical consideration for stent retrieval is to avoid the pitfalls that result in a situation where retrieval is necessary. This can largely be accomplished by gearing the

device appropriately and selecting the appropriate tools, including balloons that are resistant to scoring and pin-holing and have good stent adherence. Lastly, before making the final commitment to stent placement, be sure that excessive force is not used and that a sheath or guiding catheter is only pulled back completely once appropriate stent placement has been achieved.

RETRIEVAL DEVICES

There are several commercially available devices that can be used to retrieve lost stents or other detritus such as wire or balloon fragments from the coronary or peripheral vessels (Fig. 7.1, Table 7.1).[1] Some of these devices may not be available in all catheterization laboratories, and some operators may hesitate to use them because they are not familiar with how the devices operate. A brief description of the more commonly used devices as outlined in Table 7.1 follows.

Table 7.1 Devices for Retrieval of Lost or Retained Endovascular Equipment

- Loop snares
- Basket retrieval devices
- Biliary stone forceps
- Biopsy forceps
- Cook retained fragment retriever

LOOP SNARES
Loop snares are among the most frequently utilized retrieval devices. They consist of a movable wire contained within an outer plastic catheter (Fig. 7.1). The loops are designed to open at a 90° angle from the delivery catheter thus facilitating retrieval of the lost devices. The loop is usually made of nitinol with a diameter ranging from 2 to 35 mm, the catheter diameter ranges from 2.3F to 6F, and the length from 48 to 175 mm (Microvena Amplatz GOOSE NECK™ Snares and Microsnares; ev3, Plymouth, MN).

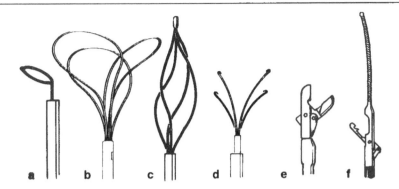

Fig. 7.1 Devices useful for recovering damaged stents or other devices lost in the peripheral vasculature.
(a) Loop snare. (b) En Snare™ three-loop retrieval system. (c) Basket retrieval device. (d) Biliary stone forceps. (e) Biopsy forceps. (f) Cook retained fragment retriever.

A more complex recently introduced snare is the 'En Snare' retrieval and manipulation system (Medical Device Technologies, Gainesville, FL) that consists of three interlaced nitinol pre-formed loops, increasing the likelihood of encircling and retrieving the lost device with at least one of the loops (see Fig. 7.1b).

If a commercial loop such as those discussed above is not available, then a snare could be made in the catheterization laboratory using an exchange length (300 cm) coronary guidewire and a 5F diagnostic coronary catheter (usually a multipurpose catheter) (Fig. 7.2). The guidewire is inserted into the catheter, and once its end exits from the distal tip of the catheter it is reinserted until it exits from the proximal end. One disadvantage of the 'homemade' snare is that the snare exits at the catheter tip in the direction of the long axis of the catheter and not at a 90° angle as seen in commercial loop snares.

BASKET RETRIEVAL DEVICE

This device consists of a set of helically arranged loops that can be expanded to collapse (see Fig. 7.1c). Originally designed to remove ureteral and biliary stones, this device can be used to trap lost or retained components within its loops. It can be used to catch a stent from the side and pull it free of a deployment balloon. This device works best if the stent has been damaged and misshapen such that a portion of the stent projects laterally away from the deployment balloon. Under some circumstances it may be possible to recover the stent without sacrificing the position of the coronary guidewire across the target lesion. Basket retrieval devices are available commercially from several companies and are available in a variety of expanded sizes and catheter lengths.

BILIARY STONE FORCEPS

Originally designed for percutaneous removal of stones from the biliary tree, this device consists of a set of curved, finger-like projections that can be expanded/extended or contracted/retracted (see Fig. 7.1d). By manipulating the 'fingers' of the device, an operator can grab hold of lost or retained components. This device is most useful in recovering partially expanded stents, or in situations in which a portion of a stent has become separated from the deployment balloon catheter. Under these circumstances it is often possible to remove a damaged stent without losing the guidewire position. Biliary forceps are available with catheter bodies of 4–5F, and in lengths of 130 cm. The retracted device has fair visibility under fluoroscopy, but the extended finger-like projections have poor radioopacity. The device should be used with great caution in the vascular system because laceration of the vessel wall can occur if it becomes entrapped in the finger-like projections of these forceps.

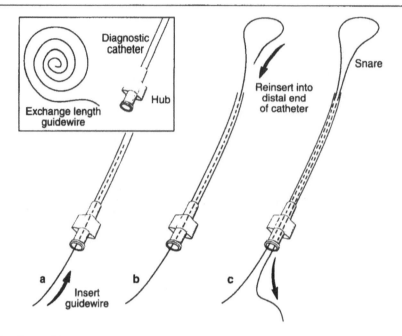

Fig. 7.2 How to make a 'homemade' snare.

An exchange length (300 cm) coronary guidewire is inserted into a 5F diagnostic coronary catheter (usually a multipurpose catheter) and once its end exits from the distal tip of the catheter it is reinserted until it exits from the proximal end of the catheter.

BIOPSY FORCEPS

These devices have distal tip modifications that allow grasping of structures through a 'biting jaws' action (see Fig. 7.1e). Myocardial biotomes are the most familiar example of such a tool. A variety of forceps is available, but most are not appropriate for vascular use because:

- the shaft diameter is very large;
- the device is too rigid to be passed safely in the arterial system; and/or
- the catheter length (often 80–90 cm) may be inadequate.

The thinner, softer, and longer disposable biotomes may be useful in stent retrieval.[2] Although biotome jaws are not meant for cutting through metal, it is possible that aggressive gripping with such a device could sever a thin metal stent.

COOK RETAINED FRAGMENT RETRIEVER

This catheter, manufactured by Cook (Bloomington, IN), has a guidewire attached to the distal end, resembling a fixed-wire angioplasty balloon catheter (see Fig. 7.1f). An articulating arm operable from the proximal hub permits grasping and retrieving of retained equipment fragments. This catheter was developed for use by vascular radiologists and is available in 80 and 145 cm lengths.

RETRIEVAL TECHNIQUES

RETRIEVAL OF A LOST STENT

Stents are the devices that are most frequently lost into the arterial circulation. Occasionally, the stent may be difficult to localize, especially if the vessel wall is calcified. In those cases intravascular ultrasound may help.[3] It is very important to leave the stent on the wire. The wire provides the essential lifeline to the stent and provides a means of retrieval that is lost if the stent is completely disengaged from the wire. In this case, the stent becomes subject to embolization which can often make stent retrieval extraordinarily difficult.

Several techniques for retrieving stents are described below.

RETRIEVING A STENT THAT IS STILL OVER A BALLOON

If stent placement is interrupted or fails, and the stent is still intact and attached to the deployment balloon catheter, then the delivery system should be withdrawn as a single unit. If a guide catheter is used, the stent may be withdrawn into it only if the guide catheter has an excellent coaxial relationship to the proximal arterial segment being approached. If this is not the case, then the guide catheter should be retracted until a favorable alignment between guide and stent delivery catheter can be achieved. On occasion, removal may require retracting the guiding catheter to the distal end of the intra-arterial sheath which results in tip straightening (Fig. 7.3). This may occur at various levels depending on the specific guiding catheter. It is usually possible to maintain the guidewire position with these maneuvers. Using high-resolution fluoroscopy, it is often possible for operators to

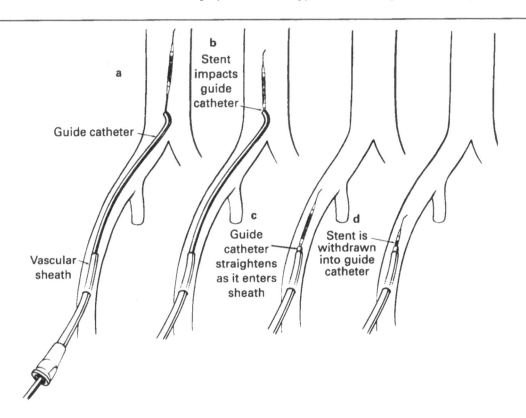

Fig. 7.3 Withdrawing an undeployed stent into the guide requires that there be an excellent coaxial relationship, otherwise the stent may be stripped off the balloon.

Achieving this coaxial relationship is dependent upon the specific guide catheter configuration and its relationship to the ostium of the target artery. In some patients the guide catheter may require withdrawal part way into the sheath to straighten it out.

determine if the stent is being displaced from the deployment balloon as the system is retracted and stents that are easily seen making this maneuver are somewhat safer.

Retraction of the stent into the guide catheter may fail if a proper alignment cannot be achieved. In this circumstance, the edge of the catheter tip may deform the stent or strip it free from the delivery catheter. If the stent cannot be withdrawn into the guide catheter, then the guide and stent catheters should be withdrawn simultaneously and the guide catheter removed from the body. With an 8F or larger vascular sheath, it is possible to advance most of the retrieval devices described above through the vascular sheath alongside the deployment catheter, and the stent may be removed whether it is attached or separated from the deployment balloon.

RETRIEVING A STENT THAT IS STILL OVER A WIRE

SMALL BALLOON TECHNIQUE

If a stent has been stripped off the deployment balloon but is still arranged coaxially over the guidewire, it may be recovered by passing a small balloon through the center of the stent, expanding the balloon and withdrawing the system (Fig. 7.4).[4] This may be used even if the stent is partially or wholly within the target artery (e.g. renal artery). Although the potential for injury exists, the diameter of an expanded 2.0 mm balloon is less than that of a 7F atherectomy catheter, and the surface of many stents, even when damaged, is relatively smooth. With the use of smaller stents, such as renal stents, this can often be quite easily accomplished, and the device can be effectively placed in the common or external iliac artery.

VARIOUS SNARE LOOP TECHNIQUES

If a stent is in a large vascular space it may be retrieved using one of the retrieval devices discussed above (see Fig. 7.1). If possible, the stent should be retracted to below the level of the renal arteries. The easiest device to use is the loop snare. If a guide catheter was used it should be withdrawn, but the stent delivery catheter is usually best left in

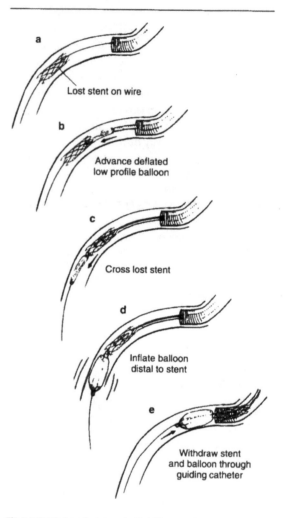

Fig. 7.4 Retrieving a lost stent that is still over a wire.

A balloon is advanced distal to the stent, and is then inflated and withdrawn pulling the stent back into the guiding catheter.

place to buttress the stent and to help identify its location. The loop snare is inserted through the hemostatic valve, alongside the stent delivery catheter, and advanced until it is superior to the damaged stent. The guidewire is retracted until it is below the level of the snare. The loop snare is opened and passed over the guidewire tip, then retracted until the stent is held (Fig. 7.5). Both the loop snare and the delivery catheter are removed as a single unit.

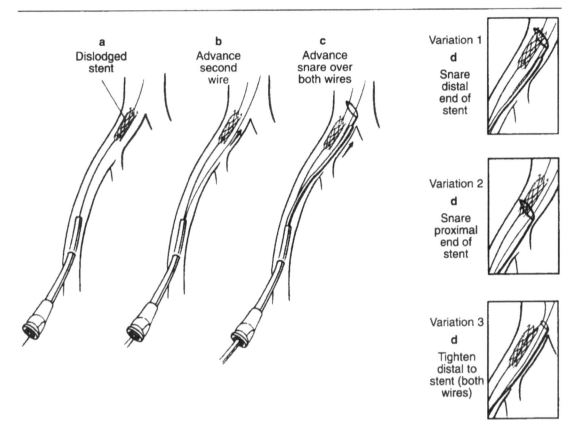

Fig. 7.5 Retrieving a lost stent using a snare.

(a) A stent is lost but is still over the guidewire. (b) A second guidewire is advanced next to the lost stent. (c) A loop snare is advanced over the second guidewire distal to the lost stent and then is pulled back in order to contain both guidewires. (d) Variation 1: the distal end of the stent is snared and withdrawn. Variation 2: the proximal end of the stent is snared and withdrawn. Variation 3: the snare is advanced distal to the stent, and is then tightened and withdrawn into the guide, maintaining the guidewire position.

One of the potential complications of using a snare is that advancing the snare towards the stent may lead to stent dislodgement. A solution to this problem is to position a second stiff angioplasty wire beside the original guidewire.[5] The snare is then widely opened and advanced over both wires distal to the stent. It can then be tightened over the distal (Fig. 7.5a) or proximal (Fig. 7.5b) part of the stent, or it can be tightened distal to the stent and withdrawn fixing the two wires (Fig. 7.5c). A disadvantage of snaring the distal part of the stent is that, during withdrawal of the stent through the femoral artery sheath, if the proximal part of the stent catches on the end of the sheath then applying force to the distal end may cause severe deformation of the stent and severe difficulty in removing it from the sheath.[6] This complication may be prevented by snaring the proximal end of the stent.

Another option is to use the snare to capture the distal end of the original guidewire, which is then withdrawn (Fig. 7.5d, Variation 1). A potential complication of this approach is that the distal end of the guidewire (which consists of a spring coil) may uncoil, and also the stent may be deformed while attempting to withdraw it into the femoral sheath. Alternatively, the second guidewire can be

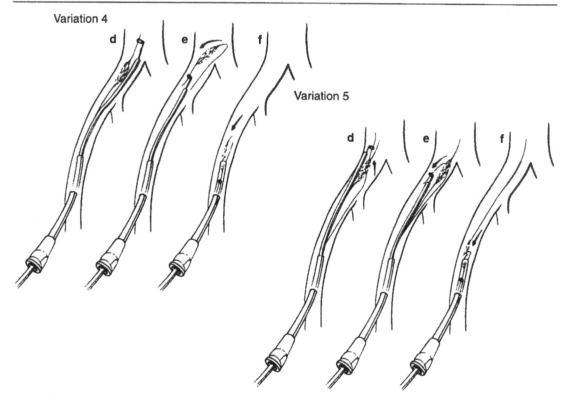

Fig. 7.5 Retrieving a lost stent using a snare – *continued*

Variation 4: (d–f) the distal end of the snare traps the end of the guidewire and is then withdrawn into the guide with the lost stent. Variation 5: (d–f) try to pass the second guidewire through the stent struts. The tip of the second guidewire is then snared using a loop snare and externalized through the femoral sheath. The second guidewire is then withdrawn, moving the lost stent without losing the original guidewire position.

advanced through the lost stent struts and then snared and withdrawn into the sheath (Fig. 7.5e, Variation 5). Using two guidewires provides a better platform to move and position the snare device without moving the dislodged stent and thus lessens the risk of stent embolization. Also, if a larger femoral sheath is needed for removing the stent, the sheath can be inserted over both guidewires.

Alternatively, the distal end of the original wire that goes through the lost stent can be snared from the contralateral femoral artery and externalized and then a small caliber catheter can be used from the ipsilateral femoral artery to push the stent out of the contralateral femoral artery (Fig. 7.6).

USING TWO WIRES
Another method for retrieving a lost stent that is still over a guidewire is to advance a second guidewire through the struts of the stent. Once distal to the lost stent the two guidewires are twisted in an attempt to intermingle the distal ends of the two wires. Both wires are then withdrawn, together with the lost stent (Fig. 7.7).

RETRIEVING A STENT WHEN THE WIRE POSITION IS LOST
If there is no wire through the unexpanded lost stent, it may be feasible to pass a fixed wire balloon (which has a very low profile) through the stent,

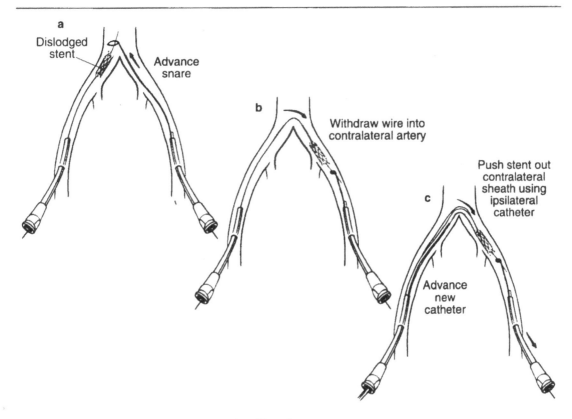

Fig. 7.6 Retrieving a lost stent using a sheath in the contralateral femoral artery.

A loop snare is advanced through the contralateral femoral sheath and is used to trap and externalize the distal tip of the guidewire over which is the lost stent. A catheter is then used to push the lost stent over the wire until it is expelled through the contralateral femoral sheath.

and then inflate the balloon distally and remove the whole system (Fig. 7.8).[6]

DEPLOYING THE LOST STENT

If retrieval is challenging, deploying the stent in an inconsequential location can be significantly easier, carries less risk of dissection or vascular access complications, and requires much less time than retrieving the stent (Fig. 7.9).[6] Kumar et al reported dislodgement of a stent during attempts to deliver it to an occluded subclavian artery; the stent migrated into the external iliac artery where it was deployed without any adverse consequences.[7] Even though this technique requires implantation of an additional iliac stent, iliac stenting carries low risk for

complications and has a low rate of restenosis. Meisel et al described a similar technique for dislodged coronary stents, which are transferred to the iliac artery, deployed locally by a peripheral balloon, and then secured by local anchoring with a peripheral stent.[8]

APPROACH TO A DEPLOYED STENT

Sometimes a deployed stent, such as an iliac stent, either migrates or is pushed into the aorta. The fully deployed stent often cannot be effectively brought back into the iliac artery using the snare balloon technique. Depending on the size of the stent, deployment with a large balloon in the infrarenal abdominal aorta is a consideration. In the event

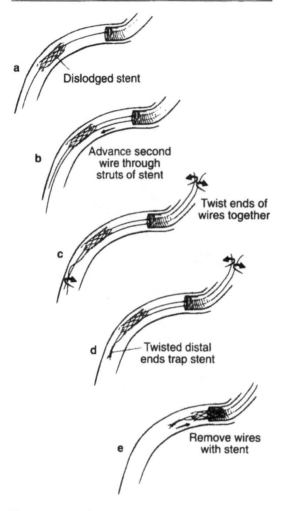

Fig. 7.7 Retrieving a lost stent that is still over a guidewire using two wires.

A second guidewire is advanced through the stent struts. Once distal to the lost stent the two guidewires are twisted in an attempt to intermingle the distal ends of the two wires. Both wires are then withdrawn, together with the lost stent.

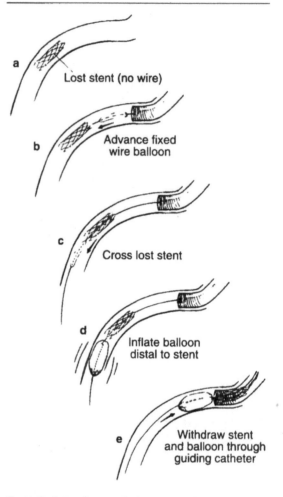

Fig. 7.8 Retrieving a lost stent that is not over a wire.

A fixed-wire balloon is advanced through the stent struts, inflated distal to the stent, and withdrawn together with the stent.

BALLOON RUPTURE DURING STENT IMPLANTATION

that this is not technically possible or the stent is too small, there is an option of snaring the stent and using the snare to squeeze or crush the stent. The crushed stent may be very difficult to remove through a sheath, even a large one (e.g. 14F). If removal is desired it may require surgical arteriotomy in order to avoid arterial laceration.

An additional area that can be problematic with peripheral artery angioplasty and stent placement involves balloon rupture during peripheral stent implantation or a situation in which the balloon becomes trapped in a partially deployed stent. This problem is clearly related to stent loss and is occasionally encountered. Frequently, the initial reaction of the operator is to pull firmly on the balloon.

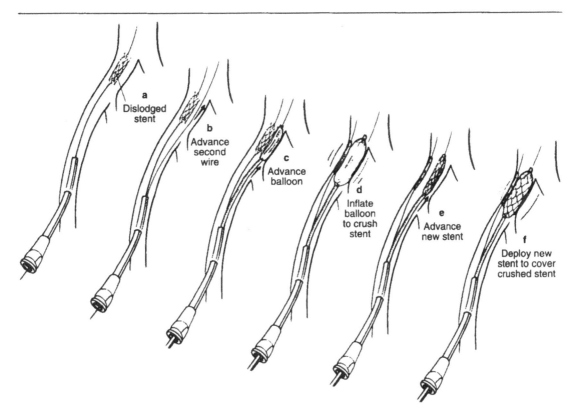

Fig. 7.9 A lost stent may not always need to be retrieved.

Sometimes a lost stent can be crushed against the vessel wall and covered using another stent.

This can often result in dislodging the stent into a position where it cannot be successfully deployed or further compromises the situation. A variety of specific techniques to resolve this problem are described below.

- *Long sheath*: This technique involves using a long sheath that can be placed up to the level of the stent which in turn holds the stent in position; the balloon is subsequently pulled into the sheath, thereby removing it.[9] Placement of a new balloon can then result in adequate deployment of the stent.
- *Balloon on a wire system*: An additional technique has been to use the balloon on a wire system. Typically a coronary balloon on a wire (e.g.

the Tegtmeyer balloon) is placed into the stent alongside the trapped balloon. This can allow sufficient expansion of the stent to enable the trapped peripheral balloon to be effectively removed.

- *High-pressure inflation*: Another solution is to use brief, rapid, high-pressure inflation designed to force the balloon to expand before it can rupture. Attaching the inflation port of a leaking balloon to a power injector and providing a brief, high-pressure, low-volume power inflation has been successful in expanding such stents further, permitting withdrawal of the damaged balloon. The best settings to use will vary according to the situation, but we have been successful using injection of 20–30 cm^3/sec over 0.5–1.0 sec, setting pressure maximums at 400–600 mmHg. Higher pressure limits may exceed the tolerance of the catheter body, thereby involving the risk of catheter (rather than balloon) rupture.

- *Snare*: The ruptured balloon could be retrieved using a snare.[10]
- *Surgery*: Finally, if all other attempts fail, the balloon should be retrieved surgically. In one case report the tip of the balloon catheter ruptured off the shaft of the catheter and was not retrieved until the patient underwent femoropopliteal bypass surgery a year after the percutaneous procedure.[11]

Rarely, a balloon catheter may rupture and a piece of balloon material may become detached and entrapped within the target vessel. If the fragment cannot be retrieved using snares or other techniques, then using a stent to trap the fragment between the stent struts and the vessel wall will allow stabilization of the fragment and avoid the need for surgery.[12] Fortunately, with the advent of newer and better constructed peripheral balloons, balloon rupture is now an infrequent occurrence.

RETRIEVAL OF A FRACTURED GUIDEWIRE

Guidewires consist of two parts: a central shaft and a distal soft tip made from a spring coil. The distal tip may fracture if caught in a coronary lesion or in a side branch of the artery being wired. Additionally, the distal tip may unravel (since it is made of a spring coil).

Leaving a guidewire fragment in the circulation is associated with low risk, especially if it is located in a small arterial branch.

Retrieval of the guidewire fragment can be accomplished by different techniques:

- *Inserting one or more wires next to the fragment and twisting those wires*. The fragment may become entrapped in those wires and the entire system can be removed en bloc.
- *Trapping the fragment between a balloon and the*

inner wall of the guiding catheter, and then removing the whole assembly.[13] This can be accomplished more easily if part of the guidewire fragment remains within the guiding catheter; if the fragment is distal, then the guiding catheter could be deeply intubated in the coronary artery in order to encase the proximal part of the fragment, which could then be removed by following the steps described above.

- *Using a retrieval device such as a snare*. This may be difficult if the fragment is located in a small coronary artery branch because the limited space may not allow the snare to expand.

CONCLUSION

Fortunately, due to advances in the design and manufacture of peripheral interventional equipment, the incidence of stent and other device loss or malfunction is very low and is decreasing continuously. Unfortunately, stent loss still occurs and can greatly complicate and lengthen a procedure; it also carries a high risk for the patient and high stress for the operator. Familiarity with the retrieval equipment and with some basic retrieval techniques can facilitate decision making, ease operator discomfort, and improve patient outcomes.

Preventing device loss is crucial and can be achieved by selecting the appropriate tools, such as score-resistant balloons, avoiding polyethylene terephthalate (PET) balloons and being careful with the amount of force exerted while placing the stent. The loop snare is probably the most consistent and user-friendly retrieval device. It is important to maintain wire access through the stent and not to hesitate in considering alternative vascular deployment.

REFERENCES

1. Foster-Smith KW, Garratt KN, Higano ST, Holmes DR Jr. Retrieval techniques for managing flexible intracoronary stent misplacement. Cathet Cardiovasc Diagn 1993;30:63–8.
2. Berder V, Bedossa M, Gras D, et al. Retrieval of a lost coronary stent from the descending aorta using a PTCA balloon and biopsy forceps. Cathet Cardiovasc Diagn 1993;28:351–3.

3. Bartorelli AL, Montorsi P, Ravagnani P, Galli S, Squadroni L. Failure of fluoroscopy and success of intravascular ultrasound to locate an intracoronary embolized Palmaz-Schatz stent. J Invasive Cardiol 1997;9:25–9.
4. Davies RP, Voyvodic F. Percutaneous retrieval of a partially expanded iliac artery stent: case report. Cardiovasc Intervent Radiol 1992;15:120–2.
5. Bogart DB, Jung SC. Dislodged stent: a simple retrieval technique. Catheter Cardiovasc Interv 1999;47:323–4.
6. Feldman T. Retrieval techniques for dislodged stents. Catheter Cardiovasc Interv 1999;47:325–6.
7. Kumar K, Dorros G, Bates MC, et al. Primary stent deployment in occlusive subclavian artery disease. Cathet Cardiovasc Diagn 1995;34:281–5.
8. Meisel SR, DiLeo J, Rajakaruna M, et al. A technique to retrieve stents dislodged in the coronary artery followed by fixation in the iliac artery by means of balloon angioplasty and peripheral stent deployment. Catheter Cardiovasc Interv 2000;49:77–81.
9. Bersin RM, Gold RS Jr. Balloon rupture during peripheral stent implantation: a new technique for balloon retrieval. Cathet Cardiovasc Diagn 1993;29:292–5.
10. Braun MA, Smith SJ, Merrill TN. Contralateral loop snare removal of a ruptured and entrapped angioplasty balloon. Cardiovasc Intervent Radiol 1996;19:428–30.
11. Gahlen J, Koeppel T, Prosst RL. Vascular occlusion by ruptured balloon after percutaneous transluminal angioplasty. J Endovasc Ther 2003;10:1117–9.
12. http://www.scvir.org/members/caseclub/0300/0300_10/ 0300_10.htm, accessed 5/23/2004
13. Patel T, Shah S, Pandya R, Sanghvi K, Fonseca K. Broken guidewire fragment: a simplified retrieval technique. Catheter Cardiovasc Interv 2000;51:483–6.

8. Aortoiliac Artery Angioplasty and Stenting

Christopher J White and Stephen R Ramee

INTRODUCTION

It is important, in the initial assessment of patients with peripheral vascular occlusive disease, to remember that there is a significant association of coronary artery disease, and that coronary artery disease is the major cause of mortality in these patients.[1,2] A complete cardiovascular assessment of the patient with aortoiliac occlusive disease should be performed, given the high incidence of associated atherosclerotic diseases. Appropriate assessment of these patients includes a complete carotid, abdominal, and lower extremity vascular examination as well as appropriate screening and assessment for coronary artery disease. A non-invasive cardiac stress test is appropriate to assess the risk of suspected coronary artery disease.

Patients with aortoiliac occlusive disease may be asymptomatic or present with a full range of symptoms from mild claudication to limb-threatening ischemia. The severity of symptoms will depend upon the severity of the occlusive lesion, the presence of collateral circulation, and the presence of multilevel vascular disease. With isolated terminal aorta stenoses, generally both legs are equally affected, although disparities in collateral circulation may render one limb more ischemic than the other.

The initial assessment should include a physical examination for signs of peripheral ischemia, distal embolization, and the status of the peripheral pulses. A rest and exercise ankle–brachial index (ABI) should be performed. A mild impairment in the resting ABI may be dramatically exaggerated with exercise. Segmental ABIs with pulse volume recordings will indicate the presence or absence of multilevel occlusive disease. Another very helpful test in the pre-procedural assessment of these patients is the duplex (Doppler and ultrasound) examination. The duplex scan will provide information regarding the presence or absence of abdominal aortic aneurysmal disease and indicate the severity of occlusive lesions. If there is doubt as to the presence of aneurysmal disease an abdominal computed tomographic (CT) scan or magnetic resonance (MR) image should be performed.

AORTOILIAC ANGIOGRAPHY

Vascular access may be obtained from either the upper extremity (radial, brachial or axillary approach) or via a femoral (ipsilateral or contra-lateral) artery. Whenever possible, we prefer to use the ipsilateral femoral artery for access. Using a standard Seldinger technique, access is obtained in the common femoral artery (the mid-level of the femoral head is a useful marker for this vessel) and a 4–6F vascular sheath is placed to ensure access. A soft, steerable, 0.035 inch Wholey guidewire is an excellent wire for crossing occlusive aortoiliac lesions. If this wire fails, we next choose an angled Glidewire™ (Terumo, Boston Scientific, Natick, MA) taking care not pass the wire subintimally across the lesion. Once the wire is across the lesion, a pigtail catheter is advanced to the level of the renal arteries (L1 or L2) and above the level of the occlusive disease. The Glidewire™ is then exchanged for an Amplatz Super Stiff™ (Cook, Bloomington, IN) 0.035 inch guidewire. It is important that once retrograde access across the aortoiliac lesion is gained, care is taken not to lose it during catheter exchanges.

A diagnostic aortogram, showing inflow and outflow of the target lesion, and run-off angiography to visualize the lower extremity circulation are performed. A 'working view' of the lesion is obtained to serve as a 'road map'. Bony landmarks or an external radiopaque ruler are helpful to guide intervention. When performing the diagnostic aortogram it is important to image the renal arteries and any collateral circulation in the pelvis. Occasionally, it is necessary to perform additional selective or angulated views of the terminal aorta and common iliac arteries to define the extent of the stenosis.

AORTOILIAC BALLOON ANGIOPLASTY

After the target lesion has been imaged it is important that an accurate assessment of the reference vessel diameter be made. This can be done with quantitative angiography (taking care to image an appropriate reference object to calibrate for any magnification errors) or intravascular ultrasound (IVUS). The duplex scan or abdominal contrast CT scan may also offer good estimates of luminal diameter of the target vessels. In our experience, visual estimation of vessel diameters in these large vessels is inaccurate and can lead to procedural complications if an oversized balloon is chosen.

Aspirin (325 mg) is given once a day several days prior to the procedure. After access has been obtained and prior to the intervention, we routinely administer 2500–5000 international units of heparin. From the ipsilateral retrograde femoral approach, we prefer to cross the lesion with an atraumatic guidewire – a soft, steerable 0.035 inch Wholey (Malinckrodt, St Louis, MO) wire. If a complete diagnostic angiogram showing inflow and outflow from the lesion has not been previously obtained, a baseline angiogram of the lesion is performed with a pigtail catheter in the best view to show the lesion. An extra-stiff guidewire (0.035 or 0.038 inch Amplatz Super Stiff™ wire; Cook, Bloomington, MN) is then advanced through the pigtail catheter above the lesion and the pigtail catheter removed. The lesion is then dilated with a balloon which is sized 1:1 with the reference vessel diameter. It is important to quantitatively measure the diameter of these large vessels, as significant errors in estimation are possible. The balloon catheter is inflated to the lowest pressure that will fully expand the balloon. The pigtail catheter is then readvanced above the dilated lesion and angiography is performed to assess the result. The

residual stenosis should be less than 30%. The presence of a potentially flow-limiting dissection should be sought. At this time a pressure gradient across the lesion should also be measured between the pigtail catheter in the aorta and the access sheath below the lesion. The gradient should be ≤5 mmHg following successful dilation. If a suboptimal angioplasty result has been obtained, the option at this time is to proceed with stent placement or to repeat the balloon inflation to either higher pressure or for longer duration.

AORTOILIAC STENT PLACEMENT

BALLOON-EXPANDABLE STENT

When deploying a balloon-expandable stent (Fig. 8.1), we prefer to use a long sheath (usually 20–30 cm long) which can be advanced across the lesion. Premounted stents have a lower profile and are less likely to embolize from the balloon catheter. The premounted stent is advanced within the sheath to the lesion site. This technique (advancing the stent to the lesion within the sheath) avoids the risk of the stent being snagged on the irregular surface of the pre-dilated lesion and minimizes the risk of stent embolization. Using bony landmarks or an external radiopaque ruler as a guide for stent placement, the sheath is then pulled

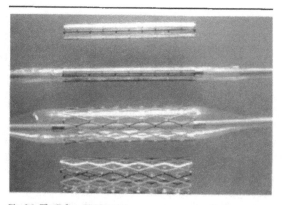

Fig. 8.1 The Palmaz™ 308 stent.

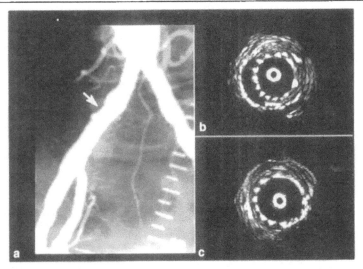

Fig. 8.2 (a) Angiography of a right common iliac stent deployment. (b) IVUS image of suboptimally expanded stent (8 mm balloon). (c) IVUS image after larger balloon (9 mm). There was no difference detectable on angiography alone.

back to uncover the stent. Contrast injections through the delivery sheath can be performed to confirm accurate stent placement. The stent is deployed by fully inflating the balloon to a minimum of six atmospheres to ensure full inflation of the balloon and adequate deployment of the stent.

It is important to assess the adequacy of stent deployment. Angiographically there should be a slight 'step-up and step-down' apparent. Intravascular ultrasound may also be used to visualize the adequacy of stent deployment (Fig. 8.2). A simultaneous pressure gradient between the distal catheter and the access sheath should be measured to confirm that the pressure gradient across the lesion is ≤5 mmHg. To deploy the stent at higher pressures, the deployment balloon is positioned so that the distal shoulder of the balloon is within the distal margins of the stent. This minimizes the chance of a distal dissection occurring during high pressure inflation. The pigtail catheter is then readvanced over the guidewire and final angiography and pressure gradient measurements are performed (Fig. 8.3).

SELF-EXPANDING STENT

It is generally recommended that a self-expanding stent with a nominal diameter ≥1 mm larger than the reference diameter and ≥1 cm longer than the lesion is placed. A long delivery sheath is not required as stent embolization is prevented by the constraining sheath. The stent is advanced over an extra-stiff guidewire (already in the aorta following angiography) to several centimeters above the lesion and approximately 25% of the stent is uncovered by retracting the constraining sheath. The stent may be withdrawn, but not advanced once it has begun to be deployed. To ensure that the distal segment of the lesion will be covered by the stent, compare the bony landmarks or an external radiopaque ruler with the diagnostic 'road map' angiogram of the lesion, and complete the deployment. The pre-dilation balloon is then readvanced within the stent and inflated to ensure full balloon expansion which further apposes the stent against the vessel wall. The pigtail catheter is then advanced over the wire and above the stented lesion for final

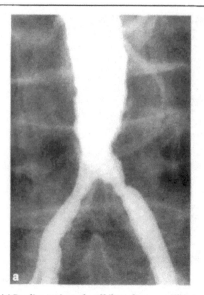
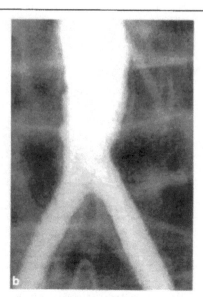

Fig. 8.3 (a) Baseline angiography of bilateral common iliac stenosis. (b) Bilateral ostial stent (Palmaz™ 308) deployment.

angiography (Fig. 8.4). A simultaneous pressure gradient between the pigtail catheter and the access sheath should be measured to confirm that the pressure gradient across the lesion is ≤5 mmHg.

Whenever possible, it is desirable to keep the inflated balloon within the stent to avoid injury to non-stented segments of the vessel wall. If the balloon is longer than the stent, then it should be withdrawn so that its distal end is within the stent. Should a dissection occur, it will be proximal to the

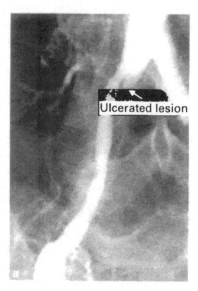
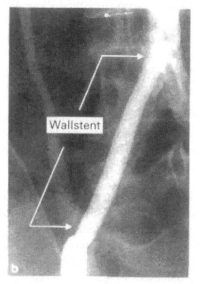

Fig. 8.4 (a) Baseline angiography showing an ulcerated segment of a long right common iliac stenosis. (b) Angiography after placement of a Wallstent™.

stent and correctable with the placement of a second stent without having to recross the deployed stent. It is important to remember that stents will shorten further with balloon expansion, so that when positioning the stent, it is ideal to center the lesion on the stent.

Following stent deployment, the balloon catheter is removed, taking care to keep the guidewire above the lesion and through the stent. The diagnostic pigtail catheter may then be readvanced through the stent and completion angiography performed. Simultaneous pressure recordings from above and below the lesion should confirm that the baseline gradient has been abolished. The target should be a zero gradient in large arteries. If there is any doubt as to the adequacy of stent implantation, intravascular ultrasound may be used to confirm stent apposition to the vessel wall.

One final note of caution is appropriate regarding angioplasty and stent placement in external iliac arteries. These arteries are particularly delicate and prone to rupture with oversized balloons: care must be taken not to oversize balloons in the external iliac arteries.

PATIENT AFTERCARE

The vascular sheath is removed when the activated clotting time (ACT) falls to <160 seconds (usually within 2 hours). When compressing the ipsilateral femoral access site, which is distal to the stent deployment, care should be taken not to occlude flow which may lead to stent thrombosis. Alternatively, one can use a femoral access site closure device. Patients are continued on oral aspirin (325 mg per day) indefinitely. Clopidogrel is not routinely administered, but may be used at the discretion of the attending physician. Prior to hospital discharge (18–24 hours following the procedure) ABIs and duplex scanning may be performed to establish a post-treatment baseline. Patients are followed in the clinic at 1, 3, and 6 months, and at 6-month intervals thereafter with non-invasive testing to document continued patency.

CLINICAL OUTCOMES OF ABDOMINAL AORTA INTERVENTION

Distal abdominal aortic disease has been conventionally treated with endarterectomy or bypass grafting.[3,4] Frequently, distal aortic occlusive disease accompanies occlusive disease of the common or external iliac arteries. The potential advantages of a percutaneous technique compared to an aortoiliac reconstruction are significant in that there is no requirement for general anesthesia or an abdominal incision, and percutaneous therapy is associated with a shorter hospital stay and lower morbidity.[5] While axillofemoral extra-anatomic bypass offers a lower risk surgical alternative for patients with terminal aorta occlusive disease and severe comorbidities, it has the disadvantages of a lower patency rate than direct surgical bypass of the lesions and requires that surgical intervention of a normal vessel be performed to achieve inflow.

Since 1980, balloon angioplasty has been used successfully, although not extensively, in the terminal aorta.[6] An extension of this strategy has been the use of endovascular stents in the treatment of infrarenal aortic stenoses. While balloon dilation of these lesions has been reported to be effective,[6-8] the placement of stents offers a more definitive treatment with a larger acute gain in luminal diameter, scaffolding of the lumen to prevent embolization of debris, and an enhanced long-term patency compared to balloon angioplasty alone.[3-5,9-12]

Ballard and co-workers[11] reported the successful use of a Wallstent™ placed from the axillary artery approach to recanalize a total occlusion of the terminal aorta and bilateral iliac arteries in a patient who was not considered a candidate for thrombolysis or surgical bypass due to severe comorbidities. They described the advantages of using a Wallstent™ in this case due to its length in covering long lesions and its flexibility. Martinez and co-workers reported excellent late follow-up (mean 48 months) in 24 patients treated with infrarenal aortic stents. They reported no in-stent restenosis.[10]

Stents are an attractive therapeutic option for the management of large artery occlusive disease to maintain or improve the arterial luminal patency after balloon angioplasty. Although the utility of stents for aortic stenoses has not been demonstrated in randomized trials, the initial clinical results are encouraging.

CLINICAL OUTCOMES OF AORTOILIAC STENT GRAFTS

It is estimated that 100,000 abdominal aortic aneurysms (AAA) are diagnosed each year and approximately 40,000 require surgical correction. The incidence of AAA appears to have risen over the past several decades. Men are affected more commonly than women and AAA is the tenth leading cause of death in men. It is generally accepted that there is clinical benefit in electively repairing aneurysms larger than 5.0 cm; in patients with hypertension and chronic obstructive lung disease aneurysms larger than 3.0 cm should be repaired.[13] In low-risk patients the operative mortality for AAA repair is estimated to be 5% compared to greater than 10% in higher risk patients. However, experience with covered stent grafts to exclude abdominal aortic and aortoiliac aneurysms is still limited, requiring surgical vascular access to introduce large diameter devices (Fig. 8.5)

Several AAA stent grafts have received US Food and Drug Administration (FDA) approval for clinical use. Using a modular bifurcated stent graft system with nitinol and polytetrafluoroethylene (PTFE) components (Excluder™; WL Gore, Flagstaff, AZ), Matsumura and colleagues reported on a prospective randomized trial in 334 patients with AAA ≥4.5 cm in diameter, comparing the stent graft procedure to conventional surgery.[14] They found no difference in survival rate between the two procedures. The 30-day mortality rate was 0% for the surgery group, and 1% for the stent graft group (p = ns). Cardiac, pulmonary and bleeding complications occurred more frequently in the surgical group (p <0.001). Endoleaks were present in 17% at 1 year and 20% at 2 years (Table 8.1). At 2 years, 14% of the stent graft aneurysms were enlarging by 5 mm or more. Aneurysm re-intervention was necessary in 14% of patients with stent graft repair in the first 2 years. The use of stent grafts for AAA repair offers a less morbid procedure than surgery, but is associated with a higher frequency of late failure requiring a commitment to long-term surveillance not necessary with conventional surgery.

The use of endovascular stent grafts to treat long-segment aortoiliac occlusive disease has been reported by Marin and co-workers in 42 patients

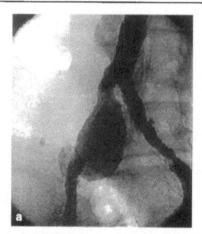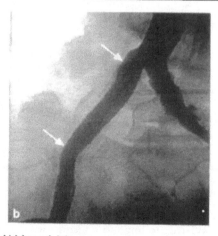

Fig. 8.5 (a) Right common iliac aneurysm. (b) Angiography following stent graft which has sealed the aneurysm.

Table 8.1 Classification of Aorta Stent Graft Endoleaks

- Type I: A separation of the graft from the vessel wall at the proximal or distal attachment site
- Type II: Filling of the aneurysm sac with retrograde flow from mesenteric arteries
- Type III: A tear in the fabric of the graft
- Type IV: Contrast blush through the porous fabric of the graft

Table 8.2 Ideal Iliac PTA Lesions

- Stenotic lesion
- Non-calcified
- Discrete (≤3 cm)
- Patent run-off vessels (≥2)
- Non-diabetic patients

Table 8.3 Contraindications (Relative) to Iliac Balloon Angioplasty

- Occlusion
- Long lesions (≥5 cm)
- Aortoiliac aneurysm
- Atheroembolic disease
- Extensive bilateral aortoiliac disease

with limb-threatening ischemia.[15] The stent grafts were hand-made and were constructed using Palmaz™ (Cordis/Johnson & Johnson, Warren, NJ) stents and 6 mm PTFE thin-walled grafts. Surgical exposure of the femoral access site was obtained and the lesion crossed with a guidewire. The stent was sewn to the proximal end of the graft and deployed with balloon inflation at the inflow site to the lesion. The distal end of the graft was surgically anastomosed at the outflow site. Procedural success was obtained in 91% (39 of 43 arteries). The 18-month patency rate was 89% and the 2-year limb salvage rate was 94%.

CLINICAL OUTCOMES OF ILIAC ARTERY INTERVENTION

Iliac artery intervention represents an important skill for the cardiovascular interventionist to master, not only to relieve patients' lower extremity symptoms, but also to preserve vascular access for what may be lifesaving cardiovascular therapies such as coronary angioplasty, management of arterial access site complications or insertion of an intra-aortic counterpulsation balloon.

Accepted indications for iliac intervention include lifestyle-limiting or progressive claudication, ischemic pain at rest, non-healing ischemic ulcerations, and gangrene. It is important that the angiographic anatomy of the inflow and outflow vessels be demonstrated prior to performing an intervention (Tables 8.2 and 8.3).

The clinical benefit of percutaneous transluminal angioplasty (PTA) versus medical therapy in iliac and femoral lesions has been demonstrated in a randomized trial with endpoints that included relief of symptoms, improvement in walking distance, and continued patency of the affected artery.[16]

A favorable procedural result is more likely with stenoses than with occlusions, with aortoiliac rather than femoropopliteal or tibioperoneal disease, and in patients with claudication rather than limb salvage situations (Table 8.4).[7,17–19] The primary success rate of angioplasty for selected iliac artery stenoses should be >90% with an expected 5-year patency rate of between 80 and 85% while iliac occlusions have a lower expected procedural success rate (33–85%).[20,21]

The long-term patency of iliac vessels treated with balloon angioplasty is influenced by both clinical and anatomic variables.[22] Restenosis rates tend to be lower in non-diabetic male patients with claudication and discrete non-occlusive stenoses with good distal run-off. Conversely, restenosis is more likely to occur in diabetic female patients with rest pain and diffuse and lengthy occlusive lesions with poor distal run-off.

Table 8.4 Patency after Iliac PTA by Clinical and Lesion Variables[22]

	1 Year (%)	3 Year (%)	5 Year (%)
ST/CL/GR	81	70	63
ST/LS/GR	65	48	38
OC/CL/PR	61	43	33
OC/LS/PR	56	17	10

CL, claudication; GR, good run-off; LS, limb-threatening ischemia; OC, occlusion; PR, poor run-off; ST, stenosis.
Reproduced from Johnston KW. Semin Vasc Surg 1989;3:117–22, with permission.

Table 8.5 Ankle–Brachial Index in Randomized Iliac Lesions

	Baseline	Post-treatment	3 Year
PTA	0.50 ± 0.01	0.78 ± 0.04	0.80 ± 0.07
Surgery	0.50 ± 0.02	0.82 ± 0.03	0.78 ± 0.05

p, ns for all.
Reproduced from Wilson et al. J Vasc Surg 1989;9:1–9,[24] with permission.

Traditional surgical therapy for iliac obstructive lesions includes aortoiliac and aortofemoral bypass, procedures reported to have a 74–95% 5-year patency which is comparable to balloon angioplasty. Ameli and co-workers[23] reported their results for a series of 105 consecutive patients undergoing aortofemoral bypass of which 58% were treated for claudication. Operative mortality was 5.7%, early graft failure rate was 5.7%, and 2-year patency was 92.8%.

A randomized trial comparing PTA to bypass surgery for 157 iliac lesions was reported by Wilson et al.[24] They found no significant difference between PTA and surgery for death, amputations, or loss of patency at 3 years (Fig. 8.6). They found no significant difference in the hemodynamic (ankle–brachial index) result of a successful procedure between the surgery group and the PTA group at 3 years (Table 8.5).

Endovascular stents have dramatically improved the success rates for PTA of the iliac arteries.[25-34] Due to the large diameter of the iliac vessels, the risk of thrombosis or restenosis after iliac placement of metallic stents is quite low. Stents may be placed 'primarily' in an iliac lesion, regardless of the balloon angioplasty result, or they may be used 'provisionally' for a suboptimal angioplasty result. Balloon expandable stents have greater radial force and allow greater precision for placement which is particularly useful in ostial lesions. Self-expanding stents are more longitudinally flexible and can be delivered more easily from the contralateral femoral access site. The self-expanding stents also allow for normal vessel tapering and are particularly suited to longer lesions in which the proximal vessel may be several millimeters larger than the distal vessel.

The overall clinical benefit of iliac stent placement has been demonstrated using a meta-analysis of more than 2000 patients from eight reported angioplasty (PTA) series and six stent series.[35] The patients that received iliac stents had a statistically higher procedural success rate and a 43% reduction in late (4-year) failures for patients treated with stents compared to those treated with balloon angioplasty alone.

Clinical results for provisional iliac stent placement with the Palmaz™ stent in 184 iliac lesions demonstrated a 91% procedural success rate and a 6-month patency rate of 99%.[36] Long-term follow-up of these iliac lesions demonstrated a 4-year primary patency rate of 86% and a secondary patency rate of 95%.[36] Results for provisional iliac stent placement with the self-expanding Wallstent™

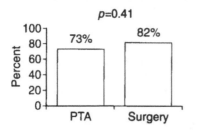

Fig. 8.6 Bar graph of the 3-year event-free survival of percutaneous transluminal angioplasty (PTA) versus surgery for iliac lesions.

(Redrawn from Wilson et al. J Vasc Surg 1989;9:1–9,[24] with permission.)

Table 8.6 Randomized Trial of Iliac PTA Versus Stents

Procedure	Technical Success (%)	Hemodynamic Success (%)	Clinical Success (%)	Complication Rate (%)	Patency 4-year (%)
Stent (n, 123)	98.4	97.6	97.6	4.1	91.6
PTA (n, 124)	91.9	91.9	89.5	6.5	74.3

Reproduced from Richter et al. In: Lierman D, ed. State of the Art and Future Developments. Morin Heights, Canada: Polyscience, 1995: 30–5, with permission.

have demonstrated patency rates of 95% at 1 year, 88% at 2 years, and 82% at 4 years in 118 treated lesions.[37]

A relatively small randomized trial comparing PTA with provisional stenting (stent placement for unsatisfactory balloon angioplasty results) to primary stenting in iliac arteries demonstrated that pressure gradients across the lesions after primary stent placement (5.8 ± 4.7 mmHg) were significantly lower than after PTA alone (8.9 ± 6.8 mmHg) but not after provisional stenting (5.9 ± 3.6 mmHg).[38] The primary technical success rate, defined as a post-procedural gradient less than 10 mmHg, revealed no difference between the two treatment strategies (primary stent = 81% vs PTA plus provisional stenting = 89%). By using provisional stenting, the authors avoided stent placement in 63% of the lesions, and still achieved an equivalent acute hemodynamic result compared to primary stenting. Longer term follow-up will be necessary to evaluate the feasibility and safety of this approach and the impact of provisional stenting on late patency.

Primary placement of Palmaz™ balloon expandable stents has been evaluated in a multicenter trial for iliac placement in 486 patients followed for up to 4 years (mean 13.3 ± 11 months).[39] Using a life-table analysis, clinical benefit was present in 91% at 1 year, 84% at 2 years, and 69% of the patients at 43 months of follow-up. The angiographic patency rate of the iliac stents was 92%. Complications occurred in 10% and were predominantly related to the arterial access site. Five patients suffered thrombosis of the stent of which four were recanalized with thrombolysis and

balloon angioplasty. A preliminary report from a European randomized trial of primary iliac (Palmaz™) stent placement versus balloon angioplasty demonstrated a 4-year patency of 92% for the stent group versus a 74% patency for the balloon angioplasty group (Table 8.6).[40]

Iliac stent placement may also be used as an adjunctive procedure to surgical bypass. Clinical results of using iliac angioplasty with or without stent placement to preserve inflow for a femorofemoral bypass over a 14 year period in 70 consecutive patients have been very encouraging.[41] This study found that those patients requiring treatment of the inflow iliac artery with angioplasty or stent placement did just as well as those without iliac artery disease at 7 years after surgery. These results suggest that percutaneous intervention can provide adequate long-term inflow for femorofemoral bypass as an alternative to aortofemoral bypass in patients at increased risk for a major operation.

CONCLUSION

Percutaneous therapy of aortoiliac disease has dramatically changed the standard of care by which these patients are currently treated. It is distinctly unusual in hospitals with qualified interventionists for a patient to undergo aortofemoral bypass surgery for aortoiliac occlusive disease if a percutaneous approach is feasible. With the maturation and development of the aneurysm exclusion devices (stent grafts) it is likely that the requirement for a major surgical procedure to correct infrarenal aortic aneurysmal disease will become an infrequent occurrence. It is the nature of surgical procedures to change. And while many surgeons feel that their specialty and livelihood are threatened by percutaneous interventions, they must accept the fact that there will be a relentless progression towards less invasive, less morbid procedures in the future.

ACKNOWLEDGMENT

The authors would like to express their appreciation to Mr James O'Meara for his assistance in the preparation of the figures and tables.

REFERENCES

1. Hertzer NR, Beven EG, Youn JR, et al. Coronary artery disease in peripheral vascular patients: a classification of 1000 coronary angiograms and results of surgical management. Ann Surg 1984;199:223–33.

2. Jamieson WRE, Janusz MT, Miyagishima RT, Gerein AN. Influence of ischemic heart disease on early and late mortality after surgery for peripheral occlusive vascular disease. Circulation 1982;66(suppl I):92–7.

3. Marin ML, Veith FJ, Cynamon J, et al. Transfemoral endovascular stented graft treatment of aorto-iliac and femoropopliteal occlusive disease for limb salvage. Am J Surg 1994;168:156–62.

4. Williams JB, Watts PW, Nguyen VA, Peterson CL. Balloon angioplasty with intraluminal stenting as the initial treatment modality in aorto-iliac occlusive disease. Am J Surg 1994;168:202–4.

5. Diethrich EB, Santiago O, Gustafson G, Heuser RR. Preliminary observations on the use of the Palmaz stent in the distal portion of the aorta. Am Heart J 1993;125:490–501.

6. Charlbois N, Saint Georges G, Hudon G. Percutaneous transluminal angioplasty of the lower abdominal aorta. Am J Radiol 1991;146:369–71.

7. Tegtmeyer CJ, Hartwell GD, Selby JB, et al. Results and complications of angioplasty in aortoiliac disease. Circulation 1991;83(suppl I):53–60.

8. Iyer SS, Hall P, Dorros G. Brachial approach to management of an abdominal aortic occlusion with prolonged lysis and subsequent angioplasty. Cathet Cardiovasc Diagn 1991;23:290–3.

9. Long AL, Gaux JC, Raynaud A. Infrarenal aortic stents: initial clinical experience and angiographic follow-up. Cardiovasc Intervent Radiol 1993;16:203–8.

10. Martinez R, Rodriguez-Lopez J, Diethrich EB. Stenting for abdominal aortic occlusive disease. Long-term results. Tex Heart Inst J 1997;24:15–22.

11. Ballard JL, Taylor FC, Sparks SR, Killen JD. Stenting without thrombolysis for aortoiliac occlusive disease: experience in 14 high-risk patients. Ann Vasc Surg 1995;9:453–8.

12. Roeren T, Post K, Richter GM, et al. Stent angioplasty of the infrarenal aorta and aortic bifurcation. Clinical and angiographic results in a prospective study. Radiologe 1994;34:504–10.

13. Cronenwett JL. Infrainguinal occlusive disease. Semin Vasc Surg 1995;8:284–8.

14. Matsumura JS, Brewster DC, Makaroun MS, et al. A multicenter controlled clinical trial of open versus endovascular treatment of abdominal aortic aneurysm. J Vasc Surg 2003;37:262–71.

15. Marin ML, Veith FJ, Sanchez LA, et al. Endovascular repair of aortoiliac occlusive disease. World J Surg 1996;20:679–86.

16. Whyman MR, Kerracher EMG, Gillespie IN, et al. Randomised controlled trial of percutaneous transluminal angioplasty for intermittent claudication. Eur J Vasc Surg 1996;12:167–72.

17. O'Keeffe ST, Woods BO, Beckmann CF. Percutaneous transluminal angioplasty of the peripheral arteries. Cardiol Clin 1991;9:519–21.

18. Wilson SE, Sheppard B. Results of percutaneous transluminal angioplasty for peripheral vascular occlusive disease. Ann Vasc Surg 1990;4:94–7.

19. Reidy JF. Angioplasty in peripheral vascular disease. Postgrad Med J 1987;63:435–8.

20. Gallino A, Mahler F, Probst P, Nachbur B. Percutaneous transluminal angioplasty of the arteries of the lower limbs: a 5 year follow-up. Circulation 1984;70:619–23.

21. Cassarella WJ. Noncoronary angioplasty. Curr Probl Cardiol 1986;11:141–74.

22. Johnston KW. Balloon angioplasty: predictive factors for long-term success. Semin Vasc Surg 1989;3:117–22.

23. Ameli FM, Stein M, Provan JL, et al. Predictors of surgical outcome in patients undergoing aortobifemoral bypass reconstruction. J Cardiovasc Surg 1990;30:333–9.

24. Wilson SE, Wolf GL, Cross AP. Percutaneous transluminal angioplasty versus operation for peripheral arteriosclerosis: report of a prospective randomized trial in a selected group of patients. J Vasc Surg 1989;9:1–9.

25. Becker GJ, Palmaz JC, Rees CR, et al. Angioplasty-induced dissections in human iliac arteries: management with Palmaz balloon-expandable intraluminal stents. Radiology 1990;176:31–8.

26. Katzen BT, Becker GJ. Intravascular stents: status of development and clinical application. Surg Clin North Am 1992;72:941–57.

27. Palmaz JC, Richter GM, Noeldge G, et al. Intraluminal stents in atherosclerotic iliac artery stenosis: preliminary report of a multicenter study. Radiology 1988;168:727–31.

28. Palmaz JC, Garcia OJ, Schatz RA, et al. Placement of balloon-expandable intraluminal stents in iliac arteries: first 171 procedures. Radiology 1990;174:969–75.

29. Sullivan TM, Childs MB, Bacharach JM, et al. Percutaneous transluminal angioplasty and primary stenting of the iliac arteries in 288 patients. J Vasc Surg 1997;25:829–39.

30. Murphy KD, Encarnacion CE, Le VA, Palmaz JC. Iliac artery stent placement with the Palmaz stent: follow-up study. J Vasc Intervent Radiol 1995;6:321–9.

31. Sapoval MR, Chatellier G, Long AL, et al. Self-expandable stents for treatment of iliac artery obstructive lesions: long-term success and prognostic factors. Am J Radiol 1996;166:1173–9.

32. Laborde JC, Palmaz JC, Rivera FJ, et al. Influence of anatomic distribution of atherosclerosis on the outcome of revascularization with iliac stent placement. J Vasc Intervent Radiol 1995;6:513–21.

33. Kichikawa K, Uchida H, Yoshioka T, et al. Iliac artery stenosis and occlusion: preliminary results of treatment with Gianturco expandable metallic stents. Radiology 1990;177:799–802.

34. Rees CR, Palmaz JC, Garcia O, et al. Angioplasty and stenting of completely occluded iliac arteries. Radiology 1989;172:953–9.

35. Bosch JL, Hunink MGM. Meta-analysis of the results of percutaneous transluminal angioplasty and stent placement for aortoiliac occlusive disease. Radiology 1997;204:87–96.

36. Henry M, Amor M, Thevenot G, et al. Palmaz stent placement in iliac and femoropopliteal arteries: primary and secondary patency in 310 patients with 2–4 year follow up. Radiology 1995;197:167–74.

37. Vorwerk D, Gunther RW, Schurmann K, Wendt G. Aortic and iliac stenosis: follow-up results of stent placement after insufficient balloon angioplasty in 118 cases. Radiology 1996;198:45–8.

38. Tetteroo E, Haaring C, van der Graaf Y, et al. Intraarterial pressure gradients after randomized angioplasty or stenting of iliac artery lesions. Dutch Iliac Stent Trial Study Group. Cardiovasc Intervent Radiol 1996;19:411–7.

39. Palmaz JC, Laborde JC, Rivera FJ, et al. Stenting of the iliac arteries with the Palmaz stent: experience from a multicenter trial. Cardiovasc Intervent Radiol 1992;15:291–7.

40. Richter GM, Noeldge G, Roeren T, et al. First long-term results of a randomized multicenter trial: iliac balloon-expandable stent placement versus regular percutaneous transluminal angioplasty. In: Lierman D, ed. State of the Art and Future Developments. Morin Heights, Canada: Polyscience, 1995: 30–5.

41. Perler BA, Williams GM. Does donor iliac artery percutaneous transluminal angioplasty or stent placement influence the results of femorofemoral bypass? Analysis of 70 consecutive cases with long-term follow up. J Vasc Surg 1996;24:363–70.

9. Stenting of the Femoropopliteal Artery

Andrej Schmidt, Dierk Scheinert and Giancarlo Biamino

INTRODUCTION

Atherosclerotic lesions arise more frequently in the femoropopliteal segment than in any other region of the lower extremity. Vascular surgery has been the standard treatment since the 1990s, but endovascular percutaneous interventions offer an attractive minimally invasive alternative therapy. Due to good long-term patency rates after stenting of iliac obstructive lesions, endovascular therapy of this arterial region is well accepted as first choice therapy prior to surgery.[1,2] In contrast, indications for percutaneous transluminal angioplasty (PTA) of femoropopliteal lesions are not well defined. In particular, long chronic occlusions of the superficial femoral artery (SFA) are still considered the province of vascular surgery.[3]

Since the clinical introduction of the pulsed excimer laser used in combination with a guidewire, long occlusions of the femoropopliteal arteries are no longer impassable obstacles for the interventionist. The most challenging aspect of endovascular treatment is, however, to maintain patency. As in iliac arteries, intravascular stents have been advocated to improve long-term patency rates in femoropopliteal lesions. Initially, only balloon expandable stents and self-expanding stainless steel stents were available, leaving peripheral interventionists with limited stent choice for infrainguinal arteries. Furthermore, using these stents, reactive intimal hyperplasia continued to be the limiting factor concerning the long-term prognosis in diffusely diseased arteries.[4] After the clinical introduction of nitinol stents, different stent designs became available. Studies comparing the different stents in terms of technical success, and short- and long-term patency are not yet published, making stent choice a difficult issue in daily practice. Whether the implantation of a stent in the superficial femoral and/or popliteal artery will be beneficial in the long term remains to be clarified.

INDICATIONS FOR ANGIOPLASTY OF THE FEMOROPOPLITEAL ARTERY

Analysis of the distribution of peripheral arterial obstructive disease shows that more than 50% of all lesions are localized in the femoropopliteal region. Corresponding to the length of this vessel, diffusely stenosed segments and long occlusions dominate over focal stenoses. The natural history of isolated SFA disease predicts a low amputation risk (0–1%) without surgical revascularization.[5] This benign natural history often drives physicians to avoid surgical or interventional treatment. However, patients who continue to smoke or who are diabetic tend to have progressive disease that may involve other arterial segments, increasing the risk of developing a critical limb ischemia. A walking program is often preferred; however, very few patients effectively improve their quality of life when sent out just to walk.[6] Supervised exercise programs have a higher success rate, but the benefit tends to be short lived after completion of the program.[7]

Endovascular treatment with balloon angioplasty is well accepted for short segmental disease of the femoropopliteal artery. The guideline for management of peripheral arterial disease, published by the TransAtlantic Inter-Society Consensus working group (TASC)[3] recommends PTA as first choice therapy in patients with lesions up to 3 cm in length, whereas those with occlusions over 5 cm in length should undergo bypass surgery. However, since bypass grafting is associated with considerable procedure-related morbidity and mortality, surgical intervention is usually reserved for patients with ischemic rest pain or very advanced claudication.[8] Consequently, many patients with SFA lesions, although in a state of relevant discomfort with limitation of quality of life, remain untreated.

Percutaneous revascularization techniques permit a lower threshold of intervention, particularly in patients with comorbidities such as coronary artery disease, where the saphenous vein should be preserved for coronary bypass grafting.

The immediate technical success of revascularization of the femoropopliteal segment by balloon angioplasty is reported by almost all working groups to be very high, reaching from 80% to more than 95%.[9-11] However, long-term results vary widely from 5-year patency rates of 68% in patients with stenosis and claudication to only 12% in patients with occlusion and critical ischemia.[12,13] Due to these unsatisfactory results improvement in endovascular recanalization techniques for treatment of the femoropopliteal tract (e.g. the introduction of stents) is particularly desirable.

STENT DESIGNS

BALLOON EXPANDABLE STENTS

The Palmaz™ stent (Cordis/Johnson & Johnson, Warren, NJ) is the prototype of balloon expandable stents and was the first device to be approved by the US Food and Drug Administration (FDA) for peripheral vascular application. The stent is a rigid laser-cut slotted tube of stainless steel, which is hand-crimped onto an appropriately sized balloon. Important characteristics of this stent include its high radial force, which makes it valuable in heavily calcified lesions, and its attribute of precise placement with limited foreshortening. Further expansion after initial deployment by balloons of incremental size is possible. One important disadvantage of this stent – a significant stiffness – has been overcome by newer articulated stainless steel stents.

Strecker™ stents (MediTech, Boston Scientific, Natick, MA) are made of knitted tantalum wire and are balloon mounted for deployment as in the Palmaz™ stent. Tantalum is radiopaque, thus helping to ensure precise placement on balloon expansion. The Strecker™ stent usually shortens by approximately 10% with full expansion. Its flexibility allows for a contralateral placement using a crossover approach.

The most important disadvantage of these stents is deformability by extrinsic compression, which can lead to restenosis and reocclusion in the femoropopliteal tract.

SELF-EXPANDING STENTS

The most important advantages of self-expandable stents over balloon expandable stents are their higher flexibility and the recoil tendency after external deformation. Self-expanding stents are therefore the stents of choice for implantation in the SFA, an artery which is subjected to compression, elongation, shortening, and distortion over its whole length.

The Wallstent™ (Meditech, Boston Scientific, Natick, MA), the first self-expanding stent, is based on a wire mesh braided from stainless steel monofilaments. When released from its delivery system, the stent tends to recoil to its preset nominal diameter. The most important disadvantage of this stent is its significant and unpredictable foreshortening of up to one-third of its unconstrained state, making an exact placement difficult. For example, a Wallstent™ with a diameter of 9 mm and a length of 40 mm shortens to 31 mm when the lumen enlarges to 10 mm. Furthermore, the radial force, which is still effective after deployment, may provoke a further enlargement with consequent ongoing foreshortening and development of gaps between initially overlapping stents.

Another concept of self-expansion uses the thermal memory characteristic of nitinol, an elastic intermetallic alloy of nickel and titanium. Preshaped at high temperatures to its nominal dimension, the stents are soft and deformable after cooling. When exposed to body temperature during deployment, the stent again tends to expand rapidly to its nominal diameter. One of its most important advantages over the Wallstent™ is its negligible foreshortening (maximum 5%), making implantation more precise. Due to the segmental design of most of the nitinol stents (except the spiral stents), accommodation to different artery diameters is potentially superior compared to the Wallstent™. Radiopacity of the nitinol stents is inferior compared to stainless steel stents, but this fact may only play a role in pelvic and not in femoropopliteal arteries, where overlying tissue is negligible. Some manufacturers have overcome this drawback by using markers at both ends of the stent.

There are several different types of nitinol stents available including the S.M.A.R.T.™ (Cordis/Johnson & Johnson, Warren, NJ), the LUMINEXX™ (CR Bard, Temple, AZ), Protégé™ (ev3, Paris, France), Sentinol™ (Boston Scientific, Natick, MA), SelfX™ (Abbott, Redwood City, CA), Absolute™ (Guidant, Santa Clara, CA), IntraCoil™ (IntraTherapeutics St Paul, MN), the Zilver™ (Cook, Bloomington, IN), Aurora™ (Medtronic AVE, Santa Rosa, CA) and several others (Table 9.1). Different in design from the above is the aSpire™ covered stent (Vascular Architects, San José, CA), which is a spiral nitinol stent completely covered by a thin layer of polytetrafluoroethylene (PTFE), which is intended to provide greater lumen wall coverage and eliminate metal-to-artery interaction.

In our opinion, balloon premounted stents are, in general, not indicated in the femoropopliteal region, perhaps with the exception of short, very calcified lesions less than 2 cm in length. Self-expanding nitinol stents have become the mainstay for the femoropopliteal tract.

INDICATIONS FOR STENTING OF THE FEMOROPOPLITEAL ARTERY

The initial hope – that the good short-term results after recanalization of stenoses and occlusions of the femoropopliteal regions could be maintained by the introduction of stents in preventing recoil and intimal hyperplasia – has been thwarted by several studies that showed long-term patency rates after stenting to be no different from PTA alone.[14–17] It must be borne in mind, however, that nearly all of these studies were carried out with balloon expandable or self-expanding stents of the first generation (Palmaz™ and Strecker™ stents, Wallstents™). It can be anticipated that the results will be different using the new generation of nitinol stents. However, until data of larger trials using these new stents are published, stenting of the femoropopliteal arteries remains controversial, and primary stenting in particular is discouraged by the majority of investigators.[18]

Accepted indications for stenting are limited to suboptimal angioplasty results such as flow-limiting dissections (Figs 9.1, 9.2), especially spiral dissections (Figs 9.3, 9.4), a residual pressure gradient >15 mmHg or a remaining stenosis >30% (Fig. 9.5), and an elastic recoil as well as failure to maintain initial patency. According to the latest meta-analysis of studies concerning interventional

Table 9.1 Different Nitinol Stents for Use in the Femoropopliteal Tract

Stent type	Diameter (mm)	Length (mm)	Minimum Sheath Size (F)	Working Length (cm)	Manufacturer
S.M.A.R.T.™ Control™	6–14	20–100	6–7	80/120	Cordis
SelfX™	6–10	32–92	7	75/135	Abbott
Absolute™	5–10	28–100	6	80/120	Guidant
LUMINEXX™	4–14	20–120	6	135	Bard
Protégé™	6–9	20–150	6–7	135	ev3
Sentinol™	5–10	20–80	6	75/135	Boston Scientific
Aurora™	6–10	20–80	6–7	75/120	Medtronic
Zilver™	6–10	40–80	5–6	80/125	Cook
aSpire™	6–12	25–100	8	50/100	Vascular Architects
Optimed Sinusstent™	4–10	10–150	5–7	45/150	Optimed
Maris™	6–12	30–120	6	80/120	Invatec

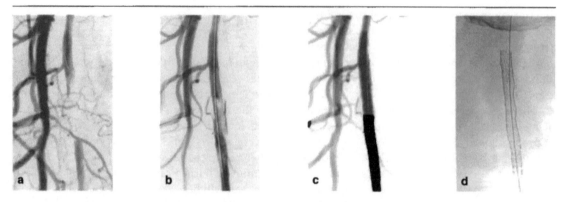

Fig. 9.1 Occlusion of the right superficial femoral artery (SFA).

(a) Short (3–4 cm) proximal occlusion of the right SFA. (b) After passing the occlusion with a guidewire and dilation of the obstruction, a relevant, flow-limiting dissection is observed. (c) After implantation of a self-expandable nitinol stent (SelfX™, 8/80 mm) and post-dilation with a 6/40 mm balloon an optimal angiographic result was achieved. (d) This frame shows the native configuration of the implanted stent.

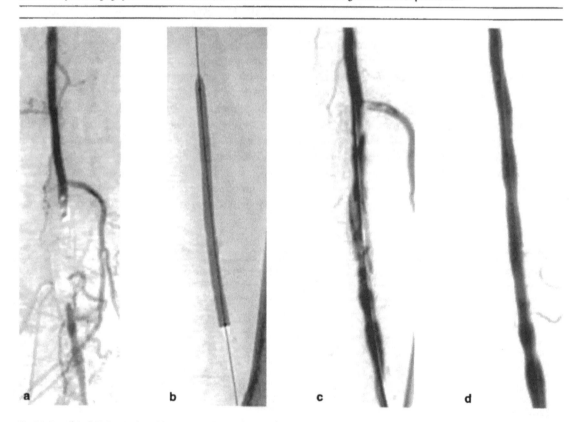

Fig. 9.2 Heavily calcified occlusion of the superficial femoral artery (SFA).

(a) Heavily calcified ca. 5 cm long occlusion of the SFA. (b) After passing the occlusion a 5/80 mm balloon was placed and inflated with 10 bars. (c) Diffuse partial spiral dissection of the obstruction. (d) After stent deployment (Dynalink™; Guidant, Santa Clara, CA; 7/80 mm) and post-dilation (5/80 mm), a good angiographic result was achieved.

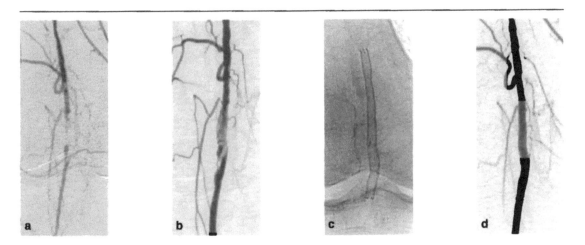

Fig. 9.3 Occlusion of the mid popliteal artery.

(a) Heavily calcified short occlusion of the mid popliteal artery. (b) The occlusion could only be passed (probably subintimal) after many attempts with different guidewires. After balloon dilation (4/40 mm) a spiral, flow-limiting dissection is observed. (c) The native frame shows the position of the delivered SMART™ stent (6/60 mm) with corresponding markers. (d) Final angiogram with optimal flow.

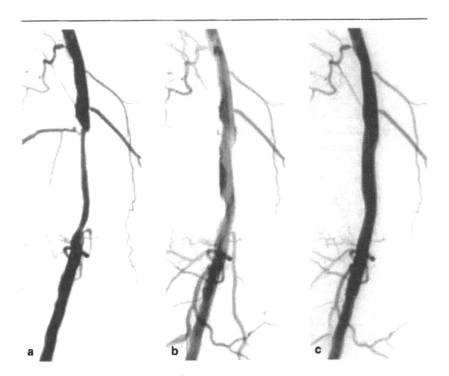

Fig. 9.4 Restenosis of a superficial femoral artery (SFA).

(a) Symptomatic restenosis of an originally occluded SFA. (b) After balloon dilation diffuse spiral dissection. (c) After implantation of a 7/100 mm nitinol stent, an excellent angiographic result was achieved.

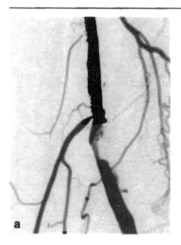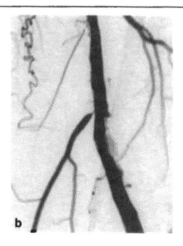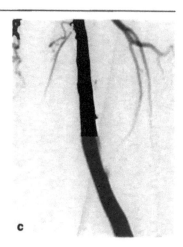

Fig. 9.5 (a–c) Recoil of a highly sclerotic stenosis after percutaneous transluminal angioplasty (6/20 mm balloon, 10 bars) and minor dissection with good result after stent implantation.

therapy of the femoropopliteal tract,[13] there may be some place for primary stenting of occlusions in combination with critical limb ischemia, yielding better results for stenting compared to balloon angioplasty alone in these patients.

When dilating long SFA segments, the placement of a stent can substantially improve the esthetic appearance. In consequence, the luminal diameters proximal or distal to the stent may appear unsatisfactory, inducing the so-called 'oculostenotic reflex' to continue stenting until the entire vessel is covered. This scenario might carry a high risk for restenosis and reocclusion. Alternative strategies would be to stent the inflow and outflow of the arterial segment leaving the middle part uncovered or spot stenting only the areas of heavy plaque burden. Which of these strategies will produce the best results remains to be clarified.

TECHNIQUE OF STENT IMPLANTATION

After balloon angioplasty, an appropriately sized stent should be chosen. The stent should cover the whole lesion, and preferably extend for some millimeters into the healthy vessel. Since collaterals almost always have their origin where occlusions start and end, stents have to be placed regardless of these vessels. The occlusion of side branches after stenting is rare. The diameter of the chosen self-expanding nitinol stent is normally 1–2 mm larger than the reference vessel; for example, in a SFA with a diameter of 5 mm, a stent with a nominal diameter of 7 mm is chosen. It is important to stress the fact that post-dilation or adaptation of the stent should never exceed the evaluated diameter of the reference segment.

If the lesion is located in the proximal SFA near the origin of the profunda artery, there seems to be an argument to use balloon premounted stents for high accuracy in exact placement. However, self-expanding stents can be placed very precisely using the following technique:

1. The delivery system of the stent is first placed a few millimeters distal to the intended region.
2. After the first struts are fully expanded, the stent is pulled to the correct level.
3. During the release maneuver nitinol stents tend to move forward slightly with initial deployment, but with gentle traction on the shaft of the delivery system (which should be maintained during the whole deployment maneuver) exact positioning is possible (Fig. 9.6).

post-interventional improvement occur, indicating the necessity for closer examination or repeat angiography and reintervention.

Color duplex sonography (CDS) is the investigation of choice in assessing the major infrainguinal arteries in patients with claudication.[24] Although the method is less sensitive than arteriography for the evaluation of iliac arteries and time consuming for the examination of crural vessels, it is generally accepted that CDS can replace diagnostic arteriography in lower limbs in over 95% of the cases, especially those concerning the femoropopliteal tract.[25] Sensitivities for detection of stenoses or occlusions in femoropopliteal arteries have been reported to be 95% with specificities of 99%.[26] Significant stenoses are easily recognized by an increase in flow velocity of at least 100%. This can be difficult and misleading in multiple or long stenoses, which are frequent in the SFA. However, taking into consideration that each consecutive stenosis leads to an additional reduction of flow velocity, even multisegmental pathology does not adversely affect the high accuracy of this method.[27]

Stents are visualized easily by B-mode sonography along the whole femoropopliteal artery. Only the area of Hunter's channel may be difficult to analyze in very obese patients. In this tract the use of transducers with lower frequencies as used for cardiac or abdominal sonography is then advisable. If a stent in this area is still not visible, examination of the popliteal artery will indirectly reveal reliable information on the patency of the stent in Hunter's channel. In cases of a high grade stenosis or occlusion, typical alterations can be obtained such as post-stenotic turbulences or a monophasic Doppler wave form (Fig. 9.8).

Color Doppler imaging in the stent permits rapid location of sites of restenosis showing the presence of lumen narrowing and a color-coded flow-jet or aliasing phenomenon (Fig. 9.9). At sites of non-laminar flow, center-stream pulsed Doppler analysis is required for precise classification of disease severity. Restenosis is mostly defined as >50% stenosis and Doppler sonographic criteria for significant stenoses are a doubling of the focal flow velocity from the proximal adjacent segment

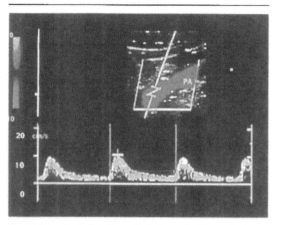

Fig. 9.8 Monophasic Doppler profile in the popliteal artery (PA) indicating a high-grade stenosis or occlusion of the superficial femoral artery.

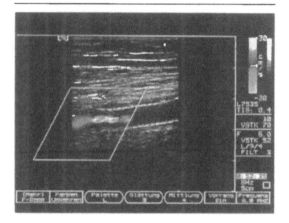

Fig. 9.9 High grade in-stent restenoses can be rapidly visualized by color Doppler showing the aliasing phenomenon

or a peak systolic velocity greater than 200–250 cm/sec[28,29] (Table 9.2).

The degree of restenosis can also be assessed by calculation of the peak systolic velocity ratio:

PSV ratio = PSV stenosis/PSV artery

A PSV ratio ≥2–2.5 is considered a criterion for hemodynamically important lesions.[30] Stenoses with a velocity ratio >3 may progress to occlusion within a relatively brief time window, so that these stenoses should be immediately considered for reintervention.[31] We recommend routine

Table 9.2 Criteria for Estimation of Stenosis of Femoropopliteal Arteries

Grade of Stenosis	Doppler Waveform Characteristics	Peak Systolic Velocity (cm/sec)
No stenosis	Triphasic or biphasic signal with minimum spectral broadening	Normal
≤20%	Normal waveform contour, spectral broadening	Normal
21–50%	PSV increased by 50–100% from the site proximal to the stenosis, marked spectral broadening	≤250
51–75%	Marked spectral broadening and post-stenotic turbulent flow	250–350
75–99%	Marked post-stenotic turbulence	>350
Occlusion	Decreased velocities proximal and monophasic waveforms distal to the occlusion	No flow

PSV, peak systolic velocity.
Modified from Bray 1995[29].

surveillance with duplex ultrasound every 3 months during the first year and twice yearly thereafter, indefinitely.

PATENCY RATES OF STENTS IN THE FEMOROPOPLITEAL REGION

REVIEW OF THE LITERATURE

Published studies about stenting of the femoropopliteal tract are difficult to compare, due to different stent designs, use of multiple versus single stents, application in short or very long lesions, and different anticoagulation regimens. Bias, due to the large proportion of cases in which stents were used after angioplasty with unsatisfactory outcome, may also have added to unfavorable results of stenting

Table 9.3 Overview of the Literature of Stenting the Femoropopliteal Tract

Author	Stent Type	Limbs (n =)	Mean Lesion Length (cm)	Mean Follow-up	Primary Patency (%)	Secondary Patency (%)
Published results of stenting short lesions of the femoropopliteal tract						
Henry et al[23]	Palmaz	111	3.8	4 years	65	95
Cejna et al[16]	Palmaz	33	2.6	2 years	53	73
Grimm et al[17]	Palmaz	30	3.0	3 years	62	90
Henry et al[17]	Nitinol (VascuCoil)	45	4.5	18 months	85	88
Jahnke et al[18]	Nitinol (IntraCoil)	37	3.6	1 year	86	100
Lugmayr et al[32]	Nitinol (Symphony)	54	3.2	3 years	76	87
Published results of stenting long lesions of the femoropopliteal tract						
Zollikofer et al	Wallstent	12	13.5	20 months	29	43
Do-Dai-Do et al[9]	Wallstent	26	8.6	1 year	59	69
Bray et al[39]	Strecker	57	6.8	1 year	79	82
Gray et al[8]	Wallstent, Palmaz	58	16.5	1 year	22	46
Conroy et al[41]	Wallstent, Palmaz	61	13.5	3 years	26	70
Gordon et al[42]	Wallstent	71	14.4	3 years	30	68
Cheng et al[43]	Wallstent, Nitinol	73	16.0	4 years	22	37
Vogel et al[44]	Nitinol (S.M.A.R.T./Precise)	41	9.6	2 years	84	90

compared to PTA alone in many of the published non-randomized studies.[15]

Several factors probably affect the outcome of stenting in the SFA. Among these, length of the diseased segment is probably the most important factor with greater likelihood of long-term patency with shorter lesions (Table 9.3).

Studies using single Palmaz™ stents in short femoropopliteal lesions showed favorable patency rates after 1 and 3 years.[17,23] Patency was reported to be significantly worse with a restenosis rate of 33% when more than four Palmaz™ stents were placed in the SFA, as compared with a 4.4% restenosis rate for a single stent.[23]

Gray et al[4] observed primary and secondary patency rates as low as 22% and 46% respectively after stenting long occlusions (mean lesion length 16.5 cm) at 1 year follow-up despite a strict surveillance program. Although other authors reported more favorable patency rates, lesion length seems to be a strong predictive factor for long-term patency (see Table 9.3).

Lesion site, according to some studies, might also be a predictor of long-term outcome. The 4.4% restenosis rate with a single Palmaz™ stent reported by Henry[23] was only seen in short lesions of the proximal SFA and increased to a rate of 18.5% for the distal SFA. This association of restenosis rate and lesion level is not confirmed by all authors.[32,33] Strecker[33] found good results after stent therapy with more flexible tantalum stents, even after implantation in the popliteal artery, with encouraging 1- and 2-year primary patency rates of 81% and 74% respectively.

In a recent review article on femoropopliteal interventions, Lammer[34] assessed the average of published long-term patency rates after stent placement in femoropopliteal artery lesions for 585 patients to be 67% and 58% at 1 and 3 years respectively. In a recent meta-analysis of long-term results after angioplasty of femoropopliteal arterial lesions collected in 19 studies, the outcome of 923 balloon dilations and 473 stent implantations were compared. The 3-year patency rates after balloon dilation were 61% for stenoses and claudication, 43% for stenoses and critical limb ischemia, and 30% for

occlusions and critical limb ischemia. The 3-year patency rates after stent implantation were 63–66% and were independent of clinical indication and lesion type.[13]

To our knowledge, five randomized clinical trials comparing balloon dilation and stent implantation in the femoropopliteal region have been published to date.[14–17,35] In contrast to the results of the meta-analysis of Muradin et al,[13] no significant difference between balloon dilation and stent implantation was found. A possible explanation could be the small size and the limited follow-up of 1 year of most of the randomized trials, or the use of balloon expandable stents, which should be avoided in the femoropopliteal tract.[35]

Different stent designs and materials could be important although little is known concerning this topic. No comparative studies have yet been conducted to assess the difference between stent types. Publications reporting on the experience with Palmaz™, Strecker™ or Wallstents™ dominate and only very few data about the use of nitinol stents in the femoropopliteal region have been available to date. The rigid stainless steel or tantalum stents may undergo external deformation, whereas nitinol is more elastic. A balloon expandable stent may give less stress to the vessel wall after initial placement than a self-expandable stent. However, Schurmann et al,[36] using an animal model, found no difference between rigid and flexible stents with regard to occurrence of neointimal hyperplasia.

In summary therefore, at present stenting seems to be superior to PTA alone only in critical ischemia and not equivocally if the lesion type is an occlusion. The most reliable predictive factor for long-term stent failure seems to be the length of the lesion. Whether stent type is also a predictor has to be clarified in randomized, prospective studies.

GERMAN MULTICENTER EXPERIENCE USING NITINOL STENTS IN THE SFA

In one multicenter study, promising improvements in clinical outcomes using nitinol stents in the treatment of long diffuse SFA lesions were observed.[45] In a sample of 329 SFA procedures stainless steel Wallstents™ were used in 166 interventions and nitinol stents in 163 procedures. The lesions were mostly complex: mean lesion length was 20 cm and 80% of these lesions were total occlusions. The reported 1-year primary patency rate was 61% in the nitinol stent group compared to 30% in the stainless steel Wallstent™ group (Fig. 9.10). One-year assisted primary patency increased to 75% in the nitinol group and 53% in the stainless steel group (Fig. 9.11). Secondary patency at 1 year was 79% in the nitinol group versus 64% in the stainless steel group (Fig. 9.12). Achieving long-term secondary patency of about 80% using nitinol stents in long lesions demonstrates that this technology is safe, clinically very effective, and comparable with reported surgical results. This, in our opinion, opens a new door for percutaneous inter-

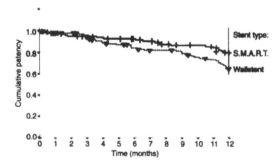

Fig. 9.12 Secondary patency at 1 year of nitinol stents compared to stainless steel Wallstents™.

vention in the femoropopliteal vascular bed to optimize clinical efficiency and durability of outcome.

TREATMENT OF IN-STENT RESTENOSIS

At present, the most common technique for treating significant intimal hyperplasia within a stent is balloon dilation, which has resulted in acceptable secondary patency rates (Fig. 9.13; see also Table 9.3). Alternatively, laser recanalization can be used for treatment of in-stent restenoses. Atherectomy has been used, but the results were discouraging, potentially also leading to strut damage.[46] A new device, the SilverHawk™ catheter (FoxHollow, Redwood City, CA), may yield better results.[47] Cutting balloons are appropriate for shorter in-stent restenoses, but data about the short- and long-term results are not yet available. In-stent stenting for treatment of dissections, residual stenoses or restenoses due to stent-fractures is possible, safe and effective; however data have yet to be published (Fig. 9.14).

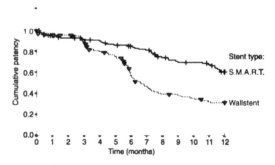

Fig. 9.10 One-year primary patency rate of nitinol stents compared to stainless steel Wallstents™.

NEW TECHNIQUES FOR ENDOLUMINAL THERAPY OF FEMOROPOPLITEAL LESIONS

Intimal hyperplasia remains the greatest limitation of long-term success after femoropopliteal stenting. Different strategies to lower this risk, including brachytherapy, stent-grafting, cryotherapy, and

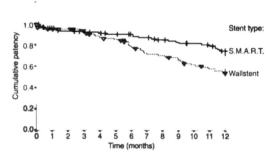

Fig. 9.11 One-year assisted primary patency rate of nitinol stents compared to stainless steel Wallstents™.

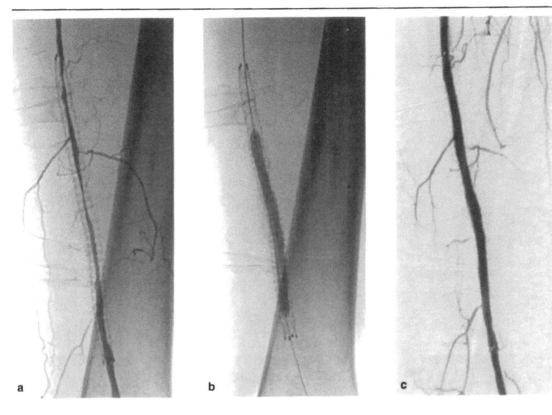

Fig. 9.13 In-stent restenosis.

(a) Typical diffuse in-stent restenosis 6 months after implantation of a 12 cm long nitinol stent in the distal superficial femoral artery. (b) After passing the subtotal occlusion, repeat inflations up to 12 bars were performed using a 5/80 mm low-profile balloon (Submarine™; Invatec, Brescia, Italy). (c) Final angiographic result without pressure gradient.

drug-eluting stents, are subjects of ongoing trials. First results with brachytherapy after angioplasty of femoropopliteal lesions with[48] or without stenting[49,50] showed a significant effect on intimal hyperplasia even in randomized study protocols. The need for a special radiation oncology-type room for the procedure because of the use of gamma radiation is a limitation, which makes other techniques for prevention of restenosis more attractive.

Endoluminal stent-grafts were introduced to prevent hypertrophic neointima formation in the SFA after angioplasty, but led to high early and late restenosis rates with a considerable rate of complications.[51]

Cryotherapy – the application of cold thermal energy during angioplasty – enhances the acute effects of conventional dilation while decreasing the likelihood of restenosis.[52] A dilation balloon is brought to the lesion and inflated by a connected NO-gas tube with a pressure of about 8 atm, delivering a balloon/artery interface temperature of approximately –10°C for a period of 30 seconds (Fig. 9.15). Data of a study using cryotherapy in the femoropopliteal region are expected in the near future.

Drug-eluting stents are the most attractive alternative to conventional stent implantation. Recent use of rapamycin and paclitaxel coating on

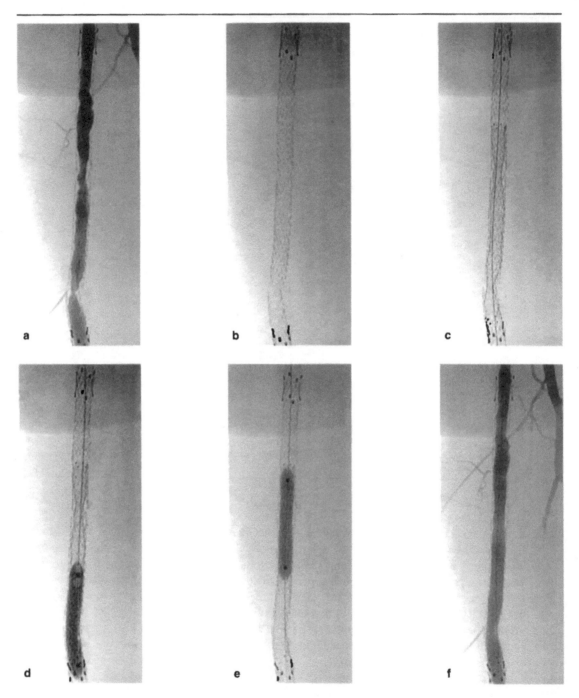

Fig. 9.14 Multiple in-stent restenoses.

(a) The angiogram shows multiple in-stent restenoses. (b) The native frame indicates that the stenoses are correlated to stent fractures. (c) After in-stent placement of a nitinol stent, (d–f) and focal post-dilation with a 6/20 mm balloon, a good angiographic result could be achieved.

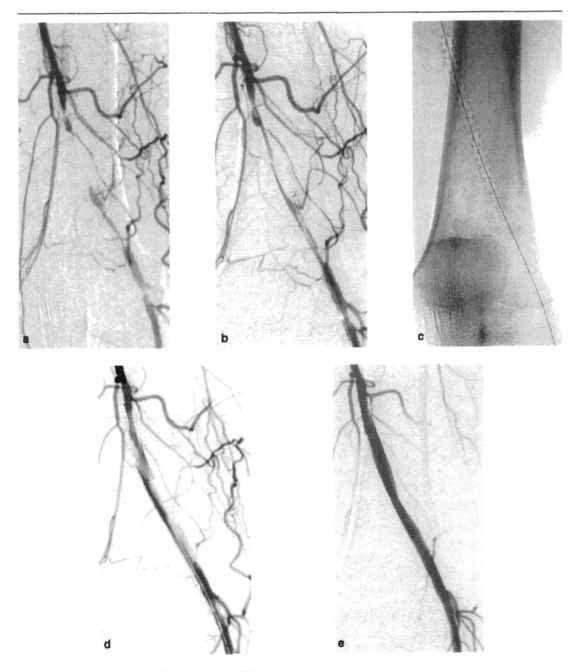

Fig. 9.15 Occlusion of the distal superficial femoral artery (SFA).

(a) Complex occlusion of the distal SFA involving the proximal popliteal artery. (b) After passing the obstruction with a 0.018 inch control wire (Boston Scientific) and repeat balloon dilations, the poor angiographic result is probably determined by subintimal wire positioning. (c) Attempt to stabilize the situation using a cryoballoon (6/60 mm). (d) After cryoplasty the result is still mediocre. (e) After delivery of a 7/100 mm SMART™ stent and post-dilation with a 5/80 mm balloon a good angiographic result was achieved.

coronary stents has shown a marked prevention of restenosis.[53] In a small pilot study (SIROCCO I trial) 36 patients with symptomatic SFA lesions with a mean lesion length of 8.5 cm were randomized to a non-coated or a sirolimus-coated S.M.A.R.T.™ nitinol stent (Fig. 9.16). At 6 months, angiographic follow-up revealed no restenosis in the sirolimus group. However, an unexpectedly low rate of restenosis of 23.5% in the control group using the uncoated nitinol stent led to a non-significant difference between the two groups in terms of restenosis (≥50%).[54] Therefore, an increased num-

ber of patients ($n = 57$) were enrolled in SIROCCO II. However, after 6-month follow-up the data of the SIROCCO I trial were confirmed, showing no restenosis for the drug-eluting stents and only a 7.7% restenosis rate for the bare S.M.A.R.T.™ stents. Regarding the primary end point – the mean stent diameter – pooled data of the two trials showed a significant difference in favor of the drug-eluting stents, even with the exceptional outcomes for the bare S.M.A.R.T.™ stent.[55] Further investigation will reveal whether these encouraging results are maintained during long-term follow-up.

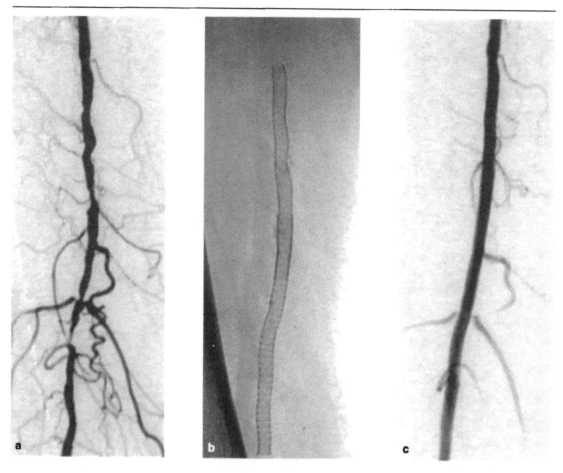

Fig. 9.16 Restenosis after percutaneous transluminal angioplasty (PTA).

(a) Diffuse restenosis 6 months after PTA of a calcified originally occluded SFA. (b) Native frame of the two implanted drug-eluting nitinol stents. Note the relatively large overlapping zone intentionally chosen in the area of a heavy calcification with tendency to recoil. (c) Final angiographic result.

CONCLUSION

Stenting of the superficial femoral artery remains a controversial topic. Guidelines for the management of peripheral arterial disease[3] recommend surgical therapy for lesions of the femoropopliteal tract longer than 5 cm and further state that stenting of the femoropopliteal artery is not indicated as a primary approach during interventional treatment of these lesions. However, endovascular therapy of even longer segments of the SFA and percutaneous stenting of the femoropopliteal artery in cases of suboptimal angioplasty has become a widely accepted therapeutic strategy. The incidence of early stent thrombosis became very low after the introduction of modern anticoagulation regimens. Patency rates after PTA and stenting are comparable to the patency rates of infrainguinal bypass surgery.[56] First experience with the use of nitinol stents is very promising. Intimal hyperplasia leading to restenosis and occlusion seems to be lower using these stents, but still remains a problem. Whether primary stenting should be liberalized for femoropopliteal arteries, as it is for iliac arteries, needs to be proven. Close surveillance by duplex sonography after stenting is mandatory. In cases of restenosis, the patients should be scheduled for early reintervention. In our opinion, endoluminal recanalization is indicated as first choice therapy in the majority of lesions of the femoropopliteal arteries before bypass operation.[57]

REFERENCES

1. Tetteroo E, van der Graaf Y, Bosch JL, et al. Randomised comparison of primary stent placement versus angioplasty followed by selective stent placement in patients with iliac-artery occlusive disease: Dutch Iliac Stent Trial Study Group. Lancet 1998;351:1153–9.

2. Scheinert D, Schroeder M, Balzer JO, Steinkamp H, Biamino G. Stent-supported reconstruction of the aortoiliac bifurcation with the kissing balloon technique. Circulation 1999;100(19 suppl): II295–300.

3. TASC Working Group TransAtlantic Inter-Society Consensus (TASC). Management of peripheral arterial disease (PAD). J Vasc Surg 2000;31(suppl):S1–S296.

4. Gray BH, Sullivan TM, Childs MB, Young JR, Olin JW. High incidence of restenosis/reocclusion of stent in the percutaneous treatment of long-segment superficial femoral artery disease after suboptimal angioplasty. J Vasc Surg 1997;25:74–83.

5. Hertzer NR. The natural history of peripheral vascular disease: implications for its management. Circulation 1991;83(suppl. 1):I-12–I-19.

6. Regensteiner JG, Meyer TJ, Krupski WC, Cranford LS, Hiatt WR. Hospital vs home-based exercise rehabilitation for patients with peripheral arterial occlusive disease. Angiology 1997;48:291–300.

7. Hiatt WR. Medical treatment of peripheral arterial disease and claudication. N Engl J Med 2001;344:1608–21.

8. Dalman RL, Taylor LM. Basic data related to infrainguinal revascularization procedures. Ann Vasc Surg 1990;4:309–12.

9. Laxdal E, Jenssen GL, Pedersen G, Aune S. Subintimal angioplasty as a treatment of femoropopliteal artery occlusions. Eur J Vasc Endovasc Surg 2003;25:578–82.

10. Johnston KW. Femoral and popliteal arteries: reanalysis of results of balloon angioplasty. Radiology 1992;183:767–71.

11. Scheinert D, Laird JR, Schröder M, et al. Excimer laser-assisted recanalization of long, chronic superficial femoral artery occlusions. J Endovasc Ther 2001;8:156–66.

12. Hunink MGM, Wong JB, Donaldson MC, Meyerovitz MF, Harrington DP. Patency results of percutaneous and surgical revascularization for femoropopliteal disease. Med Decis Making 1994;14:71–81.

13. Muradin GSR, Bosch JL, Stijnen T, Hunink MGM. Balloon dilation and stent implantation for treatment of femoropopliteal arterial disease: meta-analysis. Radiology 2001;221:137–45.

14. Cejna M, Thurnher S, Illiasch H, et al. PTA versus stent placement in femoropopliteal artery obstructions: a multicenter prospective randomized study. J Vasc Interv Radiol 2001;12:23–31.

15. Vroegindeweij D, Vos LD, Tielbeek AV, Buth J, vd Bosch HCM. Balloon angioplasty combined with primary stenting versus balloon angioplasty alone in femoropopliteal obstructions: a comparative randomised study. Cardiovasc Intervent Radiol 1997;20:420–5.

16. Zdanowski Z, Albrechtsson U, Lundin A, et al. Percutaneous transluminal angioplasty with or without stenting for femoropopliteal occlusions? A randomized controlled study. Int Angiol 1999;18:251–5.

17. Grimm J, Müller-Hülsbeck S, Jahnke T, et al. Randomized study to compare PTA alone versus PTA with Palmaz stent placement for femoropopliteal lesions. J Vasc Intervent Radiol 2001;12:935–41.

18. Lampmann LEH. Stenting in the femoral superficial artery: an overview. Eur J Radiol 1999;29:276–9.

19. Rousseau HP, Raillat CR, Joffre FG, Knight CJ, Ginestet MC. Treatment of femoropopliteal stenoses by means of self-expandable endoprostheses: midterm results. Radiology 1989;172:961–4.

20. White GH, Liew SC, Waugh RC, et al. Early outcome and intermediate follow-up of vascular stents in the femoral and popliteal arteries without long-term anticoagulation. J Vasc Surg 1995;21:270–81.

21. Strecker EP, Gottmann D, Boos IB, Vetter S. Low-molecular-weight heparin (reviparin) reduces the incidence of femoropopliteal in-stent stenosis: preliminary results of an ongoing study. Cardiovasc Intervent Radiol 1998;21:375–9.

22. Becquemin J-P. Effect of ticlopidine on the long-term patency of saphenous-vein bypass grafts in the legs. N Engl J Med 1997;337:1726–31.

23. Henry M, Amor M, Ethevenot G, et al. Palmaz stent placement in iliac and femoropopliteal arteries: primary and secondary patency in 310 patients with 2–4 year follow-up. Radiology 1995;197:167–74.

24. Davies AH, Willcox JH, Magee TR, et al. Colour duplex in assessing the infrainguinal arteries in patients with claudication. Cardiovasc Surg 1995;3:211–2.

25. Pemberton M, Nydahl S, Hartshorne T, et al. Colour-coded duplex imaging can safely replace diagnostic arteriography in patients with lower-limb arterial disease. Br J Surg 1996;83:1725–8.

26. Aly S, Jenkins MP, Zaidi FH, Coleridge Smith PD, Bishop CC. Duplex scanning and effect of multisegmental arterial disease on its accuracy in lower limb arteries. Eur J Vasc Endovasc Surg 1998;16:345–9.

27. Whelan JF, Barry MH, Moir JD. Color flow Doppler ultrasonography: comparison with peripheral arteriography for the investigation of peripheral vascular disease. J Clin Ultrasound 1992;20:369–74.

28. Cossman DV, Ellison JE, Wagner WH, et al. Comparison of contrast arteriography to arterial mapping with color-flow duplex imaging in the lower extremities. J Vasc Surg 1989;10:522–9.

29. Bray AE, Liu WG, Lewis WA, Harrison C, Maullin A. Strecker stents in the femoropopliteal arteries: value of duplex ultrasonography in restenosis assessment. J Endovasc Surg 1995;2:150–60.

30. Legemate DA, Teeuwen C, Hoeneveld H, Ackerstaff RGA, Eikelboom BC. Spectral analysis criteria in duplex scanning of aortoiliac and femoropopliteal arterial disease. Ultrasound Med Biol 1991;17:769–76.

31. Whyman MR, Ruckley CV, Fowkes FG. A prospective study of the natural history of femoropopliteal artery stenosis using duplex ultrasound. Eur J Vasc Surg 1993;7:444–7.

32. Lugmayr HF, Holzer H, Kastner M, Riedelsberger H, Auterith A. Treatment of complex arteriosclerotic lesions with Nitinol stents in the superficial femoral and popliteal arteries: a midterm follow-up. Radiology 2002;222:37–43.

33. Strecker EP, Boos IB, Gottmann D, Vetter S, Haase W. Popliteal artery stenting using flexible tantalum stents. Cardiovasc Intervent Radiol 2001;24:168–75.

34. Lammer J. Femoropopliteal artery obstruction: from the balloon to the stent graft. Cardiovasc Intervent Radiol 2001;24:73–83.

35. Becquemin J-P, Favre J-P, Marzelle J, et al. Systemic versus selective stent placement after superficial femoral artery balloon angioplasty: a multicenter prospective randomized study. J Vasc Surg 2003;37:487–94.

36. Schurmann K, Vorwerk D, Kulisch A, et al. Neointimal hyperplasia in low-profile nitinol-stents, Palmaz stent, and Wallstents: a comparative experimental study. Cardiovasc Intervent Radiol 1996;19:248–54.

37. Henry M, Amor M, Beyar R, et al. Clinical experience with a new nitinol self-expanding stent in peripheral arteries. J Endovasc Surg 1996;3:369–79.

38. Jahnke T, Voshage G, Müller-Hülsbeck S, et al. Endovascular placement of self-expanding nitinol coil stents for treatment of femoropopliteal obstructive disease. J Vasc Interv Radiol 2002;13:257–66.

39. Zollikofer CL, Antonucci F, Pfyffer M, et al. Arterial stent placement with use of the Wallstent: midterm results of clinical experience. Radiology 1991;179:449–56.

40. Do-Dai-Do, Triller J, Walpoth BH, Stirnemann P, Mahler F. A comparison study of self-expandable stents vs balloon angioplasty alone in femoropopliteal artery occlusions. Cardiovasc Intervent Radiol 1992;15:306–12.

41. Conroy RM, Gordon IL, Tobis JM, et al. Angioplasty and stent placement in chronic occlusion of the superficial femoral artery: technique and results. JVIR 2000;11:1009–20.

42. Gordon IL, Conroy RM, Arefi M, et al. Three-year outcome of endovascular treatment of superficial femoral artery occlusion. Arch Surg 2001;136:221–8.

43. Cheng SWK, Ting ACW, Pei H. Angioplasty and primary stenting of high-grade, long-segment superficial femoral artery disease: is it worthwhile? Ann Vasc Surg 2003;17:430–7.

44. Vogel TR, Shindelman LE, Nackman GB, Graham AM. Efficacious use of nitinol stents in the femoral and popliteal arteries. J Vasc Surg 2003;38:1178–84.

45. Hayerizadeh BF, Zeller T, Krankenberg H, Scheinert D, Baimino G. Superficial femoral artery stenting using nitinol stents – a German multicenter experience. The Paris Course on Revascularization 2002:451–4.

46. Tielbeek AV, Vroegindeweij D, Buth J, Landman GH. Comparison of balloon angioplasty and Simpson atherectomy for lesions in the femoropopliteal artery: angiographic and clinical results of a prospective randomized trial. J Vasc Interv Radiol 1996;7:837–44.

47. Zeller T, Krankenberg H, Reimers B, et al. Initial clinical experience with a new percutaneous peripheral atherectomy device for the treatment of femoropopliteal stenoses. Fortschr Röntgenstr 2004;176:70–5.

48. Krueger K, Landwehr P, Bendel M, et al. Endovascular gamma irradiation of femoropopliteal de novo stenoses immediately after PTA: interim results of a prospective randomized controlled trial. Radiology 2002;224:519–28.

49. Wolfram RM, Pokrajac B, Ahmadi R, et al. Endovascular brachytherapy for prophylaxis against restenosis after long-segment femoropopliteal placement of stents: initial results. Radiology 2001;220:724–9.

50. Minar E, Pokrajac B, Maca T, et al. Endovascular brachytherapy for prophylaxis of restenosis after femoropopliteal angioplasty. Results of a prospective randomized study. Circulation 2000;102:2694–9.

51. Ahmadi R, Schillinger M, Maca T, Minar E. Femoropopliteal arteries: immediate and long-term results with a Dacron-covered stent-graft. Radiology 2002;223:345–50.

52. Kataoka T, Honda Y, Bonneau HN, Yock PG, Fitzgerald PJ. New catheter-based technology for the treatment of restenosis. J Interv Cardiol 2002;15:371–9.

53. Morice MC, Serruys PW, Sousa JE, et al. A randomized comparison of a sirolimus-eluting stent with a standard stent for coronary revascularization. N Engl J Med 2002;346:1773–80.

54. Duda SH, Pusich B, Richter G, et al. Sirolimus-eluting stents for the treatment of obstructive superficial femoral artery disease: six-month results. Circulation 2002;106:1505–9.

55. Duda S. The SIROCCO study: updated results from a trial of sirolimus-eluting stents in the superficial femoral artery. Presented at TCT 2003: 15th Annual Transcatheter Cardiovascular Therapeutics. September 15–19, 2003, Washington, DC.

56. Green RM, Abbott WM, Matsumoto T, et al. Prosthetic above-knee femoropopliteal bypass grafting: five-year results of a randomized trial. J Vasc Surg 2000;31:417–25.

57. Ansel GM, Botti CF, Silver Barry S, George MJ, George BS. Why endovascular therapy should be utilized before surgical bypass for femoropopliteal occlusive disease. J Invasive Cardiol 2001;13:608–10.

10. Carotid Embolic Protection: Techniques and Results

Horst Sievert and Kasja Rabe

INTRODUCTION

Distal embolization of arteriosclerotic debris and thrombus is the most common and often the most severe complication of carotid angioplasty and stenting. It is, beside intracranial hemorrhage, the complication which has the most important impact on the outcome of the procedure. Distal emboliza-tion was the reason why the initial results of carotid angioplasty did not match the results of endarterec-tomy in many series.[1-8] From animal experiments as well as from clinical experience it is known that particles with a diameter of 200 microns may cause severe damage. Whether or not embolization results in a neurologic deficit depends upon the vascular territory to which the emboli travel. Large areas of the brain have no obvious function, and this may explain why embolism may occur without obvious clinical consequences.[9,10] Furthermore, small plaque fragments may be responsible for both stroke and more subtle neurologic dysfunction, not only during the intervention but also in late follow-up.[11,12]

For these reasons it is important to prevent embolism. Aspirin and clopidogrel are usually prescribed well in advance of angioplasty and stenting to avoid thrombus formation on the arteriosclerotic plaque. Theoretically, IIb/IIIa-receptor blocking agents may be helpful; however, it has been shown that they increase the risk of cerebral bleeding, the other major cause of severe compli-cations resulting from carotid angioplasty.[13] Another important issue is to reduce the mechani-cal manipulation inside the carotid arteries as much as possible. The introduction of low profile balloons and stent delivery systems has been a major achievement. Primary stenting (stent implantation before the first balloon inflation)

may also help to prevent distal embolization by fixation of the debris to the vessel wall.[14] However, clinically relevant embolization still occurred at a rate of between 1 and 4%.[14]

The first distal embolic protection device was developed in the 1990s by Théron et al.[15-17] This was a triple coaxial catheter with a small latex balloon at the tip of a microcatheter. With this latex balloon the internal carotid artery was occluded distal to the lesion. The dilation catheter could be advanced over the microcatheter. After the angioplasty the debris was aspirated via the guiding catheter.

In 1996 Kachel[18] developed the first proximal occlusion device which led to a retrograde flow in the internal carotid artery.

The following devices are currently available or are under evaluation in clinical trials.

FILTER DEVICES

ANGIOGUARD XP™/RX™ (CORDIS/JOHNSON & JOHNSON, WARREN, NJ)

The Angioguard filter was the first filter to become available. The Angioguard XP™ and RX™ (Fig. 10.1) are the newest versions of this filter. The device consists of the filter itself, which is mounted on a 0.014 inch wire, a delivery catheter, and a retrieval catheter. The filter comes in diameters of between 4 and 8 mm.

The filter membrane is made of polyurethane. The pores in the filter have a diameter of 100 μm. The filter has eight nitinol struts, four of which have a radiopaque marker. The delivery catheter has a diameter of 3.2–3.9F, the retrieval catheter a diameter of 5.1F.

109

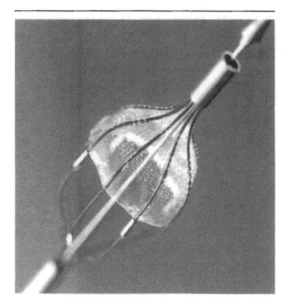

Fig. 10.1 Angioguard XP™/RX™ filter.

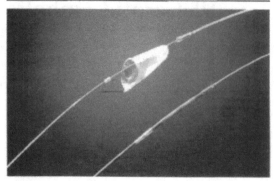

Fig. 10.2 E.P.I. FilterWire™ EZ.

We have used the Angioguard filter (old and new versions) in 49 carotid angioplasties. With the old generation device, occasionally the lesion could only be crossed after pre-dilation with a smaller balloon or could not be crossed at all. This never occurred with the new generation device which is much more flexible and has a lower profile. Arteriosclerotic debris could be captured in 84% of the cases. The Angioguard RX™ is the new rapid exchange version of this filter.

E.P.I. FILTERWIRE™ (BOSTON SCIENTIFIC, SANTA CLARA, CA)

The latest version of this filter (FilterWire™ EZ; Boston Scientific, Natick, MA; Fig. 10.2) is mounted on a 0.014 inch wire by means of a nitinol wire loop. As a result of this design, the entry of the particles into the filter is not impeded by filter struts. It has a freely rotating frame and filter to provide full vessel apposition. The membrane of the filter is made of polyurethane and has pores with a diameter of 110 μm. The delivery catheter has an outer diameter of 3.2F. The filter comes in

one size and adapts to vessel diameters between 3.5 and 5.5 mm. It can be withdrawn with a 4.1F retrieval catheter.

We have used this filter successfully in 62 procedures. With the older version of this filter it was occasionally necessary to reposition the filter to achieve full apposition to the vessel wall. This is not a problem with the new EZ version. No embolic cerebral events occurred. Deployment of this filter is very easy.

MEDNOVA EMBOSHIELD™ CEREBRAL PROTECTION SYSTEM (MEDNOVA/ABBOTT, GALWAY, IRELAND)

The third generation of this device is currently available. The fourth generation is already CE marked but has not yet been released. It consists of a 0.014 inch guidewire, a delivery catheter (3.7–3.9F), a filter basket (3–6 mm), and a retrieval catheter. Initially the lesion is crossed with the guidewire alone. Thereafter, the filter is loaded into the delivery catheter, which is advanced over the wire distal to the lesion. The device has a crossing profile of 0.038 or 0.0435 inches depending on the size used. After angioplasty and stenting the retrieval catheter is advanced over the wire and the filter. The retrieval catheter has an expansile distal section which expands upon filter retrieval and allows full recapture of the filter. In the first multicenter registry with 165 patients, a technical success rate of 94% and a procedural complication rate of 1% have been reported.[19]

SPIDER™ VASCULAR FILTRATION SYSTEM (EV3, PARIS, FRANCE)

This device consists of a nitinol basket at the tip of a 0.014 inch wire (Fig. 10.3). The diameter of the basket ranges between 4 and 7 mm. This filter is the only filter which allows usage of a wire of the operator's choice to cross the lesion. After crossing the lesion with the wire the delivery catheter of the system is introduced. The crossing profile of the delivery catheter is only 2.2F which is the lowest profile of all currently available filter devices. The wire is removed and the filter is advanced through the delivery catheter and placed distal to the stenosis. After balloon angioplasty and stenting the retrieval catheter (diameter 5F or 6F) is introduced over the wire. At the tip of the retrieval catheter a funnel made of nitinol wire mesh is opened and the filter is retracted into this funnel. Thereafter the filter, together with the funnel, is withdrawn into the retrieval catheter.

The new version of this filter is the Microvena TRAP XLP™ vascular filtration system. This is a completely new design with a windsock-type filter basket. The design of this filter has some similarities with the E.P.I. filter. However, it comes in different sizes between 3 and 7 mm. At the entrance of this filter there is a clasp to ensure a better vessel wall apposition of the opening of the filter. The profile of the delivery catheter is 2.9F; the profile of the retrieval catheter is 4.2F or 4.9F.

So far 46 patients have been treated in our center with a technical success rate of 100%. A multicenter trial with 50 patients has recently been completed.[20,21]

INTERCEPTOR™ FILTER WIRE (MEDTRONIC, MINNEAPOLIS, MN)

This device consists of a nitinol filter basket attached to a 0.014 inch guidewire. The basket diameter ranges between 4.5 and 6.5 mm. There are four entry ports in the proximal end of the filter. The pore size is 100 µm. The delivery catheter has a profile of 2.5F and the retrieval catheter of 4.5F.

ACCUNET™ EMBOLIC PROTECTION DEVICE (GUIDANT, INDIANAPOLIS, IN)

This is a polyurethane filter mounted on a nitinol basket with a diameter ranging from 4.5 to 7.5 mm (Fig. 10.4). The pore size is 115 µm. The results of the ARCHER trial were published recently.[22] The all-cause stroke, death and myocardial infarction rate after 30 days was 7.8%.

OCCLUSION DEVICES

PERCUSURGE GUARDWIRE™ (MEDTRONIC, MINNEAPOLIS, MN)

This was the first occlusion device available commercially. An elastomeric balloon is fixed at the tip of a 0.014 or 0.018 inch wire (Fig. 10.5). The

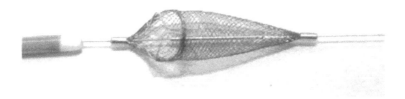

Fig. 10.3 Spider™ vascular filtration system.

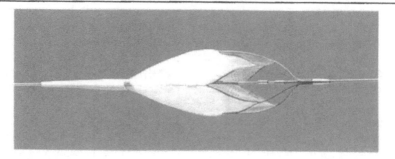

Fig. 10.4 AccuNet™ embolic protection device.

balloon can be filled through a lumen inside of the wire up to a diameter of between 3 and 6 mm. This is done via a so-called MicroSeal™ adapter. With this adapter a MicroSeal™ in the wire can be opened and closed. When the MicroSeal™ is closed, the adapter can be removed from the wire without balloon deflation. After crossing the lesion with the GuardWire™, the distal balloon is inflated distal to the stenosis to occlude the internal carotid artery. The MicroSeal™ adapter is removed and the angioplasty balloon and the stent are introduced over the wire. After stent implantation an aspiration catheter is advanced over the wire into the internal carotid artery. The debris, which may have been dislodged from the atheroma, is aspirated and

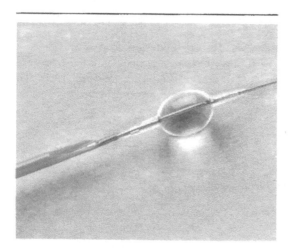

Fig. 10.5 PercuSurge GuardWire™.

removed. Thereafter, the distal occlusion balloon is deflated.

The advantage of this technique compared to filter techniques is that even very small particles can be captured. Furthermore, the crossing profile of the device is very low. However, some patients do not tolerate balloon occlusion of the internal carotid artery and it is possible in these patients to do the procedure stepwise with intermittent deflation of the balloon. Obviously this makes the procedure a little cumbersome because an aspiration is necessary before each balloon deflation. Another disadvantage is that angiography during the procedure is not possible.

In our experience the technical success of this device was 91%, and embolic complications occurred in 2%. Arteriosclerotic debris could be aspirated in 84% of the procedures. In the multi-center registry (CAFE) including 65 patients no embolic complications occurred.

PARODI AES (ARTERIA MEDICAL SCIENCE, SAN FRANCISCO, CA)

This device prevents distal embolization by establishing a retrograde flow in the internal carotid artery (Fig. 10.6). It consists of a 10F guiding catheter with a balloon at its distal tip. This balloon is inflated in the common carotid artery. To avoid blood flow from the external to the internal carotid artery, the external carotid artery is occluded with a separate balloon mounted on a wire which is introduced through the lumen of the guiding

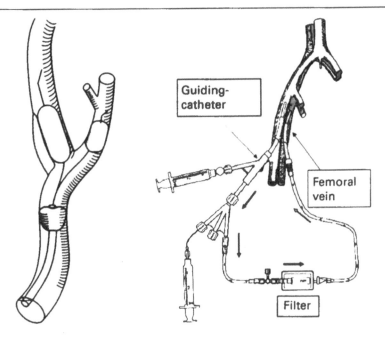

Fig. 10.6 Parodi anti-emboli system (AES).

Balloon occlusion of the common carotid and the external carotid artery allows retrograde flow in the internal carotid artery through the guiding catheter and an external filter into a venous sheath.

catheter. The proximal hub of the guiding catheter is connected with a venous sheath. Due to the pressure difference between the distal internal carotid artery and the venous system a retrograde blood flow is established. A filter located in the arteriovenous shunt prevents embolization of the debris into the venous system.

The major advantage of this technique is that because of the flow reversal during the procedure, emboli cannot move towards the brain.[23] This protection starts before crossing the lesion. This system allows usage of a wire of the operator's choice. It is important to note that only stent delivery devices of less than 7F may be used. Disadvantages of this technique are the need for a 10F sheath and intolerance of balloon occlusion in some patients. In contrast to the distal balloon occlusion technique (PercuSurge), angiography during the procedure is possible. To perform the procedure in a stepwise fashion is easier and faster than with the

PercuSurge technique because it is not necessary to introduce an aspiration catheter before deflating the balloon. We have used this technique in more than 50 patients without embolic complications. Recently, the results of the world registry were presented: in 302 lesions the procedural stroke and death rate was only 1%.[24]

MO.MA (INVATEC, RONCADELLE, ITALY)

The MO.MA is a 'proximal flow blockage' cerebral protection device. Cerebral protection occurs by interruption of antegrade blood flow from the common carotid artery and retrograde blood flow through the ipsilateral external carotid artery. This is achieved by balloon occlusion of the two vessels by means of a single (one-piece) device integrating the two occlusive balloons and a working channel for the delivery of interventional devices (dilation

113

balloons, stents, etc.) to the target lesion. Debris is thus stopped at the carotid bifurcation and prevented from traveling to the brain. Removal of debris is performed by spot (active) syringe aspiration which can be performed at any time during the intervention. Similar to the ArteriA device, the MO.MA has the advantage of establishing protection before crossing of the lesion. Furthermore, as it comes as a single unit with two fixation points, it has a high stability. In cases of intolerance the procedure may be performed step by step with intermittent balloon deflation without losing device fixation. The operator may use any kind of wire and angiography is possible at any time during the procedure. Obviously the external carotid artery has to be open and not severely stenosed, and the fixed distance between the balloon at the guiding catheter and the external occlusion balloon has to be suitable for the anatomy of the individual patient. It is mandatory to occlude not only the external carotid artery itself but also all proximal side branches of this vessel to prevent any distal flow. The MO.MA is particularly indicated for fresh thrombus, highly friable subocclusive lesions or when internal carotid artery anatomy reasonably prevents passage of an alternative, built-in wire type protection device.

Embolic protection devices, especially the first generation of these devices, may also cause problems. All devices placed distally in the internal carotid artery may cause spasm or dissection. It may be difficult to retrieve these devices through the implanted stent. It may be that the filter is not fully apposed to the vessel wall. In contrast, the major disadvantage of occlusion devices is intolerance in patients with occlusion or high-grade stenosis of the contralateral internal carotid artery or patients with poorly developed intracranial collaterals. A specific disadvantage of the MO.MA and the ArteriA devices is the need for a large sheath which may cause vascular access problems.

An open question is: do even very small particles (less than 80 μm diameter) cause significant damage? If so, occlusion techniques may be more effective than filter techniques.

CLINICAL TRIALS

Several observational studies have shown a lower complication rate after the introduction of embolic protection devices.[25-30] For several reasons no randomized trials examining angioplasty and stenting without embolic protection devices versus with embolic protection devices have been done. One of these reasons is that because the complication rate of angioplasty without embolic protection devices is already very low (less than 5%) a very large number of procedures would be necessary to statistically prove the benefit of these devices. On the other hand, it is impressive how often and how much debris can be captured (Figs 10.7, 10.8).[31,32] Whether or not this debris causes stroke depends on which vascular territory in the brain it goes to. Therefore, for most investigators it seems unethical to conduct a randomized trial. Also for these reasons the majority of the ongoing trials designed to compare stenting and surgery include the use of an embolic protection device. The preliminary results of the first of these trials, the SAPPHIRE study, were recently presented.[33] In this trial 307 high-risk patients were randomized to endarterectomy or angioplasty and stenting under protection with the Angioguard filter. The 30-day major complication rate (death, stroke, myocardial infarction) was

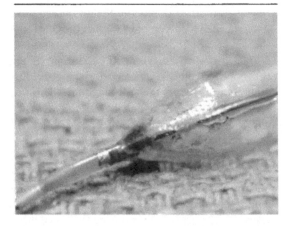

Fig. 10.7 Arteriosclerotic debris captured during a procedure with the MedNova EmboShield™ cerebral protection system.

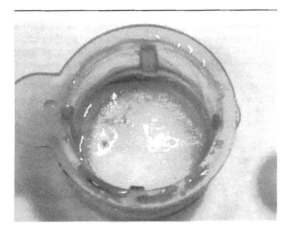

Fig. 10.8 Arteriosclerotic debris captured during a procedure with the Parodi AES.

12.6% in the surgical group compared to only 5.8% in the angioplasty group ($p <0.05$).

CONCLUSION

Cerebral protection devices most likely decrease the rate of embolic complications during carotid stenting and therefore should be used whenever possible. Depending upon the anatomy of the individual patient, filter devices or distal or proximal occlusion devices may be preferable.

REFERENCES

1. Bockenheimer SAM, Mathias K. Percutaneous transluminal angioplasty in arteriosclerotic internal carotid artery stenosis. Am J Neuroradiol 1983;4:791–2.
2. Wiggli U, Gratzl O. Transluminal angioplasty of stenotic carotid arteries: case reports and protocol. Am J Neuroradiol 1983;4:793–5.
3. Tsai FY, Matovich V, Hieschima G, et al. Percutaneous transluminal angioplasty of the carotid artery. Am J Neuroradiol 1986;7:349–58.
4. Kachel R, Basche S, Heerklotz I, Frossmann K, Endler S. Percutaneous transluminal angioplasty of supra-aortic arteries, especially the internal carotid artery. Neuroradiology 1991;33:191–4.
5. Sievert H, Rubel C, Ensslen R, et al. Initial experience with stent implantation of the internal carotid artery [Erste Erfahrungen mit der Stentimplantation in der Arteria carotis interna]. Herz/Kreislauf 1996;28:359–61.
6. Yadav JS, Roubin GS, Iyer S, et al. Elective stenting of the extracranial carotid arteries. Circulation 1997;95:376–81.
7. Dietrich EB, Ndiaye M, Reid DB. Stenting in the carotid artery: initial experience in 110 patients. J Endovasc Surg 1996;3:42–62.
8. Wholey MH, Wholey M, Jarmolowski CR, et al. Endovascular stents for carotid occlusive disease. J Endovasc Surg 1997;4:326–38.
9. Ohki T, Marin ML, Lyon RT, et al. Ex vivo human carotid artery bifurcation stenting: correlation of lesion characteristics with embolic potentials. J Vasc Surg 1998;27:463–71.
10. Jordan WD Jr, Voellinger DC, Doblar DB, et al. Microemboli detected by transcranial Doppler monitoring in patients during carotid angioplasty versus carotid endarterectomy. Cardiovasc Surg 1999;7:33–8.
11. Rapp JH, Pan XM, Sharp FR, et al. Atheroemboli to the brain: size threshold for causing acute neuronal cell death. J Vasc Surg 2000;32:68–76.
12. Ackerstaff RG, Moons KG, van de Vlasakker CJ, et al. Association of intraoperative transcranial Doppler monitoring variables with stroke from carotid endarterectomy. Stroke 2000;31:1817–23.
13. Qureshi AI, Fareed M, Suri K, et al. A prospective evaluation of intravenous abciximab as an adjunct to high-risk carotid angioplasty and stent placement. Am J Cardiol 2000;86(suppl 8A):28i.
14. Sievert H, Pfeil W, Bösenberg I, et al. Primary stent implantation in the internal carotid artery [Primäre Stent-Implantation in der Arteria carotis interna]. Dtsch Med Wochenschr 1999;124:1262–6.
15. Théron J, Courtheoux P, Alachkar F, Bouvard G, Maiza D. New triple coaxial catheter system for carotid angioplasty with cerebral protection. AJNR Am J Neuroradiol 1990;11:869–74.
16. Théron JG, Payelle GG, Coskun O, Huet HF, Guimaraens L. Carotid artery stenosis: treatment with protected balloon angioplasty and stent placement. Radiology 1996;201:627–36.
17. Théron J, Kachel R. Cerebral protection during carotid angioplasty. J Endovasc Surg 1996;3:484–6.
18. Kachel R. Results of balloon angioplasty in the carotid arteries. J Endovasc Surg 1996;3:22–30.
19. Al-Mubarak N, Colombo A, Gaines PA, et al. Multicenter evaluation of carotid artery stenting with a filter protection system. J Am Coll Cardiol 2002;39:841–6.
20. Cremonesi A, Castriota F, Sievert H, et al. Embolic protection during carotid artery stent implantation: European experience with the ev3 Embolic Protection Device. Am J Cardiol 2002;90(suppl 6A):57H.
21. Rabe K, Sievert H, Cremonesi A, et al. Emboli protection during carotid angioplasty with the SPIDER emboli protection system: results of the European multicenter trial [Embolie-Protection bei der Carotis-Angioplastie mit dem SPIDER-Embolie- Protektions-System: Ergebnisse der Europäischen Multicenter-Studie]. Kardiol 92; Suppl. 1:408
22. Wholey M. ARCHER Trial. Transcatheter Cardiovascular Therapeutics, 15th Annual Symposium, Washington, USA. September 15–19, 2003.
23. Parodi JC, Bates MC, Schonholz C, et al. International Multi-center Parodi Anti-Embolic System Study: preliminary results. Am J Cardiol 2000;86(suppl 1 8A):33i.
24. Sievert H, Bates MC, Rabe K. Carotid stenting with flow reversal with the ArteriA System. 14th Annual Symposium, Transcatheter Cardiovascular Therapeutics, Washington, Sept 24–28, 2002.
25. Wholey MH, Wholey M, Mathias K, et al. Global experience in cervical carotid artery stent placement. Catheter Cardiovasc Interv 2000;50:160–7.
26. Roubin GS, New G, Iyer SS, et al. Immediate and late clinical outcomes of carotid artery stenting in patients with symptomatic and asymptomatic carotid artery stenosis. A 5-year prospective analysis. Circulation 2001;103:532–7.
27. Al-Mubarak N, Roubin GS, Vitek JJ, et al. The effect of the distal-balloon protection system on microembolization during carotid stenting. Circulation 2001;104:1999–2002.

28. Henry M, Amor M, Klonaris C, Henry I, Hugel M. Endovascular management of carotid artery stenosis. The impact of cerebral protection. In: Veith FH, Amor M, eds. Endovascular Therapies: Current Status of Carotid Bifurcation Angioplasty and Stenting. New York: Marcel Dekker, 2001: 95–117.

29. Al-Mubarak N, Colombo A, Gaines P, et al. Multicenter evaluation of carotid artery stenting with filter protection system. J Am Coll Cardiol 2002;39:841–6.

30. Reimers B, Corvaja N, Moshiri S, et al. Cerebral protection with filter devices during carotid artery stenting: Circulation 2001;104:12–15.

31. Ohki T, Roubin GS, Veith FJ, Iyer SS, Brady E. Efficacy of a filter device in the prevention of embolic events during carotid angioplasty and stenting: an ex vivo analysis. J Vasc Surg 1999;30:1034–44.

32. Tübler T, Schlüter M, Dirsch O, et al. Balloon-protected carotid artery stenting: relationship of periprocedural neurological complications with the size of particulate debris. Circulation 2001;104:2791–6.

33. Yadav JS. Stenting and angioplasty with protection in patients at high risk for endarterectomy (The SAPPHIRE Study). AHA Scientific Sessions, Chicago, November 19, 2002.

11. Renal Artery Stent Placement

Christopher J White and Stephen R Ramee

INTRODUCTION

Atherosclerotic renal artery stenosis is the most common cause of secondary hypertension, being present in some degree in <5% of the general population of hypertensive patients.[1] There are, however, several clinical subsets of patients in which atherosclerotic renal artery stenosis is much more common, such as those with hypertension and renal insufficiency,[2] and in patients with associated coronary or peripheral vascular disease (Table 11.1).[3-6]

In patients undergoing angiography for suspected coronary artery or peripheral vascular disease, the incidence of renal artery stenosis ranges from 11 to 18%.[3-5] The frequency of asymptomatic, unsuspected renal artery stenosis is increased in patients with multivessel coronary disease.[3] In patients with known aneurysmal or occlusive peripheral vascular disease, one study demonstrated associated renal artery stenosis in 28%.[7] In patients with renal insufficiency the incidence of unsuspected renal artery stenosis has been reported to be 24%.[8]

There is general agreement among investigators that the natural history of renal artery stenosis is for the lesions to progress over time. The incidence of renal artery lesion progression in angiographic serial studies ranges from 39 to 49%.[9 12] Many of these lesions progress to total occlusion, with the majority of these patients suffering loss of renal function manifested by increasing serum creatinine and decreasing renal size.[11]

In a prospective study of patients with renal artery stenosis treated medically, progression occurred in 42% (11% progressed to occlusion) of the patients over a 2-year period.[13] Of particular importance is the recognition that progression of renal artery stenosis and loss of renal function is *independent* of the ability to control blood pressure medically.[14] Renal artery stent placement can significantly slow the progression of renal failure.[15] By calculating the mean slope of the reciprocal of serum creatinine values before and after stent placement, investigators were able to demonstrate a four-fold slowing in the progression of renal insufficiency after renal artery stent placement.

A consensus is now developing that patients with symptomatic renal artery stenosis are appropriate candidates for percutaneous revascularization. Patients on hemodialysis whose parenchyma is supplied by stenotic renal arteries, and those with renal artery stenosis and refractory congestive heart failure or unstable angina, should also be considered candidates for revascularization.[16-22]

Table 11.1 Hypertensive Patients at Increased Risk of Renal Artery Stenosis

- Abdominal bruit (systolic and diastolic)
- Onset of hypertension >55 years
- Malignant hypertension
- Azotemia with angiotensin-converting enzyme inhibitors
- Atrophic kidney
- Refractory hypertension
- Multivessel coronary atherosclerotic disease
- Unexplained renal insufficiency in a patient with known atherosclerotic disease

---

TECHNIQUE OF RENAL ARTERY STENT PLACEMENT

BRACHIAL APPROACH

The initial decision facing the interventionist is to select the appropriate vascular access site. For renal arteries that are oriented cephalad, it is often easier to approach them from the brachial artery. A 6F or 7F long sheath or coronary angioplasty guiding catheter may be advanced to the descending aorta. After 2000–5000 international units of heparin are administered, the target renal artery is selectively engaged with a diagnostic catheter. Baseline angiography is performed and quantitative angiographic diameter measurements of the reference segment are taken. The lesion is crossed with a steerable, exchange length 0.014 or 0.018-inch angioplasty guidewire. It is desirable that a steerable, soft wire is used to cross the lesion to minimize the risk of dissection and distal perforation of the renal artery. We recommend not using a Terumo Glidewire™ (Boston Scientific, Natick, MA) because of the danger of inadvertent perforation or dissection.

An angioplasty balloon sized to match the measured diameter of the reference segment is used to pre-dilate the lesion and ensure that the lesion is expandable. As the balloon is deflated, the sheath or guiding catheter is advanced atraumatically across the lesion over the balloon. This will allow the stent to be easily positioned at the lesion site without risking its edges catching on the plaque, thereby reducing the risk of stent embolization.

A balloon expandable (biliary) stent, long enough to fully cover the target lesion, is advanced to the lesion. For ostial lesions we attempt to have approximately 0.5–1 mm of the stent protrude into the aorta to ensure that the ostium of the renal artery lesion is covered. We inflate the balloon gradually to ensure that the ends of the balloon (which are uncovered by stent) create a 'dumb-bell' effect. This prevents the stent from being pushed off the balloon during asymmetric balloon inflation. The stent is fully deployed with inflation of the balloon to 6–8 atm. The balloon is deflated and withdrawn into the sheath. Contrast angiography is performed to judge the adequacy of deployment. If the lesion has not been adequately dilated, the balloon may be reinserted and inflated to a higher pressure, or a larger balloon may be used. We attempt to produce a final stent diameter slightly larger than the reference segment of the renal artery which angiographically appears as a 'step-up' and 'step-down' effect.

FEMORAL APPROACH

When the renal artery origin is oriented horizontally or caudally with respect to the aorta, a femoral approach is preferred. Retrograde femoral artery access is obtained and a 6–8F sheath is inserted. After 2000–5000 international units of heparin are administered, a 4–6F diagnostic catheter (internal mammary, cobra, or Judkins right configuration) is advanced to engage the ostium of the renal artery. We use diagnostic catheters to locate the renal artery ostium to avoid trauma and potential cholesterol embolization from scraping the aorta that may occur with larger angioplasty guiding catheters. Baseline angiography is performed and on-line quantitative angiographic measurement of the reference vessel diameter is performed. The lesion is then crossed with a 0.014 or 0.018 inch steerable guidewire. We recommend against routinely using a Glidewire™ because of the danger of inadvertent perforation or dissection with this relatively stiff wire. The diagnostic catheter is then exchanged over the guidewire for a renal angioplasty guiding catheter or sheath.

An angioplasty balloon, sized to match the measured diameter of the reference segment, is advanced through the guiding catheter to pre-dilate the lesion and ensure that the lesion is expandable. As the balloon is deflated, the guiding catheter is advanced across the lesion over the balloon. This will allow the stent to be advanced to the lesion site without risking its edges catching on the plaque, thereby lowering the risk of stent embolization.

A balloon expandable (biliary) stent, long enough to fully cover the target lesion, is then advanced within the guiding catheter or long sheath to the lesion site. For ostial lesions we attempt to leave approximately 1–2 mm of the stent protruding into the aorta to ensure that the aorto-ostial segment of the renal artery is covered. We inflate the balloon gradually to create a 'dumb-bell' effect. This ensures that the stent will not be pushed off the balloon during asymmetric balloon inflation. The stent is fully deployed with inflation of the balloon to 6–8 atm. The balloon is deflated and withdrawn. With the balloon withdrawn completely into the stent, the ostium of the stent may be flared with a high-pressure (10–12 atm) inflation. Contrast angiography is performed to judge the deployment. If the lesion has not been adequately dilated, the balloon may be reinserted and inflated to higher pressure, or a larger balloon may be used. We attempt to produce a final stent diameter slightly larger than the reference segment of the renal artery which angiographically appears as a 'step-up' and 'step-down' effect.

MEDICATION

Patients are pretreated with 325 mg of aspirin per day, commencing at least one day prior to the procedure; this regimen is continued indefinitely. The use of other platelet inhibitors has not been tested in this vascular distribution. The use of adenosine diphosphate (ADP) inhibitors such as clopidogrel is at the discretion of the operator. Antihypertensive medications are withheld immediately following the procedure and the patients observed for several hours before resuming or adjusting their medications.

INTRAVASCULAR ULTRASOUND

Intravascular ultrasound (IVUS) is an adjunctive tool which can facilitate accurate stent placement and help to optimize the stent result. The quantitative cross-sectional images provide precise information regarding the diameter of the target vessel. IVUS imaging is also capable of determining if the stent struts are appropriately deployed and properly apposed to the vessel wall. Finally, IVUS may visualize distal dissections not seen by angiography which could possibly jeopardize patency of the stent.

PRESSURE WIRE MEASUREMENT

In situations where the angiographic stenosis is not clearly visualized or there is need for confirmatory evidence of the severity of the stenosis, we measure pressure gradients across the stenosis. This can be done with small catheters (3F) or with a pressure wire. A systolic gradient of ≥ 20 mmHg or a mean gradient of ≥ 10 mmHg is considered significant.

CLINICAL OUTCOMES OF RENAL ARTERY INTERVENTION

Balloon angioplasty is an accepted treatment for renal artery stenosis (RAS) causing renovascular hypertension, renal insufficiency, and cardiac disturbance syndromes,[23–28] and is the treatment of choice for RAS caused by fibromuscular dysplasia.[24,29–32] However, balloon angioplasty alone is associated with a lower success rate for atherosclerotic lesions,[25,33–39] and a restenosis rate of approximately 50% over 6 months.[40] Aorto-ostial renal artery lesions are particularly difficult to treat effectively with balloon dilation alone. They are especially prone to restenosis due to vascular recoil caused by confluent plaque from the wall of the aorta extending into the ostium of the renal artery, and are considered by many as unsuitable lesions for balloon angioplasty alone.[41–43]

The use of balloon expandable stents, which have the capacity to scaffold the renal artery and prevent elastic recoil after balloon expansion, offers a major advantage for treatment of aorto-ostial renal artery lesions. Other lesions, such as recurrent lesions following previous angioplasty, and lesions with a significant residual stenosis ($\geq 30\%$ diameter stenosis) after balloon angioplasty are also suitable for stent placement.

Quantitative angiographic measurements have shown that vascular recoil may account for the loss of up to 50% of the cross-sectional area initially gained after coronary balloon angioplasty.[44,45] Following balloon angioplasty, there is fibrointimal proliferation in response to the controlled injury resulting from balloon inflation, which results in tissue ingrowth at the site of the angioplasty. Elastic recoil and intimal proliferation are responsible for the late loss in luminal area resulting in restenosis following balloon angioplasty. Clinical results with renal artery stent placement have documented superior hemodynamic and angiographic results when compared to balloon angioplasty alone.[46–49] Endovascular stenting enables a greater acute gain in lumen diameter than balloon angioplasty, largely defeating vascular recoil, thereby diminishing the impact of intimal hyperplasia on long-term patency.[50,51]

PATIENT SELECTION AND INDICATIONS

A presumptive diagnosis of renovascular hypertension may be made in a patient with hypertension and an angiographically demonstrated diameter narrowing of ≥50%. Jean and co-workers[4] published their experience in 196 patients undergoing cardiac catheterization for suspicion of coronary artery disease. Some degree of renal artery stenosis was demonstrated in one-third of the patients and was significant (>50% diameter stenosis) in 18%. Of those patients found to have coronary atherosclerosis (*n* = 152), 22% had significant renal artery stenosis. Univariate analysis revealed that the presence of coronary disease and renal insufficiency correlated with the presence of significant renal artery stenosis, but that the presence of hypertension did not. In our cardiology practice, screening renal angiography is routinely performed in patients at increased risk of having renal artery stenosis at the time of cardiac catheterization for atherosclerotic heart disease.

Patients with renal failure and associated renal artery stenosis may benefit from percutaneous revascularization. Two reports have demonstrated that renal artery stent placement improved or slowed the progression of renal insufficiency in a group of patients with impaired renal function and atherosclerotic renal artery stenosis.[15,52] The patients had their renal function analyzed by plotting the slopes of the reciprocal serum creatinine values before and after successful stent placement. Progression of renal failure was significantly slowed after stent placement.

Finally, treatment of isolated renal artery stenotic lesions which do not cause uncontrolled hypertension or renal insufficiency has been debated as a means to preserve renal function. The natural history of atherosclerotic renal artery stenosis is to progress with time.[9–13] Timely intervention and correction of these lesions may prevent progressive narrowing of the vessel and loss of renal function.

RENOVASCULAR HYPERTENSION

Renal artery stent placement is an effective therapy for renovascular hypertension. Dorros et al[47] demonstrated that renal artery stent placement was more effective than balloon angioplasty alone in improving or abolishing pressure gradients across renal artery lesions treated. In 76 patients (92 renal arteries) undergoing primary renal artery stent placement the technical success rate was 100% and the angiographic restenosis rate at 6 months was 25%.[48] Clinical follow-up demonstrated that 78% of the patients had stable or improved renal function, with a significant decrease in blood pressure and number of antihypertensive medications for the entire group.

RENOVASCULAR HYPERTENSION AND LESIONS DIFFICULT TO TREAT WITH BALLOON ANGIOPLASTY ALONE

We have recently reported our experience in 100 consecutive patients with renovascular hypertension and lesions difficult to treat with balloon angioplasty alone.[53] Our patient population consisted of 58% females with an overall mean age of 67 ± 10 years. All of the patients had poorly controlled hypertension (systolic ≥150 mmHg and/or diastolic >90 mmHg) while taking at least two antihypertensive drugs. The average number of antihypertensive medications they were taking before renal stent placement was 2.6 ± 1.0. Renal artery stenosis (>50% diameter stenosis) was bilateral in 33% (both arteries stented) and unilateral in 67%, with five patients having a solitary renal artery treated with a stent.

We placed a total of 149 stents in 133 arteries of 100 consecutive patients. Angiographic success (≤30% residual diameter stenosis) was obtained in 99% (132/139) of arteries attempted (Fig. 11.1). Clinical success, defined as normalization of blood pressure on the same or fewer medications, was achieved in 76% of the patients at the 6-month clinic visit.

COMPLICATIONS

One major complication – stent thrombosis 3 days following placement – occurred in this series. The patient was immediately taken to the catheterization laboratory and the occlusion reopened with balloon dilation. The renal artery remained patent at the 6-month follow-up angiogram. Several

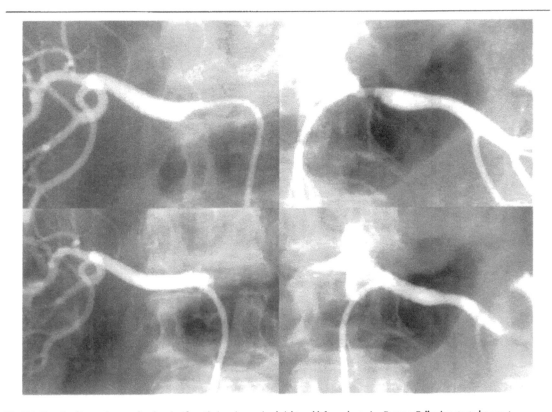

Fig. 11.1 Top: Baseline angiogram showing significant lesions in proximal right and left renal arteries. Bottom: Following stent placement.

minor complications occurred. There were no renal artery perforations or need for emergency surgery in any patient. Two patients experienced transient contrast nephropathy which resolved without the need for dialysis. There were seven access site complications including groin hematomas in five patients, one femoral pseudoaneurysm which resolved with ultrasound-guided compression, and one brachial artery occlusion which occurred following sheath removal and was resolved with a percutaneous balloon dilation from a femoral access site. One patient suffered a sudden cardiac death several days following stent implantation which was unrelated to the stent procedure.

FOLLOW-UP RESULTS

At 6-month follow-up, there continued to be a statistically significant improvement in blood pressure control (Fig. 11.2), the average number of anti-hypertensive medications per patient was reduced from 2.6 ± 1.0 to 2.0 ± 0.9 ($p < 0.001$), and the angiographic restenosis rate (>50% diameter stenosis) was 18.8% (15/80) in the 67 patients undergoing follow-up angiography. Quantitative angiographic analysis of the restenosis lesions demonstrated that the only procedural variable associated with angiographic restenosis was the immediate post-stent minimal lumen diameter (MLD). We found that the post-stent MLD following stent placement was significantly higher in the patients with continued patency (4.9 ± 0.9 mm) versus those with angiographic restenosis (4.3 ± 0.7 mm, $p = 0.025$). We identified a non-significant trend for higher systolic blood pressure in those patients with angiographic restenosis but there was no difference in diastolic blood pressures.

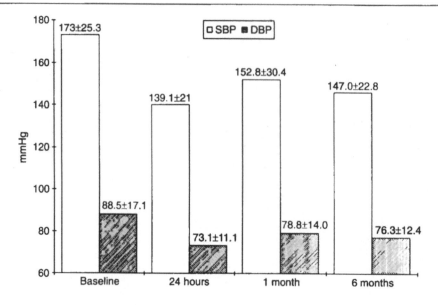

Fig. 11.2 Blood pressure results at baseline, post-stent, and at 6 months.

DBP, diastolic blood pressure; SBP, systolic blood pressure.

UNSTABLE ANGINA AND CONGESTIVE HEART FAILURE

We have analyzed the results of renal artery stent placement in another group of 48 patients with unstable angina ($n = 23$) or congestive heart failure ($n = 25$) who had hypertension refractory to medical therapy and $\geq70\%$ stenosis of one ($n = 30$) or both ($n = 18$) renal arteries.[21] Results of renal artery stenting for each subgroup are shown in Table 11.2. For the entire cohort of patients hypertension control was achieved within 24 hours in 87% and a sustained benefit was seen in 74% at 6 months.

PRESERVATION OF RENAL FUNCTION

In our series of 100 consecutive patients receiving renal stents for refractory hypertension, there were 44 patients with renal insufficiency (serum creatinine >1.5 mg%) with a mean serum creatinine of 2.4 ± 1.6 mg/dl.[53] There was no significant change in renal function following stent placement for the entire group. However, nine (22.5%) of the patients with renal failure did normalize their serum creatinine values (1.8 ± 0.1 mg/dl to 1.4 ± 0.1 mg/dl) following successful stent placement.

A recent study has shown that renal artery stent placement slowed the progression of renal artery stenosis in a group of patients with impaired renal function and atherosclerotic renal artery stenosis.[15] A group of 23 patients had their renal function analyzed by plotting the slopes of the reciprocal serum creatinine values before and after successful stent placement. The authors found that the progression of renal failure was significantly slowed after stent placement.

CONCLUSION

In patients with atherosclerotic cardiovascular disease and poorly controlled hypertension, the incidence of renal artery stenosis is higher than previously suspected and should be looked for in patients at increased risk (see Table 11.1). Superior

Table 11.2 Outcome Results for Renal Stents in Hypertensive Patients with Unstable Angina and Congestive Heart Failure

	Unstable Angina (n = 23)			Heart Failure (n = 25)		
	Pre-stent	24 hr	6 months	Pre-stent	24 hr	6 months
Survival	–	100%	96%	–	100%	88%
Event-free	–	100%	96%	–	100%	84%
Sx improved	–	91%	82%	–	76%	75%
Functional class	3.1 ± 0.7	1.5 ± 0.8*	1.5 ± 1.3*	3.2 ± 0.8	1.8 ± 0.9*	1.4 ± 1.4*
SBP (mmHg)	176 ± 24	133 ± 20*	151 ± 24*	163 ± 31	128 ± 19*	146 ± 28*
DBP (mmHg)	90 ± 13	70 ± 11*	81 ± 11	83 ± 17	71 ± 7*	75 ± 15*
Serum Cr (mg%)	1.5 ± 0.4	1.6 ± 0.8	1.7 ± 0.8	1.8 ± 0.4	1.8 ± 0.3	2.0 ± 0.6

DBP, diastolic blood pressure; SBP, systolic blood pressure.
* = p <0.05 at 24 hours or 6 months versus pre-stent value.
Reproduced from Khosla et al. Am J Cardiol 1997;80:363–6,[11] with permission.

results after stent placement compared to balloon angioplasty for reducing the pressure gradient across the renal artery lesion have been demonstrated.[47] The advantage of stents is their ability to scaffold the lumen of the renal artery to defeat the inherent vascular elastic recoil of the target lesion. This is particularly important for the aorto-ostial lesions in which elastic recoil is difficult for balloons to overcome.

Percutaneous revascularization of renal arterial obstructive disease has been dramatically enhanced by the addition of vascular stents to the interventionist's armamentarium. We believe that stent placement enhances both safety and long-term efficacy compared to balloon angioplasty alone, but requires a higher level of operator skill to achieve optimal results. To date no randomized studies have been performed comparing balloon angioplasty alone with renal stent placement.

Surgical revascularization of atherosclerotic renal artery stenosis is an effective treatment for renovascular hypertension.[28] However, renovascular surgery is associated with the morbidity and hospital stay of a major operation as well as complications including bypass graft thrombosis and nephrectomy in up to 4% of patients and operative mortality rates of up to 3%.[54,55]

We successfully placed stents in lesions which historically have been difficult to treat successfully and durably with balloon angioplasty alone. Our patients were not randomized and therefore we cannot directly compare our results to balloon angioplasty alone; however, given the historically poor results in this group of lesions, we did not believe we could ethically randomize our patients to balloon angioplasty versus stent placement.

Our experience with renal stenting in patients with renovascular hypertension and refractory unstable angina or congestive heart failure is also very encouraging. These patients were unmanageable with medical therapy alone. The placement of renal stents successfully reduced afterload and allowed these patients to be stabilized and managed medically.

Improvement or stabilization of renal function appears to be possible with intervention in patients with atherosclerotic renal artery stenosis. The goals of therapy include reversing the relentless progression of the renal artery stenosis and preservation of renal function. In our series of patients with renovascular hypertension, the initial benefit in blood pressure reduction was sustained in the majority of patients for at least 6 months with a reduction in the number of antihypertensive medications required to control blood pressure. The 6-month restenosis rate was <20%, which is a marked improvement over the reported restenosis rates for balloon angioplasty in atherosclerotic lesions. Quantitative angiographic analysis demonstrated that the main determinant of restenosis is intimal proliferation, and that a larger post-stent minimal lumen diameter correlated with 6-month patency. When considering the treatment strategies for renal artery stenosis causing medically refractory hypertension, we believe that the percutaneous placement of renal artery stents is the treatment of choice.

ACKNOWLEDGMENT

The authors would like to express their appreciation to Mr James O'Meara for his assistance in the preparation of the figures and tables.

REFERENCES

1. Simon N, Franklin SS, Bleifer KH, Maxwell MH. Clinical characteristics of renovascular hypertension. JAMA 1972;220:1209–18.
2. Jacobsen HR. Ischemic renal disease: an overlooked clinical entity? Kidney Int 1988;34:729–43.
3. Weber-Mzell D, Kotanko P, Schumacher M, et al. Coronary anatomy predicts presence or absence of renal artery stenosis. Eur Heart J 2002;23:1684–91.
4. Jean WJ, al-Bitar I, Zwicke DL, et al. High incidence of renal artery stenosis in patients with coronary artery disease. Cathet Cardiovasc Diagn 1994;32:8–10.
5. Harding MB, Smith LR, Himmelstein SI, et al. Renal artery stenosis: prevalence and associated risk factors in patients undergoing routine cardiac catheterization. J Am Soc Nephrol 1992;2:1608–16.
6. Olin JW, Melia M, Young JR, Graor RA, Risius B. Prevalence of atherosclerosis renal artery stenosis in patients with atherosclerosis elsewhere. Am J Med 1990;88:46N–51N.
7. Valentine RJ, Clagett GP, Miller GL, et al. The coronary risk of unsuspected renal artery stenosis. J Vasc Surg 1993;18:433–40.
8. O'Neil EA, Hansen KJ, Canzanello VJ, Pennell TC, Dean RH. Prevalence of ischemic nephropathy in patients with renal insufficiency. Am Surg 1992;58:485–90.
9. Meaney TF, Dustan HP, McCormack LJ. Natural history of renal arterial disease. Radiology 1968;91:881–7.
10. Greco BA, Breyer JA. The natural history of renal artery stenosis: who should be evaluated for suspected ischemic nephropathy? Semin Nephrol 1996;16:2–11.
11. Schreiber MJ, Pohl MA, Novick AC. The natural history of atherosclerotic and fibrous renal artery disease. Urol Clin North Am 1984;11:383–92.
12. Wollenweber J, Sheps SG, Davis GD. Clinical course of atherosclerotic renovascular disease. Am J Cardiol 1968;21:60–71.
13. Zierler RE, Bergelin RO, Isaacson JA, Strandness DE Jr. Natural history of atherosclerotic renal artery stenosis: a prospective study with duplex ultrasonography. J Vasc Surg 1994;19:250–8.
14. Dean RH, Kieffer RW, Smith BM, et al. Renovascular hypertension: anatomic and renal function changes during drug therapy. Arch Surg 1981;116:1408–15.
15. Harden PN, MacLeod MJ, Rodger RS, et al. Effect of renal artery stenting on progression of renovascular renal failure. Lancet 1997;349:1133–6.
16. Novick AC, Pohl MA, Schreiber M, Gifford RW Jr, Vidt DG. Revascularization for preservation of renal function in patients with atherosclerotic renovascular disease. J Urol 1983;129:907–12.
17. Kaylor WM, Novick AC, Ziegelbaum M, Vidt DG. Reversal of end stage renal failure with surgical revascularization in patients with atherosclerotic renal artery occlusion. J Urol 1989;141:486–8.
18. Pickering TG, Herman L, Devereux RB, et al. Recurrent pulmonary edema in hypertension due to bilateral renal artery stenosis: treatment by angioplasty or surgical revascularisation. Lancet 1988;2:551–2.
19. Messina LM, Zelenock GB, Yao KA, Stanley JC. Renal revascularization for recurrent pulmonary edema in patients with poorly controlled hypertension and renal insufficiency: a distinct subgroup of patients with arteriosclerotic renal artery occlusive disease. J Vasc Surg 1992;15:73–82.
20. Tami LF, McElderry MW, al-Adli NM, Rubin M, Condos WR. Renal artery stenosis presenting as crescendo angina pectoris. Cathet Cardiovasc Diagn 1995;35:252–6.
21. Khosla S, White CJ, Collins TJ, et al. Effects of renal artery stent implantation in patients with renovascular hypertension presenting with unstable angina or congestive heart failure. Am J Cardiol 1997;80:363–6.
22. Scoble JE. Is the 'wait-and-see' approach justified in atherosclerotic renal artery stenosis? Nephrol Dial Trans 1995;4:588–9.
23. Tegtmeyer CJ, Brown J, Ayers CA, Wellons HA, Stanton LW. Percutaneous transluminal angioplasty for the treatment of renovascular hypertension. JAMA 1981;246:2068–70.
24. Derkx F, Schalekamp M. Renal artery stenosis and hypertension. Lancet 1994;344:237–9.
25. Losinno F, Zuccala A, Busato F, Zucchelli P. Renal artery angioplasty for renovascular hypertension and preservation of renal function: long-term angiographic and clinical follow-up. AJR Am J Roentgenol 1994;162:853–7.
26. Ying CY, Tifft CP, Gavras H, Chobanian AV. Renal revascularization in the azotemic hypertensive patient resistant to therapy. N Engl J Med 1984;311:1070–5.
27. Russo D, Iaccarino V, Conte G, et al. Treatment of severe renovascular hypertension by percutaneous transluminal renal angioplasty in patients with solitary functioning kidney. Nephron 1988;50:315–19.
28. Weibull H, Bergqvist D, Bergentz SE, et al. Percutaneous transluminal angioplasty versus reconstruction of atherosclerotic renal artery stenosis: prospective randomized study. J Vasc Surg 1993;18:841–52.
29. Archibald GR, Beckmann CF, Libertino JA. Focal renal artery stenosis caused by fibromuscular dysplasia: treatment by percutaneous transluminal angioplasty. AJR Am J Roentgenol 1988;151:593–6.
30. Cluzel P, Raynaud A, Beyssen B, Pagny JY, Gaux JC. Stenosis of renal branch arteries in fibromuscular dysplasia: results of percutaneous transluminal angioplasty. Radiology 1994;193:227–32.
31. Soulen MC. Renal angioplasty: underutilized or overvalued? Radiology 1994;193:19–21.
32. Ramsay LE, Waller PC. Blood pressure response to percutaneous transluminal angioplasty for renovascular hypertension: an overview of published series. BMJ 1990;300:569–72.
33. Greminger P, Steiner A, Schneider E, et al. Cure and improvement of renovascular hypertension after percutaneous transluminal angioplasty of renal artery stenosis. Nephron 1989;51:362–6.
34. Sos TA, Pickering TG, Sniderman K, et al. Percutaneous transluminal renal angioplasty in renovascular hypertension due to atheroma or fibromuscular dysplasia. N Engl J Med 1983;309:274–9.

35. Libertino JA, Beckmann CF. Surgery and percutaneous angioplasty in the management of renovascular hypertension. Urol Clin North Am 1994;21:235–43.

36. Canzanello VJ, Millan VG, Spiegel JE, et al. Percutaneous transluminal renal angioplasty in management of atherosclerotic renovascular hypertension: results in 100 patients. Hypertension 1989;13:163–72.

37. Klinge J, Mali WP, Puijlaert CB, et al. Percutaneous transluminal renal angioplasty: initial and long-term results. Radiology 1989;171:501–6.

38. Plouin PF, Darne B, Chatellier G, et al. Restenosis after a first transluminal percutaneous renal angioplasty. Hypertension 1993;21:89–96.

39. Martin LG, Cork RD, Kaufman SL. Long-term results of angioplasty in 110 patients with renal artery stenosis. J Vasc Interv Radiol 1992;3:619–26.

40. Weibull H, Bergqvist D, Jonsson K, et al. Long term results after percutaneous transluminal angioplasty of atherosclerotic renal artery stenosis: the importance of intensive follow up. Eur J Vasc Surg 1991;5:291–301.

41. Sos TA, Pickering TG, Sniderman K, et al. Percutaneous transluminal renal angioplasty in renovascular hypertension due to atheroma or fibromuscular dysplasia. N Engl J Med 1983;309:274–9.

42. Brawn LA, Ramsay LE. Is improvement real with percutaneous transluminal angioplasty in the management of renovascular hypertension? Lancet 1987;2:1313–16.

43. Cicuto KP, McLean GK, Oleaga JA, et al. Renal artery stenosis: anatomic classification for percutaneous angioplasty. AJR Am J Roentgenol 1981;137:599–601.

44. Rensing BJ, Hermans WR, Beatt KJ, et al. Quantitative angiographic assessment of elastic recoil after percutaneous transluminal coronary angioplasty. Am J Cardiol 1990;66:1039–44.

45. Rensing BJ, Hermans WR, Strauss BH, Serruys PW. Regional differences in elastic recoil after percutaneous transluminal coronary angioplasty: a quantitative angiographic study. J Am Coll Cardiol 1991;6(suppl B):34B–38B.

46. van de Ven PJG, Beutler JJ, Kaatee R, et al. Transluminal vascular stent for ostial atherosclerotic renal artery stenosis. Lancet 1995;346:672–4.

47. Dorros G, Prince C, Mathiak L. Stenting of a renal artery stenosis achieves better relief of the obstructive lesion than balloon angioplasty. Cathet Cardiovasc Diagn 1993;29:191–8.

48. Dorros G, Jaff M, Jain A, Dufek C, Mathiak L. Follow-up of primary Palmaz-Schatz stent placement for atherosclerotic renal artery stenosis. Am J Cardiol 1995;75:1051–5.

49. Rees CR, Palmaz JC, Becker GJ, et al. Palmaz stent in atherosclerotic stenoses involving the ostia of the renal arteries: preliminary report of a multicenter study. Radiology 1991;181:507–14.

50. Serruys PW, de Jaegere P, Kiemeneij F, et al. A comparison of balloon-expandable-stent implantation with balloon angioplasty in patients with coronary artery disease. N Engl J Med 1994;331:489–95.

51. Fischman DL, Leon MB, Baim DS, et al. A randomized comparison of coronary-stent placement and balloon angioplasty in the treatment of coronary artery disease. N Engl J Med 1994;331:496–501.

52. Watson PS, Hadjipetrou P, Cox SV, et al. Effect of renal artery stenting on renal function and size in patients with atherosclerotic renovascular disease. Circulation 2000;102:1671–7.

53. White CJ, Ramee SR, Collins TJ, et al. Renal artery stent placement: utility in difficult lesions for balloon angioplasty. J Am Coll Cardiol 1997;30:1445–50.

54. Hansen KJ, Starr SM, Sands RE, et al. Contemporary surgical management of renovascular disease. J Vasc Surg 1992;16:319–31.

55. Novick AC, Ziegelbaum M, Vidt DG, et al. Trends in surgical revascularization for renal artery disease. Ten years experience. JAMA 1987;257:498–501.

12. Stent-Graft Repair of Aortic Aneurysms

Gregory S Domer, Brendan P Girschek and Frank J Criado

ABDOMINAL AORTIC ANEURYSMS

Modern surgical treatment of abdominal aortic aneurysms (AAA) – by aneurysm resection or graft replacement – has been performed since the early 1950s.[1] With improvements in peri-operative care and refined surgical techniques, the operation became quite effective, offering AAA patients a sound and generally successful therapeutic approach. Unfortunately, operative therapy is not without risks and problems. Post-operative recovery tends to be difficult and prolonged, and operation-related morbidity is significant. Worse yet, there are high-risk cases where standard open surgery carries inordinate or unreasonable dangers; some in fact are truly 'inoperable'. Addressing such challenges became the main driving force for the development of less invasive treatment options. In 1991, Parodi reported the first series of patients undergoing endovascular aneurysm repair (EVAR).[2] It signaled the true beginning of a new era in vascular surgery and catheter-based technology. Since then, more than 25,000 stent-graft devices have been implanted and many devices were created, leaving no doubt that EVAR is feasible and of clear-cut benefit to many patients. Experienced endovascular teams are reporting that 60% (or more) of patients with AAA can be treated with currently available devices.[3] It has become a critical treatment tool, especially for the management of high-risk individuals who may not have another reasonable therapeutic option.

There are presently (January 2004) three commercially available, Food and Drug Administration (FDA)-approved devices in the United States. These are the AneuRx™ (Medtronic AVE, Santa Rosa, CA), the Excluder™ (WL Gore, Flagstaff, AZ), and the Zenith™ (Cook, Bloomington, IN) stent-grafts (Figs 12.1, 12.2). The Ancure™ device (Guidant, Menlo Park, CA) was also approved, but

it has been withdrawn from the market. Many more choices exist in Europe and other parts of the world, with the Talent™ stent-graft (Medtronic AVE) representing perhaps the most 'popular' device overall (Fig. 12.3).

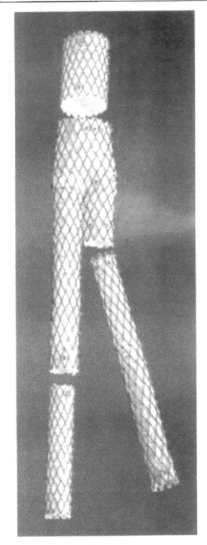

Fig. 12.1 AneuRx™ stent-graft.

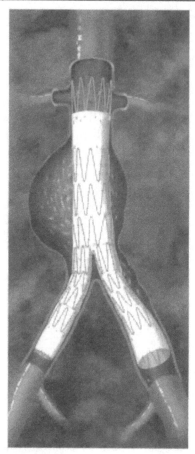

Fig. 12.2 Zenith™ stent-graft.

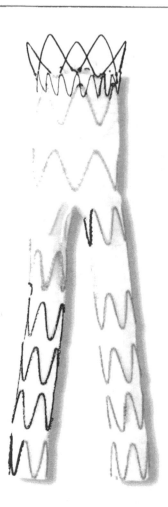

Fig. 12.3 Talent™ stent-graft.

ANATOMIC AND CLINICAL CONSIDERATIONS

Decision making vis-à-vis endovascular therapy is influenced by device type, but is largely determined by anatomy. In general, appropriate candidates should have an infrarenal neck of at least 10–15 mm in length, and with a diameter not to exceed 26 mm. Other aspects of the 'ideal neck' (Fig. 12.4) are listed in Table 12.1. Neck angulation and configuration are particularly important, as are combinations of two or more unfavorable features. The distal aorta and bifurcation should be large enough to allow deployment of a bifurcated device

with passage of two limbs side by side across the region of the bifurcation.[4]

Iliac artery anatomy and disease are the second most common limitation to EVAR. Generally, at least one external iliac artery of ≥7.5 mm is necessary for successful access and delivery of the device. The common iliac arteries should be free of aneurysmal dilation or marked ectasia (<20 mm diameter), and there should be a landing zone of 10–15 mm or more for distal endograft limb fixation. Focal iliac stenoses are best managed with

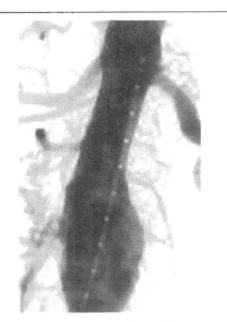

Fig. 12.4 Angiographic example of 'ideal' AAA neck.

Table 12.1 The 'Ideal' Abdominal Aortic Aneurysm Neck

- >15 mm length
- <26 mm diameter
- Cylindrical
- <45° angulation
- Little or no calcification
- Little or no mural thrombus

angioplasty at the time of stent-graft intervention; placement of a self-expanding stent within the endograft limb at the site of narrowing may become necessary in such situations. Persistent stenosis of the limb from extrinsic compression or angulation must be treated aggressively to avoid limb thrombosis and the need for secondary procedures. Performance of angioplasty and stenting ahead of time, before the stent-graft procedure, should generally be avoided since the stent might interfere

with transluminal passage of the endograft delivery system. We have found probing of questionable (borderline small) access iliac arteries with Coons dilators very useful. Iliac artery tortuosity, in the absence of significant calcification, is no longer a major technical issue as stiff guidewires (such as the Lunderquist™ wire; Cook, Bloomington, IN) can straighten such pathways relatively easily.[5,6]

MORPHOLOGY ASSESSMENT AND EVAR PLANNING

Axial and three-dimensional contrast-enhanced computed tomography (CT) imaging are the most useful means of assessing the anatomy and determining suitability for EVAR.[7] Pre-operative angiography (with a calibrated diagnostic catheter) continues to be used but less frequently. Our group finds it helpful, especially in combination with IVUS imaging and measurements. The importance of and difficulties with length measurements have clearly been underestimated in the past. It is a crucially important feature with great potential impact on device choice and design as well as outcome. Magnetic resonance angiography (MRA) has not yet achieved the diagnostic 'stature' of CT for this assessment but it can be helpful. Its main limitation relates to the availability of commonly used MR-incompatible devices (i.e. the Zenith™ stent-graft) where it cannot be used for post-implantation follow-up.

PRINCIPLES OF DEVICE CHOICE AND IMPLANTATION

In most cases, the choice will be for a modular bifurcated device, such as one of the three endografts that are currently approved and available in the US. The distinguishing feature of the Zenith™ (and Talent™) stent-graft is that it incorporates suprarenal fixation, and anchoring barbs at the top end. Aneurysm exclusion requires the achievement of secure anchoring and a hemostatic seal at all fixation sites. Selection of a particular device for a given case is dependent on several factors, including – perhaps most powerfully –operator's choice and personal experience. Some degree of diameter oversizing (<20%) is necessary with all endografts, especially important to achieve adequate fixation and seal at the proximal neck. However, it must be emphasized that excessive oversizing can be counterproductive and lead to poor apposition and endoleak.[8]

ENDOLEAKS

Endoleaks, or continued arterial flow within the aneurysm sac but outside of the endograft, are complications that are unique to EVAR. They imply 'failure' to attain complete circulatory isolation of the sac.

- Type 1 (proximal or distal attachments) and type 3 (modular disconnections or graft defects) endoleaks are directly related to device or implantation issues.
- Type 2 (branch back flow) endoleaks are perhaps only partially influenced by endograft type, but are mostly dependent on anatomic characteristics.
- Type 4 endoleaks reflect transgraft flow and porosity; they tend to occur during the procedure only, especially while the patient is anticoagulated.

Overall, endoleak rates vary widely (10–30%). Management guidelines continue to evolve. Definitive diagnosis of endoleak type is paramount, usually requiring a combination of CT and angiographic techniques. Ultrasound can also be helpful.

Most leading investigators agree that a type 2 endoleak requires careful follow-up and observation only, but would consider intervention in case of sac growth. On the other hand, type 1 and type 3 leaks signify that the sac is still pressurized and at risk for rupture. These types of endoleak must be repaired; this usually involves placement of cuff extensions, but even surgical conversion may have to be considered depending on the individual case.[9,10] Type 4 endoleaks are not clinically significant and typically resolve spontaneously.

MIGRATION

Device migration has been reported in the literature to range from 2.95 to 45%. It was found in 96 of 3251 EUROSTAR patients (2.95%).[10] Data analysis showed migration to be an independent predictor of late rupture with a risk ratio of 5.3.[11] The reasons attributed to migration were inadequate anchorage, deterioration of stent-graft integrity, and proximal neck dilatation. Morphologic studies have shown a progressive increase in the cross-sectional area of the infrarenal neck by more than 10% by 6 months and by more than 15% by 1 year after endovascular repair. Suprarenal fixation and active anchoring with barbs and hooks are felt to enhance stability and to minimize or prevent migration, but there is no scientific proof that such is the case.[12]

OVERVIEW

EVAR has rapidly become a very important tool in the treatment of many AAA patients. We can now offer patients a less invasive approach that compares favorably with standard surgical repair in terms of morbidity, length of hospitalization and recovery time, and with an equally low mortality.[13] More importantly perhaps, it provides high-risk individuals and inoperable cases with a viable treatment option. But it is not without challenges and unresolved issues, mainly continuing concern regarding device integrity and durability of the repair, high device costs, the need for life-long surveillance, and a 10% rate of secondary interventions over time. Future technological evolutions will undoubtedly result in further device refinements and better techniques. It is likely that, in the near future, surgical treatment's role will be limited to those situations that prove unsuitable for EVAR.

THORACIC AORTIC ANEURYSMS

Surgical repair of thoracic aortic aneurysms (TAA) is associated with significant morbidity and mortality. This, in turn, has led to surgeons' reluctance to offer treatment to many patients. In addition, there are indeed 'inoperable' cases because of major co-morbidities, making the risks of thoracic aortic surgery truly prohibitive. The need for a less invasive treatment alternative was thus imperative and rather clear, resulting in the current evolution of endovascular stent-graft techniques. Such interventions can offer TAA patients hope where none existed before. They carry the promise to revolutionize the whole field of thoracic aortic surgery, and will have a major impact on management paradigms and therapeutic indications for several pathologic conditions affecting the aortic arch and descending thoracic aorta.

INCIDENCE AND NATURE

The incidence of TAA is estimated to be 8 per 100,000 per year.[14] Men appear to be exposed to an incidence that is three times that of women's, and tend to be younger (62 versus 76 years of age for women). The risk factors that have been associated with the development of TAA are the same as those for atheromatous disease, namely age, gender, smoking, hypertension, and hypercholesterolemia. The incidence of TAA appears to have doubled over the last two decades; this is most likely related to the aging of our population, and also because of a significant increase in the rate of discovery through the more common use of better imaging – CT, chest x-rays, and fluoroscopy in particular.

Most TAAs are considered to represent atherosclerotic lesions; they tend to be fusiform, and be more common in older males with multiple co-morbidities such as hypertension, coronary artery disease, and coronary obstructive pulmonary disease. Most importantly, they often (30%+) coexist with an infra-abdominal aortic aneurysm (AAA).[15] Chronic type B dissection is the second most common cause of TAA ('dissecting aneurysm'). Post-traumatic aneurysms associated with deceleration injuries are most often located at the isthmic portion of the aorta. Other less common etiologies include dystrophic aneurysms (Marfan's disease, Ehlers–Danlos syndrome, tuberous sclerosis, etc.), false aneurysms (found at points of surgical anastomosis), congenital aneurysms, and inflammatory aneurysms secondary to aortitis (Takayasu's, Behçet's and Horton's diseases).

NATURAL HISTORY

Like AAAs, TAAs tend to enlarge progressively and eventually rupture. The risk of rupture grows with aneurysm size. The 5-year life expectancy of untreated TAA is <20%.[16,17] The most common cause of death associated with TAA is rupture with exsanguinating hemorrhage that tends to be rapid and beyond repair, even when occurring in the hospital setting. TAA size >6.0 cm is generally regarded as particularly ominous in this regard. Other potential morbid consequences include fistulization into and compression of neighboring organs, and distal embolization to visceral and lower extremity vascular beds.

SURGICAL TREATMENT

Surgical repair involves segmental graft replacement of the aneurysmal aorta through a thoracotomy or thoracoabdominal incision. It is attended by many significant risks and technical difficulties. The in-hospital surgical mortality has ranged from 3 to 15% for elective procedures. Prolonged respiratory support is required by at least 15% of all patients and up to 20% develop renal failure.[18–20] Nearly 20% of patients have experienced aneurysm rupture at a different location from the one that was previously repaired. In addition, the need for 'redo' operations for the correction of residual or recurring aneurysms is relatively common. Nonetheless, a 70% 5-year survival has been reported.[21]

ENDOVASCULAR STENT-GRAFT INTERVENTION

The avoidance of a thoracotomy incision and of aortic cross-clamping are the most obvious advantages of the endovascular approach, making it a safer and much more appealing form of therapy. Moreover, the occurrence of spinal cord ischemia and paraplegia, renal failure, and myocardial infarction has been minimized in comparison with the surgical outlook. As a result, need for ICU care and length of hospitalization and recovery can be reduced significantly. All of these reasons combined make it possible to offer treatment to many more TAA patients, even those considered at high surgical risk.

Only a few devices are available for endovascular intervention in the thoracic aorta. The most extensive experiences have been accumulated with the Talent™ and Zenith™ stent-grafts. Newer designs and further refinements of existing thoracic endografts will undoubtedly emerge in the near future.

ANATOMY AND CASE SELECTION STRATEGIES

Optimal results and technical ease can be anticipated when favorable anatomy is present, such as a (relatively) straight thoracoabdominal aorta, soft access iliac arteries of large diameter, and a target focal lesion in the mid-descending thoracic aorta. Unfortunately, in real-life practice, a majority of patients offer more challenging situations. As at any other location, stent-graft intervention is designed to segmentally exclude the aneurysm-bearing portion of aorta. This requires the availability of proximal and distal fixation and seal zones that should be >20 mm in length. Some have advocated the use of a simple guideline for optimal anatomical suitability: the length (for fixation and seal) of the proximal (and distal) neck should match the aortic diameter at that segment.

Aneurysmal disease is often extensive and multifocal, with consequent need for endograft coverage of long segments of the thoracic and thoraco-abdominal aorta. Frequently, the proximal fixation site is within the distal or mid aortic arch. Coverage (occlusion) of the origin of the left subclavian artery is often necessary to achieve good fixation and seal in the more likely normal distal arch area. Our experience and that of others has demonstrated the safety of this technique; about one-third of these patients develop left arm claudication which tends to be self-limited and non-incapacitating. Better yet, the arm claudication improves or resolves spontaneously in approximately 70% of the cases. However, the potential for serious complications (i.e. vertebrobasilar insufficiency, brainstem and cerebellar strokes) is real when the contralateral vertebral artery is occluded, or when a prior left internal mammary artery (LIMA) procedure has been performed. Such conditions would demand the performance of preliminary left subclavian transposition or bypass to avert serious adverse events.

In all other situations, we have found endograft coverage/occlusion of the vessel to be safe and very well tolerated. The need for more proximal graft attachment (i.e. to the innominate artery origin), however, would dictate the performance of left carotid artery transposition bypass, typically in the form of a retropharyngeal carotid–carotid crossover bypass with proximal ligation of the left common carotid artery. At the distal end, the celiac artery signals the caudad boundary of present-day endovascular grafting techniques. Crossing of this vessel with a naked stent is considered safe, but coverage/occlusion of the celiac artery should be avoided if possible because of several anecdotal reports of serious ischemic consequences to the liver and pancreas.

As with endovascular treatment of AAA, TAA patients need to be tested and evaluated for life following stent-graft repair. Long-term device failures and metal frame and stent fractures have been reported with essentially every device. Clinical consequences have been few, if any.[22][24] Imperatives for re-intervention would include the finding of a type 1 (attachment site) or type 3 (modular disconnection) endoleak, device migration with loss of fixation, and a progressively enlarging aneurysm sac (in spite of stent-graft 'exclusion'). Both CT scans and plain chest x-rays constitute excellent imaging tools in this regard.

UNRESOLVED ISSUES AND COMPLICATIONS

The long-term durability of stent-graft devices and endovascular aneurysm repair are a continuing concern. Unlike surgical replacement, endovascular aneurysm exclusion does not 'cure' the disease. The aneurysm sac remains and can be re-pressurized or 'recur' in the face of device failure or migration. These considerations apply to both AAAs and TAAs. Although short-term and even mid-term results are quite encouraging, serious complications – such as paraplegia, strokes and aortic rupture – have all been described.[22] The risk of spinal cord ischemia seems to be considerably lower than that of conventional surgical repair.[25] Patients at increased risk have been identified, especially those with a history of prior infrarenal AAA repair. Prophylactic use of a cerebrospinal fluid (CSF) drainage catheter (kept in place for 2–3 days post-operatively), the empiric use of steroids, and the prevention of hypotension have all been shown in various publications (and anecdotal reports) to be helpful.[23] Other possible procedure and device-related complications include visceral artery and lower extremity embolization, renal failure, aortic rupture – especially that involving the false lumen in acute dissection cases – and the 'post-implant syndrome'. The last is relatively frequent after stent-graft repair in the thoracic aorta, causing low-grade fevers, back pain, leukocytosis and other changes.[24,26] It tends to be self-limited, resolving spontaneously in several days without sequelae.

SUMMARY AND OVERVIEW

Endovascular repair of thoracic aortic pathology has emerged as the most promising and (perhaps) best clinical application of stent-graft technology. Many such patients are often treated with 'benign neglect', so these newer techniques may represent their only hope for survival. Early and mid-term results are encouraging, but longer follow-up of a larger group of patients will be necessary before more definitive statements on durability and clinical efficacy can be made. Further refinements of current technologies and new devices are but a sure development in the near future. Clinical indications will probably expand and, in the end, the standards of care and various treatment paradigms for thoracic aortic lesions are likely to change sig-

nificantly as these endovascular options continue to evolve.

REFERENCES

1. Dubost C, Allary M, Oeconomos N. Resection of an aneurysm of the abdominal aorta: establishment of the continuity by a preserved human arterial graft, with result after five months. Arch Surg 1952;64:405–8.

2. Parodi JC, Palmaz C, Barone HD. Transfemoral intraluminal graft implantation for abdominal aortic aneurysm. Ann Vasc Surg 1991;5:491–9.

3. Tanquilut EM, Ouriel K. Current outcomes in endovascular repair of abdominal aortic aneurysms. J Cardiovasc Surg 2003;44:503–9.

4. Sternbergh WC III, Carter G, York JW, Yoselevitz M, Money SR. Aortic neck angulation predicts adverse outcome with endovascular abdominal aortic aneurysm repair. J Vasc Surg 2002;35:482–6.

5. Criado FJ, Barnatan MF, Lingelbach JM, et al. Abdominal aortic aneurysm: overview of stent-graft devices. J Am Coll Surg 2002;194(1 Suppl.):S88–97.

6. Amesur NB, Zajko AB, Orons PD, Makaroun MS. Endovascular treatment of iliac limb stenosis or occlusions in 31 patients treated with the Ancure endograft. J Vasc Interv Radiol 2000;11:421–8.

7. White RA, Donayre CE, Ealot I, et al. Computed tomography assessment of abdominal aortic aneurysm morphology after endograft exclusion. J Vasc Surg 2001;33(2 Suppl.):S1–10.

8. Prinssen M, Wever JJ, Mali WP, Eikelboom BC, Blankensteijn JD. Concerns for the durability of the proximal abdominal aortic aneurysm endograft fixation from a 2-year and 3-year longitudinal computed tomography angiography study. J Vasc Surg 2001;33(2 Suppl.):S64–9.

9. Chaikof EL, Blankenstein JD, Harris PL, et al. Reporting standards for endovascular aortic aneurysm repair. J Vasc Surg 2002;35:1048–60.

10. Mohan IV, Laheju RJ, Harris PL. Risk factors for endoleak and the evidence for stent-graft oversizing in patients undergoing endovascular aneurysm repair. Eur J Vasc Endovasc Surg 2001;21:344–9.

11. Wever JJ, de Nie AJ, Blankensteijn JD, et al. Dilatation of the proximal neck of infrarenal aortic aneurysms after endovascular AAA repair. Eur J Vasc Endovasc Surg 2000;19(2):197–201.

12. Conners MS III, Sternbergh WC, Carter G, et al. Endograft migration one to four years after endovascular abdominal aortic aneurysm repair with the AneuRx device: a cautionary note. J Vasc Surg 2002;36:476–84.

13. Zarins CK, White RA, Schwarten D, et al. AneuRx stent graft versus open surgical repair of abdominal aortic aneurysms: multicenter prospective clinical trial. J Vasc Surg 1999;29:292–305.

14. Bickerstaff LK, Pairolero PC, Hollier LH, et al. Thoracic aortic aneurysms: a population based study. Surgery 1982;92:1103–8.

15. Pressler V, McNamara JJ. Improved prognosis of thoracic aortic aneurysms: natural history and treatment. J Thorac Cardiovasc Surg 1980;79:489–98.

16. Perko MJ, Norgaard M, Herzog TM, et al. Unoperated aortic aneurysm: a survey of 170 patients. Ann Thorac Surg 1995;59:1204–9.

17. Coady MA, Rizzo JA, Hammond GL, et al. What is the appropriate size criterion for resection of thoracic aneurysms? J Thorac Cardiovasc Surg 1997;113:476–91.

18. Verdant A, Cossette R, Page A, et al. Aneurysms of descending thoracic aorta: three hundred sixty-six consecutive cases resected without paraplegia. J Vasc Surg 1995;21:385–91.

19. Coselli JS, Konstadinos AP, La Francesca S, Cohen S. Results of contemporary surgical treatment of descending thoracic aortic aneurysms: experience with 198 patients. Ann Vasc Surg 1996;10:131–7.

20. Hayashi J, Eguchi S, Yasuda K, et al. Operation for non-dissecting aneurysm in the descending thoracic aorta. Ann Thorac Surg 1997;63:93–7.

21. Lawrie GM, Earle N, Debakey ME. Evolution of surgical techniques for aneurysms of the descending thoracic aorta: twenty-nine years of experience with 659 patients. J Card Surg 1994;9:648–61.

22. Dake MD, Miller DC, Mitchell RS, et al. The 'first generation' of endovascular stent-graft for patients with aneurysms of the descending thoracic aorta. J Thorac Cardiovasc Surg 1998;116:689–703.

23. Gowda RM, Misra D, Tranbaugh RF, Ohki T, Khan IA. Endovascular stent grafting of descending thoracic aortic aneurysms. Chest 2003;124:82–6.

24. Ohki T, Veith FJ. Endovascular grafts and other image-guided catheter-based adjuncts to improve the treatment of ruptured aortoiliac aneurysm. Ann Surg 2000;232:466–79.

25. Gravereaux EC, Faries PL, Burks JA, et al. Risk of spinal cord ischemia after endograft repair of thoracic aortic aneurysms. J Vasc Surg 2001;34:997–1003.

26. Criado FJ, Barnatan MF, Rizk Y, et al. Technical strategies to expand stent-graft applicability in the aortic arch and proximal descending thoracic aorta. J Endovasc Ther 2002;9:493–4.

13. Role of Covered Stents in Peripheral Arterial Diseases

Michel Henry, Isabelle Henry and Michèle Hugel

INTRODUCTION

The number of patients who have peripheral diseases is steadily increasing worldwide, primarily as a result of the aging of the population.

It is estimated that 10–20% of individuals more than 70 years of age sustain some degree of chronic lower extremity ischemia. This percentage is greater in some subgroups of patients, such as those having diabetes or end stage renal failure.

Patients may suffer from claudication or critical limb-threatening ischemia, with a different prognosis: better for patients with claudication, worse for those with more advanced stages of ischemia. These patients should be offered relatively aggressive therapy.

During the past 40 years, surgery has been established as a reliable treatment for peripheral disease in all regions. Endovascular therapy is a relatively new field of vascular medicine and has continued to expand over the past two decades, thanks to the advancement of technical developments. This new concept has become widely recognized and accepted. The applications of endovascular procedures have been expanded dramatically throughout the human body for both occlusive and aneurysmal diseases, not only at iliac and femoropopliteal levels but also at aortic, renal, and supra-aortic levels.

Angioplasty is now the first treatment proposed for peripheral vascular diseases and the treatment of choice for simple arterial lesions. However, angioplasty alone is limited and has several complications (dissections, acute thromboses, etc.). The problem of restenosis remains, and for long lesions the initial success and the long-term results are not as good as they are for short lesions, particularly in femoropopliteal arteries, in which surgery is often preferred.[1–3]

The concept of vascular stenting originated with Charles Dotter in 1969,[4] but it did not become a clinical reality until the late 1980s. Expandable metallic stents have proved their usefulness in the management of complications related to angioplasty and possibly restenosis;[5–7] for the latter, however, this benefit is debated. The process of restenosis starts when a stent is placed, with a vascular injury that is induced by percutaneous transluminal angioplasty (PTA) and/or stent placement; such injuries include deposits of plasma proteins, platelets, and leukocytes on the stent struts.[8–10]

Stenting is controversial and particularly at infrainguinal locations.[11–18] Its use is considered acceptable in the aortoiliac vessels and in the majority of published series in the literature, the immediate and long-term results are encouraging.[19–26]

A primary or a direct stenting could be envisaged for these lesions if we consider the meta-analysis reported by Bosch and Hunink.[27] Nevertheless, Tetteroo et al[28] did not find any difference between primary and selective stent placement. Stenting is more in dispute for the femoropopliteal vessels and the results in the literature are very disparate,[11–18,25,29–37] with a primary patency between 22 and 77%. Three randomized trials[38–40] showed no difference between PTA alone versus PTA and stent and, according to TASC recommendation 36,[41] femoropopliteal stenting as a primary approach to the interventional treatment of intermittent claudication or arterial limb ischemia is not indicated. Stents may have a limited role in salvage of acute PTA failure or complications. These recommendations were based on studies performed with the old generation of stents and it is the same with the randomized studies. New stents are now available: nitinol stents which seem to give better results[42,43] and covered stents.

Endoluminal stent-grafts and covered stents are now being investigated for treatment of both aneurysmal and occlusive peripheral arterial diseases.[44-57] For occlusive diseases, it is postulated that an endoluminal bypass with a stent-graft may limit the ingrowth of intimal hyperplasia along the length of the treated segment, thereby improving patency as compared to conventional angioplasty and stenting. For an aneurysmal disease, the stent-graft may be used to bridge the aneurysmal segment and therefore occlude the aneurysm from the native circulation.

Several covered stents are either currently available or are in clinical experiment:

- The Cragg Endopro System 1/Passager™ (Boston Scientific, Natick, MA);
- The Corvita™ endoluminal graft (Boston Scientific);
- The Hemobahn™ or the new Viabahn™ (WL Gore, Flagstaff, AZ);
- The Wallgraft™ (Boston Scientific);
- The Jostent™ (Jomed International AB, Helsingborg, Sweden);
- The aSpire™ covered stent (Vascular Architects, San José, CA).

We describe below these different covered stents, the results obtained, and their clinical applications in different locations.

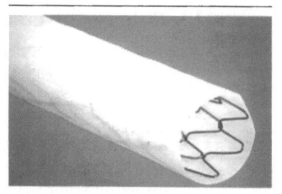

Fig. 13.1 Cragg Endopro System 1/Passager™.
Nitinol stent covered with polyester fabric.

with ultrathin woven polyester fabric (Fig. 13.1). It has the property of shape memory.[14,45] The design and construction of the stent have been previously described.[15,46,58-60] The fabric is of low porosity and is attached to the stent framework by polyester ligatures. The stent-graft is presented in a compressed form in a loading cartridge. Stent-grafts range from 5 to 12 mm in diameter and from 3 to 10 cm in length. They are delivered through 50 cm long introducer sheaths ranging in diameter from 7F to 10F, depending on the size of the stent-graft to be implanted.

THE DIFFERENT LOCATIONS FOR COVERED STENTS

ILIOFEMOROPOPLITEAL ANGIOPLASTY AND STENTING: RESULTS WITH THE DIFFERENT COVERED STENTS

CRAGG ENDOPRO SYSTEM 1/PASSAGER™

STENT-GRAFT CONSTRUCTION

The Cragg Endopro System 1/Passager™ consists of a flexible, self-expandable nitinol stent covered

STENT-GRAFT INTRODUCTION TECHNIQUE

Device delivery is usually accomplished using an ipsilateral retrograde or antegrade femoral artery approach. A retrograde popliteal approach has been used in cases in which femoral artery access was not possible. The rigidity of the delivery device limits the possibilities of implantation using the contralateral access. For occlusive disease, balloon angioplasty is always performed first in order to enlarge the arterial lumen. Occasionally, debulking techniques such as rotational atherectomy are used. The stent-graft is delivered through the 50 cm long introducer sheath, which is placed across the lesion to be treated. The stent-graft diameter is usually selected to be equal to or 1 mm greater than the nominal arterial diameter.

The stent-graft is positioned fluoroscopically across the treated segment. Platinum markers at each end of the stent assist in positioning the device. Once the stent-graft is in position, the sheath is withdrawn, and an internal positioning catheter is used to fix the stent-graft in place. The stent-graft expands using the thermal memory characteristics of its nitinol frame. The graft is usually then dilated with an angioplasty balloon at high pressure (14–16 atm); this fixes the graft against the arterial wall and helps to unwrinkle the fabric. When several grafts are needed to cover a long lesion, it is important to overlap the prostheses by at least 5 mm so that the fabric portion of the graft covers the entire arterial lumen. In the middle part of the femoral artery, an overlap of 1 cm may be better to avoid disjunction of the stents.

OUR EXPERIENCE

PATIENT POPULATION

One hundred and fifty-six patients (134 males, 22 females), mean age 63.4 ± 10.5 years (range 38–88 years) were selected for treatment with the stent-graft. Risk factors included smoking (78), hypertension (57), dyslipidemia (41), and diabetes (21). Sixty-three patients had multiple vascular symptoms including cerebral, cardiac, or renal diseases, 37 had prior surgical vascular intervention, and 48 had prior angioplasty. According to Rutherford's classification, 136 patients were in grade I (8 in category 2, 128 in category 3), 12 patients in grade II, and 8 in grade III (category 5). The mean ankle–brachial index (ABI) was 0.56 ± 0.11. Three tibial vessels were patent in 72, two in 74, and one in 10 patients.

RESULTS

Table 13.1 shows the locations and the types of lesions. We treated 64 iliac arteries (33 for stenoses, 18 for occlusions, and 13 for aneurysms), 82 femoral arteries (28 for stenoses, 46 for occlusions, and 8 for aneurysms), and 10 popliteal arteries (4 for occlusions, 1 for stenosis, and 5 for aneurysms) (Figs 13.2–13.4). Ninety-three lesions were heavily calcified (21 were treated with rotational atherectomy), and 17 ulcerated.

Tables 13.2 and 13.3 detail the lesion characteristics including the mean lesion length, the mean percent stenosis before angioplasty and graft placement, and the mean arterial diameter. Occlusions were recanalized using either a hydrophilic guidewire (33) or Holmium laser (35). Eleven patients had a combination of Holmium laser treatment and rotational atherectomy.

Table 13.1 Lesion Characteristics (1)

Location	No.	Stenoses	Occlusions	Aneurysms	Calcified	Ulcerated
Iliac	64	33	18	13	27	10
Femoral	82	28	46	8	63	6
Popliteal	10	1	4	5	3	1
Total	156	62	68	26	93	17

Table 13.2 Lesion Characteristics (2): Mean Lesion Length

Location	Stenoses	Occlusions	Aneurysms	Range
Iliac	52.2 ± 26.4	86.7 ± 36.1	38.5 ± 13.9	20–150
Femoral	112.5 ± 69.8	161.1 ± 85.3	125 ± 93.3	20–300
Popliteal	80	67.5 ± 15	114 ± 80.5	30–200

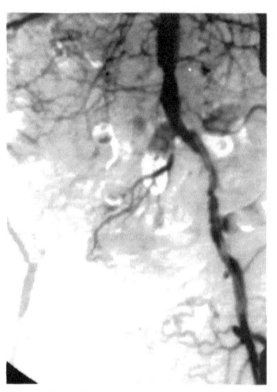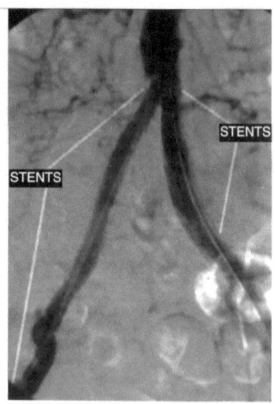

Fig. 13.2 Left: Right iliac artery thrombosis. Right: Left iliac artery polystenosis.
Placement of Cragg Endopro System 1/Passager™ stents.

Table 13.3 Lesion Characteristics (3)

Mean percent stenosis before PTA		
SFA	93 ± 4.1%	(70–100%)
Iliac	89 ± 3.7%	(70–100%)
Popliteal	92 ± 4.6%	(75–100%)
Mean arterial diameter		
SFA	5.95 ± 0.6 mm	(5–7)
Iliac:		
Stenosis	7.8 ± 1.1 mm	(6–10)
Occlusion	7.9 ± 1.1 mm	(7–10)
Popliteal	5.5 ± 0.6 mm	(5–6)

PTA, percutaneous transluminal angiography;
SFA, superficial femoral artery.

The arterial approaches were as follows: retrograde femoral 64, antegrade femoral 68, and popliteal access 24. In 21 cases, the popliteal access was initially used to approach an otherwise inaccessible superficial femoral lesion. In three cases, the popliteal access was used after failure of the antegrade access.

A total of 266 stent-grafts were placed. Lengths ranged from 3 to 10 cm and diameters ranged from 5 to 10 mm. In 33 patients, two stent-grafts were placed in the same artery: 7 at the iliac, 25 at the femoral, and 1 at the popliteal level. In 17 patients, three stent-grafts were placed in the same superficial femoral artery to treat long occlusions or aneurysms. In one patient, four stent-grafts were placed to treat a 35 cm long femoral aneurysm.

Indications for stent-graft placement were post-angioplasty residual stenoses ($n = 70$), dissections ($n = 22$), restenoses ($n = 21$), ulcerated lesions ($n = 17$), and aneurysms ($n = 26$).

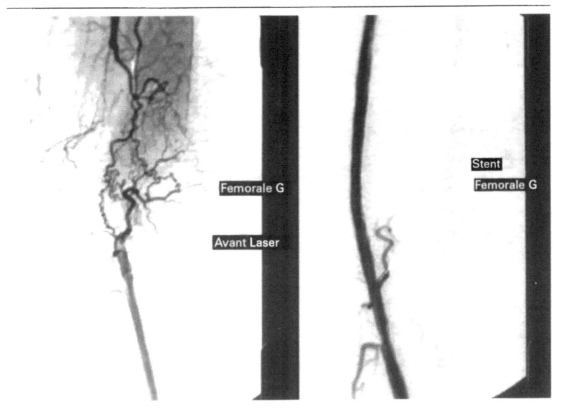

Fig. 13.3 Femoral artery thrombosis.
Result after recanalization and placement of Cragg Endopro System 1/Passager™ stents.

Technical success was achieved in all cases but one at the iliac level (98%) and the femoropopliteal level (99%) (83 cases of 84). In this one case, the patient had a large femoral aneurysm, and partial success was achieved but with a persistent arterial leak at the distal part of the aneurysm. This patient was in poor general condition and died of an acute myocardial infarction 4 days after the procedure.

Post-angioplasty percent stenoses decreased from 43 ± 3.9% to 0.6 ± 3% after stent-graft implantation, with no significant difference in the iliac and femoropopliteal location (Table 13.4). No significant residual stenosis was seen even in

Table 13.4 Results (1)

	Stenosis Before PTA	Stenosis After PTA	Stenosis After Stent
Global population	92 ± 3.7	43 ± 3.9	0.6 ± 0.3
Iliac	89 ± 3.7	48 ± 4.3	0
Femoral	93 ± 4.3	45 ± 3.8	0.8 ± 0.8
Popliteal	92 ± 4.6	37 ± 2.7	0.5 ± 0.3

PTA, percutaneous transluminal angiography.

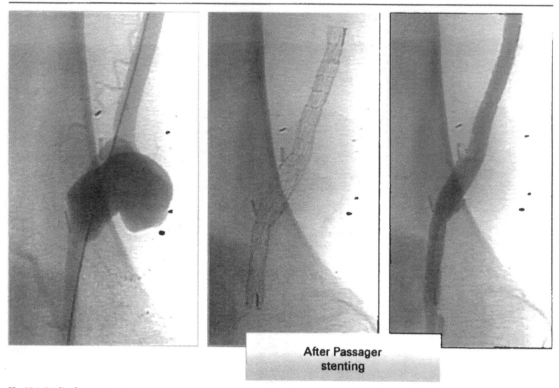

After Passager
stenting

Fig. 13.4 Popliteal artery aneurysm.
Result after placement of a Cragg Endopro System 1/Passager™ stent.

calcified lesions. The mean length of stent segments was significantly greater at the femoropopliteal level in comparison with the iliac level for occlusions and stenoses (Table 13.5). The mean stent-graft length for all lesions was 114.7 ± 65.7 mm. Immediate clinical success was obtained in all uncomplicated cases with an increase in the ABI from 0.56 ± 0.11 to 0.95 ± 0.14. All patients were given ticlopidine (250 mg/day) and aspirin (100 mg/day) for 1 month, and aspirin alone thereafter.

Table 13.5 Results (2)

	Lesion Length Before Stent (mm)	Stented Lesion Length (mm)	Mean Percent of Covering
Global population	104.1	114.7	110.2
Iliac	59.2	63.8	107.8
Femoral	140.9	155.2	110.1
Popliteal	92	112	121.7

COMPLICATIONS

In the first 30 days there were 18 major complications. At the puncture site, five complications occurred:

- two hematomas, one requiring surgery;
- two pseudoaneurysms, both requiring surgery;
- one local thrombosis treated by thrombolysis.

At the iliac level, four complications occurred (6.2%):

- one stent-graft thrombosed within 24 hours (this was associated with distal embolization, treated by surgical thrombectomy);
- one patient who had two stent-grafts placed for treatment of a right iliac occlusion presented 15 days post-procedure with left leg claudication (angiography demonstrated partial obstruction of the left common iliac artery by one of the stent-grafts, which protruded slightly into the aorta; a new stent-graft was placed in the left common iliac artery with a good result);
- two arteries thrombosed and were treated with success by new PTA.

At the femoropopliteal level:

- one patient developed distal embolization after recanalization of an 8 cm long femoral occlusion, treated by thrombolysis and thromboaspiration (this patient died of an acute myocardial infarction on the third postoperative day);
- seven stent-graft thromboses occurred within 24 hours of the procedure (three were treated by thrombolysis and thromboaspiration and four required surgical bypass; five of the lesions were longer than 15 cm);
- one stent-graft thrombosis occurred on day 8, requiring surgical bypass.

Finally, a complication that appears to be directly linked with this type of endoprosthesis is the rapid development of fever along with pain in the region of the implant that can last from 2 to 3 weeks. However, no infection has been found in these cases and consequently the etiology of this phe-nomenon is still uncertain. This was observed 29 times (18.6%): 25 times at the femoropopliteal level (occlusion, $n = 15$; stenosis, $n = 7$; aneurysm, $n = 3$) and four times at the iliac level (occlusion, $n = 1$; stenosis, $n = 3$). There could be a relation between this phenomenon and lesion length, as it appears to be more frequent as the lesion length increases; however, the condition appears to be self-limiting.

FOLLOW-UP

All patients were followed up by duplex scan on day 180 and every 6 months thereafter. At 6 months, a follow-up angiography was performed. The maximum follow-up was 60 months, the mean follow-up 36.9 ± 17.9 months.

RESTENOSIS

- At the iliac level, one restenosis occurred outside the stent and was treated with success by new PTA.
- At the femoropopliteal level, eight patients (8.6%) developed a restenosis, regardless of the stents placed at this extremity. Restenosis inside the stent was not observed. Of these eight restenoses, seven were treated by new angioplasty and three had an additional stent-graft placement. One patient was treated surgically with a bypass.

PSEUDOANEURYSMS

In three patients small pseudoaneurysms were detected at the end of the stent-graft. In two cases they were treated by the placement of an additional short stent-graft. The third patient, however, was only monitored medically due to the small size of the aneurysm.

LATE THROMBOSIS

- At the iliac level, no late thrombosis was observed.
- At the femoropopliteal level, 18 patients (19.6%) had graft thrombosis. One was recanalized percutaneously, 3 were treated by surgical thrombectomy, 10 required bypass graft placement, and 4 refused surgery and were treated medically. Of these lesions, 12 were longer than 15 cm.

LONG-TERM FOLLOW-UP

The long-term patencies at 60 months are shown in Figs 13.5–13.11 and Tables 13.6–13.13 (primary and secondary patencies).

IN THE LITERATURE

Several series were published with the Cragg Endopro System 1/Passager™. Scheinert et al[61] analyzed the primary and long-term results of 48 endoprostheses implanted in the iliac artery in 39 patients for long iliac occlusions ($n = 22$), aneurysms ($n = 16$), perforation ($n = 1$). The primary patency was 89.7% at 6 months, 87.1% at 12 months and 84.2% at 24 months. The secondary patency was 94.9% at 6, 92.1% at 12 and 24 months, respectively.

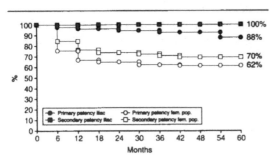

Fig. 13.5 Primary and secondary patencies: iliac–femoropopliteal.

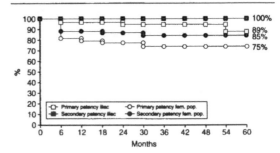

Fig. 13.8 Primary and secondary patencies (lesions <100 mm): iliac–femoropopliteal.

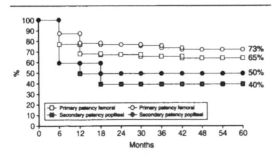

Fig. 13.6 Primary and secondary patencies: femoral–popliteal.

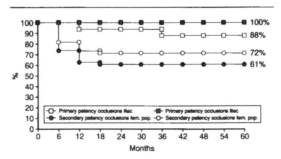

Fig. 13.9 Primary and secondary patencies (occlusions): iliac–femoropopliteal.

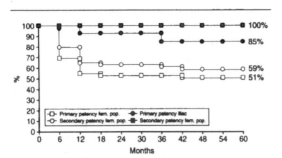

Fig. 13.7 Primary and secondary patencies (lesions ≥100 mm): iliac–femoropopliteal.

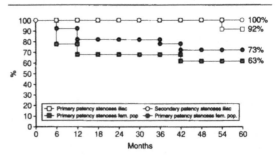

Fig. 13.10 Primary and secondary patencies (stenoses): iliac–femoropopliteal.

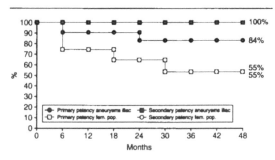

Fig. 13.11 Primary and secondary patencies (aneuryms): iliac–femoropopliteal.

Table 13.6 Primary and Secondary Patencies: Iliac–Femoropopliteal (60 months)

Iliac
Primary patency: 88%   Secondary patency: 100%

Femoropopliteal
Primary patency: 62%   Secondary patency: 70%

Table 13.7 Primary and Secondary Patencies: Femoral–Popliteal (60 months)

Femoral
Primary patency: 65%   Secondary patency: 73%

Popliteal
Primary patency: 40%   Secondary patency: 50%

Table 13.8 Primary and Secondary Patencies (Lesions ≥100 mm): Iliac–Femoropopliteal (60 months)

Iliac
Primary patency: 85%   Secondary patency: 100%

Femoropopliteal
Primary patency: 51%   Secondary patency: 59%

Table 13.9 Primary and Secondary Patencies (Lesions <100 mm): Iliac–Femoropopliteal (60 months)

Iliac
Primary patency: 89%   Secondary patency: 100%

Femoropopliteal
Primary patency: 75%   Secondary patency: 85%

Table 13.10 Primary and Secondary Patencies (Occlusions): Iliac–Femoropopliteal (60 months)

Iliac
Primary patency: 88%   Secondary patency: 100%

Femoropopliteal
Primary patency: 61%   Secondary patency: 72%

Table 13.11 Primary and Secondary Patencies (Stenoses): Iliac–Femoropopliteal (60 months)

Iliac
Primary patency: 92%   Secondary patency: 100%

Femoropopliteal
Primary patency: 63%   Secondary patency: 73%

Table 13.12 Primary and Secondary Patencies (Aneurysms): Iliac–Femoropopliteal (48 months)

Iliac
Primary patency: 84%   Secondary patency: 100%

Femoropopliteal
Primary patency: 55%   Secondary patency: 55%

Table 13.13 Long-Term Patencies at 60 Months

	Primary Patency (%)	Secondary Patency (%)
Iliac		
Global	88	100
Lesions ≥10 cm	85	100
Lesions <10 cm	89	100
Occlusions	88	100
Stenoses	92	100
Aneurysms	84	100
Femoropopliteal		
Global	62	70
Lesions ≥10 cm	51	59
Lesions <10 cm	75	85
Occlusions	61	72
Stenoses	63	73
Aneurysms	55	55
Femoral	65	73
Popliteal	40	50

Link et al[62] treated an iliac occlusion and 15 high grade iliac stenoses with a cumulative patency rate of 71% at 12 months.

Dorffner et al[63] reported a series of 14 aneurysms in 13 patients (common iliac artery = 6; external iliac artery = 1; hypogastric artery = 1; femoral artery = 2; popliteal artery = 4). In all cases, the aneurysm was successfully occluded after stent implantation. The primary and secondary patency rates at 6 months were 93% and 100% respectively.

An arterial rupture of the external iliac artery during balloon angioplasty was treated successfully with the prosthesis by Formichi et al.[64]

Beregi et al[65] reported a series of 19 aneurysms (iliac = 7; subclavian = 5; femoral = 3; popliteal = 3; carotid = 1) treated with the same prosthesis with a successful aneurysm occlusion in 18 of the 19 patients. At 1 year, the stent was patent in 13 patients (68%) and the aneurysm excluded in 17 (89%).

Scheinert et al[66] reported a series of 48 iliac aneurysms treated with 53 endoprostheses. Complete occlusion of the aneurysm was achieved in 47 of the 48 cases (97.9%). Primary patency rates were 100% after 1 year, 97.9% after 2 years, 94.9% after 3 years and 87.6% after 4 years. No secondary leaks were observed.

Cormier et al[67] treated 34 iliac aneurysms (mean diameter 42 mm); three procedures were carried out under emergency conditions after acute rupture. The technical success was 97.6%

Scheinert et al[68] reported a series of 20 catheter-included iliac artery injuries treated with these covered stents. An immediate exclusion of the lesion was achieved in all cases, but within 24 hours fever (55%), elevations in white blood cell count (50%) and C-reactive protein (65%) were seen in the majority of patients. Two restenoses appeared at the outlet of the endografts, successfully treated with balloon angioplasty. Primary and secondary patency rates of 87% and 100% respectively were achieved for a median 21 months' follow-up.

Muller-Hulsbeck et al[69] treated 23 patients with stenoses or occlusions of the pelvic or femoral arteries with 31 stent-grafts. Angiography and intravascular ultrasound (IVUS) of the stented artery were performed 13.9 ± 9.7 months after stent implantation. The maximum in stent restenosis was 53.2 ± 26.5% for femoral and 14.2 ± 10.1 for pelvic arterial stent-grafts. Pre-dilation sites of maximum neointimal tissue accumulation were the edges of the femoral stent-grafts in contrast to pelvic stent-grafts.

THE CORVITA™ ENDOLUMINAL GRAFT[70-72]

STENT-GRAFT CONSTRUCTION

The Corvita™ endoluminal graft (Fig. 13.12) is a self-expanding endoluminal vascular prosthesis with an introducer system that makes it a low-profile device and permits percutaneous delivery and deployment.

The integrated endoluminal graft consists of two components: a self-expanding cylindrical wire structure and a highly porous and elastic coating of spun 13 µm thin Corethane™ (polycarbonate urethane; The Polymer Technology Group, Berkeley, CA) fibers in which blood can coagulate and seal

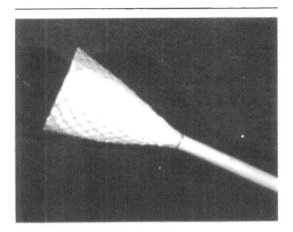

Fig. 13.12 Corvita™ endoluminal graft.

the Corvita™ endoluminal graft to form a new blood-tight vessel wall. The Corethane™ coating is glued on the inside of the metallic structure.

STENT-GRAFT IMPLANTATION

The endoluminal graft can be cut to length with surgical scissors and mounted in the tip of an introducer sheath. For that purpose, the Corvita™ endoluminal graft is manually compressed to one-fifth or one-sixth of its original expanded diameter and inserted into the introducer sheath. It is then loaded into and deployed from a delivery system consisting of an internal sheath and a coaxial catheter which is introduced inside the sheath and therefore helps to release the endoluminal graft precisely at the predetermined placement site. The introducer sheath with the compressed Corvita™

endoluminal graft in the tip can be introduced transfemorally as well as over a guidewire into the arterial system and advanced under continual fluoroscopic visualization to the site of the lesion. The Corvita™ endoluminal graft can be released from the introducer sheath at the intended site by coaxial introduction of a holding catheter and by slowly withdrawing the introducer sheath. The exact placement of the Corvita™ endoluminal graft can still be corrected during the initial release process. The flexibility of this device allows its implantation using various approaches such as the ipsilateral femoral, the contralateral or the popliteal approach, and in tortuous arteries.

OUR EXPERIENCE

PATIENT POPULATION

Sixty-four patients (51 males, 13 females), mean age 65.1 ± 9.8 years (range 39–86 years) were treated with the Corvita™ endoluminal graft. All patients presented with lower limb arterial disease. According to Fontaine's classification, 10 were in stage IIa (patients with aneurysms), 52 were in stage IIb, and 2 were in stage III. At the distal arterial level, 6 patients had only one patent leg vessel, 36 had two patent vessels, and 22 had three patent vessels.

LESION CHARACTERISTICS

Table 13.14 summarizes the localization of the lesions following their etiology. We treated 27 stenoses (iliac, $n = 18$; femoropopliteal, $n = 9$), 20 occlusions (iliac, $n = 8$; femoropopliteal, $n = 12$),

---

Table 13.14 Corvita™ Endoluminal Graft: Lesion Characteristics (1)

Location	No.	Stenoses	Occlusions	Aneurysms
Iliac	38	18	8	12
Femoral	22	8	12	2
Popliteal	3	–	–	3
Bypass	1	1	–	–
Total	64	27	20	17

and 17 aneurysms (iliac, $n = 12$; femoropopliteal, $n = 5$) (Figs 13.13–13.16). The mean length of the lesions was 80.5 ± 55.2 mm (range 20–300 mm). At the iliac level, the mean length was 60.5 ± 28.3 mm (range 20–150 mm) and at the femoropopliteal level it was 109.7 ± 70.7 mm (range 20–300 mm).

Table 13.15 shows the average percent stenoses and the mean arterial diameter before PTA.

REASONS FOR STENTING

- Long residual stenoses: 31;
- Dissections: 7;

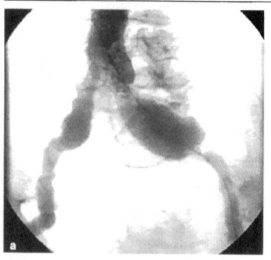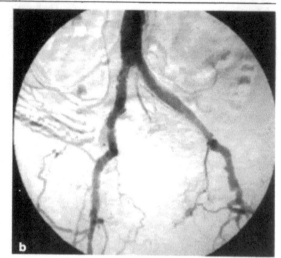

Figs 13.13 (a, b) Bilateral iliac aneurysms.
Result after placement of a Corvita™ stent.

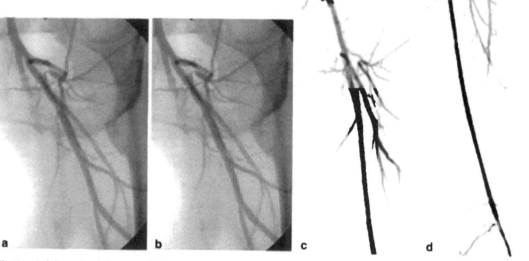

Fig. 13.14 Left femoral occlusion: recanalization.
Result after placement of a Corvita™ stent.

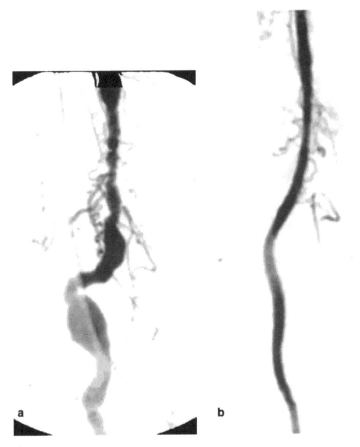

Fig. 13.15 Femoropopliteal aneurysm.

Result after placement of a Corvita™ stent.

Table 13.15 Corvita™ Endoluminal Graft: Lesion Characteristics (2)		
Mean percent stenosis before PTA		
Overall population	77.9 ± 8.4%	(50–100)
Iliac	75.5 ± 8.6%	(50–100)
Femoropopliteal	83.3 ± 5.0%	(80–100)
Mean arterial diameter		
Overall population	8.1 ± 1.5 mm	(5–14)
Iliac	8.5 ± 1.6 mm	(7–14)
Femoropopliteal	7.4 ± 1.2 mm	(5–10)

PTA, percutaneous transluminal angioplasty.

- Restenoses: 6;
- Ulcerated lesions: 3;
- Aneurysms: 17.

TECHNIQUE

The lesion was always treated by the percutaneous approach with an 8–12F introducer through the following approaches:

- Ipsilateral: 52 patients;
- Contralateral: 12 patients.

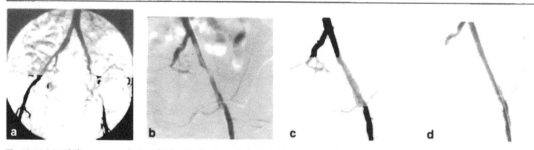

Fig. 13.16 (a) Left iliac artery occlusion. (b) Result after thrombolysis. (c) Result after balloon angioplasty. (d) Final result.

TREATMENT OF THE LESION

Twenty occlusions were treated either with a hydrophilic guidewire ($n = 11$) or an excimer laser fiber ($n = 9$). Balloon angioplasty was always performed with a balloon diameter equal to that of the artery. Twenty-seven stenoses were treated with balloon angioplasty. Seventeen aneurysms were treated. In six cases, an associated stenosis was treated with balloon angioplasty after placement of the Corvita™ endoluminal graft.

IMPLANTED STENTS

Seventy-five stents were implanted (length 40–230 mm, diameter 5–14 mm). Two stents were implanted in the same artery in five femoral and two iliac arteries, and three stents in two iliac arteries.

The diameter of the stent was chosen so that it was 10–20% larger than the diameter of the artery. Its length was at least equal to the length of the lesion, because it is important to cover the entire length of the lesion. Also, the stent should be implanted on a safe segment.

The stent was always dilated at the end of the procedure so as to obtain a good expansion and a good anchorage to the arterial wall. An endovascular ultrasound study was performed during and at the end of the procedure in several cases to check the expansion of the stent and to look for residual lesions.

FOLLOW-UP

All patients were followed up by echo Doppler the day after the procedure, on day 30, on day 180, and every 6 months thereafter. At 6 months, follow-up angiography was performed.

ADJUNCT TREATMENT

All of our procedures were performed using 5000–10,000 units of intravenous heparin as bolus. The patients were given ticlopidine (250 mg/day) and aspirin (100 mg/day) for 1 month. Thereafter, they were given aspirin alone (250 mg/day).

RESULTS

- *Immediate results:* Immediate technical success was obtained in all patients (100%). The ABI increased from 0.60 ± 0.05 to 0.98 ± 0.03. Table 13.16 shows the mean percent stenosis at the iliac and the femoropopliteal level before and after PTA and after stenting. Significant stenosis still persisted after PTA, but there was no significant stenosis after stent placement.
- *Early complications:* We reported:
  — seven early thromboses:

    (a) two at the iliac level: one after treatment of a large aneurysm, which was treated using a Fogarty™ catheter (Edwards Lifesciences, Irvine, CA) and patency was rapidly restored, the other after treatment of a long stenosis, which was successfully treated by new PTA;

    (b) four at the femoral level after treatment of lesions longer than 15 cm: three were treated by bypass and one by new PTA;

    (c) one at the popliteal level after treatment of an aneurysm; it was successfully treated by thromboaspiration and repeat angioplasty.

Table 13.16 Corvita™ Endoluminal Graft: Immediate Results

	Mean Percent Stenosis Before PTA	Mean Percent Stenosis After PTA	Mean Percent Stenosis After Stenting
Overall population	77.9 ± 8.4	39 ± 3.7	3.1 ± 1.9
Iliac	75.5 ± 8.6	41 ± 4.2	3 ± 2.6
Femoropopliteal	83.3 ± 5.0	35 ± 4.9	2 ± 1.9

PTA, percutaneous transluminal angiography.

— one distal embolism in the deep femoral artery after treatment of an iliac aneurysm, successfully treated using a Fogarty catheter;

— two hematomas at the puncture site that resolved spontaneously;

— one patient with two 12 cm long prostheses in the superficial femoral artery developed a fever along with pain in the leg for 3 weeks; these prostheses thrombosed at 2 months.

LONG-TERM FOLLOW-UP

The maximum follow-up period of our patients was 32 months, mean follow-up period was 20.3 ± 10 months.

RESTENOSIS

We reported four restenoses:

• two at the iliac level: one was treated by bypass and the other was treated successfully by new PTA;
• one at the femoral level treated by bypass;
• one at the popliteal level treated by a new PTA and successful placement of an Instent™ (Medtronic, Minneapolis, MN) stent.

In three patients, restenoses were located at the extremities of the endoprosthesis, and one inside the prosthesis (iliac).

LATE THROMBOSIS

We reported five late thromboses:

• one at the iliac level treated by bypass;
• three at the femoral level: two were treated by new PTA with success and one surgically (bypass);
• one at the popliteal level after treatment of an aneurysm; this patient refused surgery and was treated medically.

PATENCY RATES

Primary and secondary patency rates at 3-year follow-up are listed in Table 13.17.

Table 13.17 Primary Patency and Secondary Patency at 3-Year Follow-Up

	Primary Patency (%)	Secondary Patency (%)
Global	74	86
Iliac		
Global	87	95
Lesions ≥10 cm	100	100
Lesions <10 cm	85	94
Stenosis	83	94
Occlusion	88	88
Aneurysm	92	100
Femoropopliteal		
Global	55	72
Lesions ≥10 cm	55	64
Lesions <10 cm	54	82
Stenosis	78	78
Occlusion	31	64
Aneurysm	57	78

THE HEMOBAHN™ STENT

The prograft Hemobahn™ (Fig. 13.17) is a self-expanding endovascular stent-graft composed of 30 μm internodal ultrathin-wall polytetrafluoroethylene (PTFE) graft on the inner surface and a self-expanding nitinol stent on the outer surface. These devices have excellent flexibility in both the deployed and the non-deployed state, excellent kink resistance, and good radial stiffness. Devices available in the initial study ranged from 4.5 to 12 mm in diameter with lengths from 5 to 15 cm. An initial feasibility study[73] addressing iliac and femoral artery occlusive disease was performed at 3 investigational sites in the US and in 12 European centers. In total, 93 patients had 100 lesions treated (iliac 58, femoral 42). The current mean implant duration was 5.4 months. The primary technical success in this group was 99%. The primary and secondary iliac patency at 1 month ($n = 49$), 3 months ($n = 43$), and 6 months ($n = 24$) was 96% at all intervals. The primary patency for treated femoral arteries at 1 month ($n = 37$), 3 months ($n = 24$) and 6 months ($n = 7$) was 100%, 91%, and 80%, respectively. The corresponding secondary patency in the femoral region was 100%, 94%, and 82% at 1 month, 3 months, and 6 months of follow-up.

Procedure-related complications have included distal embolization in 5%, groin hematoma in 2%, and iliac artery rupture in 1%. The last case was successfully managed with deployment of a second stent-graft without clinical sequelae.

Lammer et al[74] reported a study of 127 patients treated for symptomatic peripheral arterial occlusive disease (iliac, $n = 61$ limbs; femoral, $n = 141$ limbs). Endoprosthesis deployment was successful in all patients. Primary patency rates in iliac arteries were 98 ± 3% and 91 ± 4% at 6 and 12 months respectively, and at femoral level 90 ± 3% and 79 ± 5% at 6 and 12 months respectively. Secondary patency rates were 95% and 93% for iliac and femoral arteries respectively at 12 months.

Bauermeister[75] treated 25 patients with long segment occlusions of the femoropopliteal arteries with the Hemobahn™ stent-graft (median occlusion length 22 cm). Primary and secondary patency rates were 73.2% and 82.6% respectively at 1 year.

Bleyn[76] reported a series of 65 patients (67 limbs) with a mean femoral occlusion length of 14.3 cm. The primary patency rates were 80% at 1 year and 55.6% at 4 years; secondary patency rates were 88.7% at 1 year and 77.8% at 4 years. The new generation of this endoprosthesis (Viabahn™) could give better results.

THE WALLGRAFT™ STENT

This prosthesis consists of a Wallstent coated with polyester yarn (PET) (Figs 13.18, 13.19). The

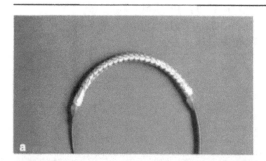
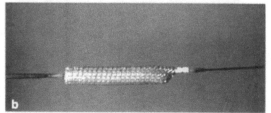

Fig. 13.17 (a, b) The Hemobahn™ stent.

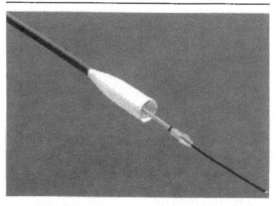

Fig. 13.18 The Wallgraft™ stent.

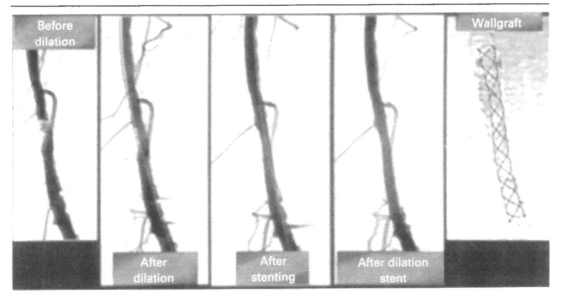

Fig. 13.19 Ulcerated, calcified stenosis of the left superficial femoral artery.
Result after dilation and placement of a Wallgraft™ stent.

available diameters range from 6 to 12 mm, and the lengths from 5 to 7 cm. Its flexibility allows use in tortuous arteries and even through a contralateral approach. Its shortening, however, may render precise placement difficult.

We have used this prosthesis in 10 patients to treat occlusive or aneurysmal diseases in the iliac ($n = 3$), femoral ($n = 3$), popliteal ($n = 2$), radial ($n = 1$), and carotid ($n = 1$) arteries. All prostheses remain patent at a mean of 16 months' follow-up (3–41 months).

Steinkamp et al[77] implanted 24 prostheses in 16 patients in iliac arteries to treat large dissections ($n = 9$), arterial perforations ($n = 4$), and aneurysms ($n = 3$). The secondary patency rate was 94.1%.

Kumins et al[78] successfully treated three iliac embolic lesions responsible for blue toe syndrome with no recurrence after 16 months.

THE JOSTENT™ STENT

The Jostent™ stent (Figs 13.20, 13.21) is a balloon expandable prosthesis. It is available in lengths ranging from 28 to 58 mm and its expansion diam-

eter ranges from 5 to 10 mm. It consists of a double thin stainless steel prosthesis. There is a PTFE coating between the two prostheses.

We have implanted this stent with success in the iliac and femoral arteries in 20 patients with the same indications as for other covered stents. A popliteal implantation in a flexion area such as the popliteal artery should be avoided because of potential compression.

Liistro et al[79] reported a case of a thrombus-containing iliac lesion treated with a Jostent™ stent with good follow-up at 6 months.

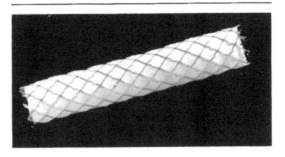

Fig. 13.20 The Jostent™ covered stent.

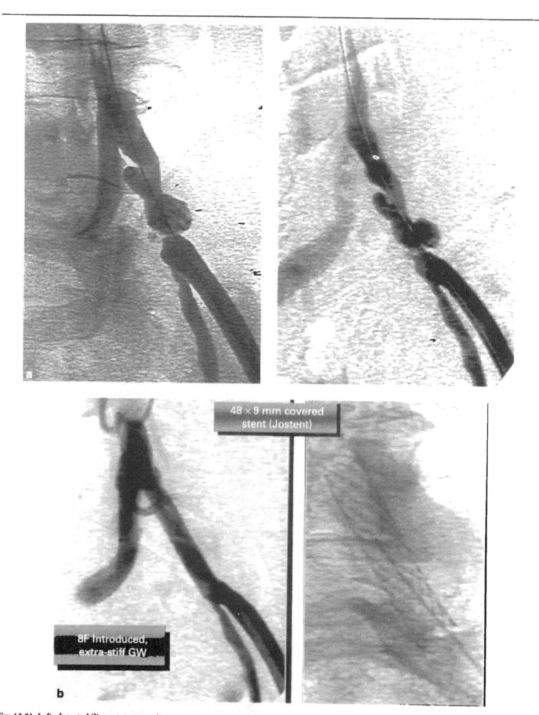

Figs 13.21 Left ulcerated iliac artery stenosis.

(a) Before angioplasty. (b) Result after placement of a Jostent™ stent. GW, guidewire.

THE ASPIRE™ COVERED STENT

The aSpire™ stent (Vascular Architects, San José, CA) (Fig. 13.22) is shaped into a spiral design and is fully covered by PTFE. It provides good radial strength, flexibility, and conformability. The spiral design preserves smooth laminar flow, maintains natural compliance, withstands torsional stress, and protects side branches of the lumen.

In a multicenter study published by Martin et al,[80] 34 patients (36 lesions) were treated with this stent for total occlusion or critical stenosis of the common or external iliac artery or the superficial femoral artery. The average length of the lesions was 16.7 cm (range 1–33 cm). Sixty-two stents were successfully deployed. Mean follow-up was 5 months with a primary patency rate of 94%.

The early results of this study confirmed the safety and early efficacy of the aSpire™ stent.

CAROTID ANGIOPLASTY AND STENTING: INDICATIONS FOR COVERED STENTS

Self-expandable stents have been providing excellent results when treating most cases of carotid stenosis. With cerebral protection, the neurologic complication rate is reduced by 60%. However, brain embolisms may occur even with brain protection, and delayed embolic post-procedure events

may also occur. With soft plaques there may be herniation of cholesterol material through the net of the metallic stent. The migration of the plaque material through the mesh may go on for several days after the insertion of the stent and thus produce these delayed embolisms and strokes.

Covered stent-grafts have been proposed to treat these high-risk embolism plaques.[81] They can seal the plaque completely and also eliminate the risk of the stent being crossed by the cholesterol material. Covered stents can also exclude thrombi from the lumen of a vessel.[79]

Several covered stent-grafts may be used. The Jostent™ stent-graft is a balloon expandable stent and its precise delivery makes it preferable when treating lesions at the ostium of the common carotid and brachiocephalic trunk.

Self-expandable stents such as the Wallgraft™ are more resistant to external compression and adapt better to areas where flexion may occur such as carotid bifurcation. Moreover, if this stent is delivered across the bifurcation, the flow of the external carotid artery may be jeopardized. To address this, designs are currently being developed to provide partial covering of the stent which will maintain the flow toward the external carotid artery, while sealing the internal carotid plaque.[81]

Covered stents have also been proposed in other indications:

- carotid aneurysms with their risk of brain embolism;[82]
- carotid pseudoaneurysms which are more common than true aneurysms, being usually iatrogenic or post-traumatic.[83–86]

A covered stent has also been used to seal a pseudoaneurysm which had developed at the site of an infected anastomosis between the carotid and the subclavian artery[87] as well as in the following situations:

- severe or extensive disruption of the vessel wall;[88]
- arteriovenous carotid to jugular fistula;[89]
- aneurysms in Behçet's disease;[86]
- dissection which may occasionally follow iatrogenic catheter injury or spontaneous trauma.

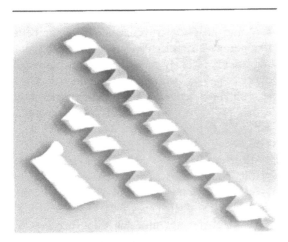

Fig. 13.22 The aSpire™ covered stent.

SUBCLAVIAN AND VERTEBRAL ANGIOPLASTY AND STENTING: INDICATIONS FOR COVERED STENTS

Covered stents may be indicated to treat specific lesions of the subclavian and vertebral arteries:

- aneurysm[90] or pseudoaneurysm;[91]
- traumatic artery injury;[92]
- spontaneous arterial rupture or dissection.[93]

OTHER INDICATIONS FOR COVERED STENTS

Covered stents may be indicated in the following situations.

- *Renal arteries* in cases of aneurysms not involving a large collateral branch, or pseudoaneurysm or arteriovenous fistula, or in cases of arterial rupture during renal angioplasty. We have used a Jomed covered stent to treat successfully two cases of rupture of a renal artery avoiding surgery.
- *Digestive arteries* with the same indications as for renal arteries.
- *Hemodialysis access.* Covered stents (e.g. Cragg stents[94]) are effective in controlling angioplasty-induced rupture and sometimes for maintaining patency after restenosis in another stent such as the Wallstent™, but they do not prevent restenosis for de novo lesions. Aneurysm or pseudoaneurysm of hemodialysis access may also be treated with covered stents.

DISCUSSION

PTA is the first treatment to be proposed for peripheral vascular diseases but before offering a patient with intermittent claudication the option of any invasive therapy, we must take into account the following considerations of TASC recommendation 21:[41]

- A predicted or observed lack of adequate response to exercise therapy and risk factor modification;

- Presence of severe disability, either being unable to perform normal work, or having a very serious impairment of other activities important to the patient;
- Absence of other disease that would limit exercise even if the claudication is improved (e.g. angina or chronic respiratory disease);
- The individual's anticipated natural history and prognosis;
- The morphology of the lesion must be such that the appropriate intervention would have low risk and high probability of initial and long-term success.

Multiple clinical risk factors have been identified to increase the risk of restenosis or occlusion following angioplasty.[95-97] In general, PTA is more successful with short lesions in large vessels (>6 mm diameter). It is also known that patients with long lesions (>10 cm), especially in the femoral artery, or patients with poor initial angioplasty results (significant residual stenosis, irregular lesion) do much worse, with patency rates as low as 20% at 5 years. Restenosis rates are also lower with concentric lesions instead of markedly eccentric, non-ostial stenosis, and stenoses versus occlusions (given equal lesion length) and for claudication than limb salvage. Clark et al in the STAR registry[98] identified important promoting factors for long-term patency after femoral global angioplasty. The absence of diabetes is a significant predictor of long-term success, and may be partly accounted for the better tibioperoneal runoff. Patients with renal failure were twice as likely to occlude following angioplasty as patients without renal failure. Clark et al also observed better results in patients presenting with short lesions, non-calcified lesions, and good runoff. With poor runoff, the 3-year patency rate is 40%, with good runoff, 92% (p <0.001).

The number of sites dilated is also an important predicting factor. If one or two sites are dilated, the 3-year patency rate is 87%, but is 74% if more than three sites are dilated (p = 0.04). In their studies, Clark et al did not find any difference between stenosis and occlusion; however, the post-angioplasty results seem to play a role. Residual stenosis and dissection affect the long-term results. For Dutzel et al[99] predictors of restenosis at femoral level included lesion length and tobacco use. Alternative revascularization methods such as laser and atherectomy have not in general improved the long-term patency of occlusive lesions.

Endoprostheses have been proposed and implanted at different levels, not only to deal with acute problems of an angioplasty (dissection, residual stenosis, poor cosmetic results, recoil, occlusive threat, etc.) but also to try to improve the long-term results. These stents are not equivalent and all have different properties and characteristics which may influence the long-term results.

STENT SELECTION

Many factors must be considered during stent selection for patients in different clinical situations. Knowledge of the various stent types and their individual properties is a necessity. In addition, selection depends on adequate peri-procedural evaluation of the lesion, the access site, the use of primary direct stenting or selective stent placement, the lesion location and characteristics, the stent availability, and the experience of the operator.

ILIAC LEVEL

At the iliac level, with PTA alone, we can expect a 5-year patency rate of 70%.[100] Stent implantation may improve these results. After performing a meta-analysis of 14 studies that included more than 2000 patients, Bosch and Hunink[27] concluded that PTA with stent placement lowered the risk of long-term failure by 39% compared with the risk of PTA alone.

In the majority of the published series of iliac stenting, the long-term results are encouraging and similar to those of surgery with a mean primary patency rate of 75% and a mean secondary patency rate of about 90%.[6–10,15,16,40–45] Current data indicate no obvious differences with the use of different types of stent with regard to technical success rates and follow-up.[101] All stents can be implanted at iliac level, but some specific indications must be emphasized. Long lesions seem a good indication for covered stents. In our series, the iliac lesions were longer (5–9 cm) than those of series that are usually reported with more covered stents. Despite the length of the segments, primary and secondary patencies were excellent, regardless of the prosthesis used.

Ulcerated lesions, long dissections, and catheter-induced traumatic lesions are perhaps better treated with covered stents. Obviously aneurysms are the best indications for covered stents. To treat an external iliac artery lesion we have to choose flexible, self-expandable stents due to the anatomy of the artery and the risk of compression.

FEMOROPOPLITEAL LEVEL

At the femoropopliteal level, stenting is controversial. According to the 1994 American Heart Association (AHA) guidelines, surgery is the preferred therapy for lesions in categories 3 and 4, as well as PTA for lesions in categories 1 and 2. PTA could be proposed for category 3 lesions for poor surgical patients only. According to the TASC recommendations,[41] type A lesions may be treated by interventional procedures and type D by surgery; however, for types B and C more evidence is needed to make recommendations.

Bypass surgery gives a 5-year patency rate of 60–70% for claudicants, 21–58% for limb salvage and is always at risk particularly for elderly patients. Hunink et al[102] used a decision analysis model based on reported success rates of surgery and angioplasty to determine optimal treatment in a hypothetical cohort of men with femoropopliteal disease. In patients with stenosis and claudication or chronic critical ischemia, angioplasty was superior to surgery in increasing quality adjusted life expectancy and decreasing lifetime expenditures. Surgery was the preferred initial treatment only when chronic critical ischemia was due to an occlusion. However, the authors noted that angioplasty would always be preferable to surgery when 5-year patency rates of at least 30% could be achieved.

Several studies were published with PTA alone.[96,97,102–107] The mean primary patency rate is 51% at 3 years, and 48% at 5 years.

Different stents have been used to treat femoropopliteal lesions and the published data are very disparate, as we reported previously,[101] primary patency ranging from 22% at 1 year[35] with the Wallstent™ to 77% at 2 years with the Palmaz™ stent.[108]

Three randomized studies were published comparing PTA alone and PTA and stent:

- Céjna et al[38] reported a 12-month patency rate of 63.7% with PTA, 62.7% with PTA and stent ($p = 0.31$).
- Vroegindeweij et al[39] reported rates of 74% and 62% respectively ($p = 0.22$).
- Zdanowski et al[40] treated 32 patients with occlusion and reported a restenosis rate of 25% after PTA, 50% after stenting ($p = 0.03$).

If these studies do not support femoropopliteal stenting as a primary approach and lead to the same conclusions as the TASC consensus document,[41] stents may have a limited role in salvage of acute PTA, failure or complications. However, we must point out that these studies were carried out with Palmaz™, Wallstent™ and Strecker™ stents and not with the new generation of stents, particularly nitinol stents and those for short lesions.

The stent design greatly influences outcome and the superficial femoral and the popliteal artery have some particularities. Flexion and elongation of the artery occurs constantly in association with movement of the leg. The common femoral artery and the popliteal artery cross a joint. In these locations and at the Hunter canal level, there is a risk of stent fatigue, fracture and compression. The ideal stent might be self-expanding stent (no external compression) which should bend in concert with the artery (joint flexion), respond to flexion and elongation and reduce the risk of stent fatigue and fracture (absence of joints or bonding points). Covered stents except Jostent™ (balloon expandable) have some of these characteristics.

In femoropopliteal arteries, covered prostheses were used for long lesions greater than 10 cm (three to four times longer than non-covered endoprostheses). The results obtained with these long covered endoprostheses in femoropopliteal arteries are still linked with high thrombotic complication rates. These complications were usually treated by an interventional technique (thrombolysis or angioplasty). The secondary patency therefore remains satisfactory with regard to the treated lesions. However, the results seem more favorable for lesions smaller than 10 cm, and also more favorable for femoral lesions than for popliteal lesions. The use of covered endoprostheses in femoropopliteal arteries is therefore crucial: first, in the interest represented by the use of the stent itself, and second, for the surface it covers. The stent portion of the device provides mechanical enlargement of the arterial lumen. The stent-graft is flexible and expandable so that compression and moderate bending in the femoropopliteal segment do not compromise the integrity of the graft. Since the stent is fully supported, kinking and external compression (which can occur with a rigid stent) do not happen with these prostheses. The graft covering acts as a barrier to smooth muscle ingrowth. In this fashion, a true endoluminal bypass can be created.

Nevertheless, restenosis is still possible despite this type of stent. With the Cragg Endopro System 1 or Passager™, we have only seen restenoses at the extremities of the prosthesis, which could be easily dilated, whereas with the Corvita™ endoluminal graft, in-stent restenoses were possible due to its greater porosity.

TECHNIQUES AND TREATMENT

Our technique for graft placement has evolved with practice. The following are important points that we have learned during our initial stent-graft experience.

Prior to stent-graft implantation, the target lesion should be pre-dilated with a balloon approximately 1 mm larger than the nominal arterial diameter. In some cases, such as calcified lesions, rotational atherectomy may be useful to debulk the arteries. It is important to cover the entire lesion with the stent-graft and, if possible, to implant a sufficiently long stent-graft so that both ends are implanted in a relatively normal segment of the artery. Angioplasty should not be performed outside the target lesion to avoid restenosis. Accurate placement of the endoprosthesis can be obtained with the Cragg Endopro System 1/Passager™ and the Hemobahn™, due to the minimal shortening, but can sometimes be difficult with the Corvita™ endoluminal graft since its distal end may be precisely placed but its proximal end may not because of significant shortening during expansion. After stent implantation, it is important to dilate the stent-graft to its nominal diameter. This helps to fully expand the stent and to remove any wrinkles in the fabric that may have occurred during compression and delivery of the graft. When long lesions must be treated with several prostheses, grafts should overlap by approximately 5–10 mm to prevent them from separating from each other. Separation may lead to a false aneurysm that could thrombose, as occurred in one of our cases with the Corvita™ endoluminal graft.

In our experience, better results were obtained with the placement of the stent-graft in the iliac artery versus the femoropopliteal arteries. A number of short- and mid-term thrombotic episodes have occurred that may be related to the thrombogenic nature of the graft, poor flow during ipsilateral compression after sheath removal, inadequate anticoagulation, or other factors. Generally, these episodes were readily treated with a secondary interventional technique such as thrombolysis, mechanical thrombectomy, and PTA. The global secondary patency for these endoprostheses may be considered as encouraging due to the length of the lesions, regardless of the graft used. Nonetheless, significant improvements must be made in the short- and mid-term patency of longer endoluminal grafts. Issues that must be addressed include the short-term thrombogenicity of the implanted graft and the development of restenosis at the ends of the graft. A powerful antiaggregant protocol associating ticlopidine or clopidogrel and aspirin given several days before the procedure seems to have limited early thromboses. In the future, pharmacologic or radiation inhibitors of intimal hyperplasia may allow a broader application of these devices for long-term segment revascularization of the peripheral arterial circulation.

The treatment of aneurysms with covered stents in the iliac and femoropopliteal arteries seems rather easy. The results of our series are very favorable at the iliac level but less favorable at the femoropopliteal level, regardless of the graft used. The simplicity of their use should make these covered grafts the treatment of choice for aneurysmal lesions. We wish to insist that even after a stent occlusion at the femoropopliteal level, there have been no serious ischemic complications or limb loss in our experience.

The phenomenon of pain and fever encountered after implantation of Cragg Endopro System 1/Passager™ is a complication that we still do not fully understand. The phenomenon does not seem to be related to local infection, but it is clearly an inflammatory response to graft implantation.[109] It is likely that the stent-graft itself or one of its fabric or metal components may be an inducer of cytokinins from neutrophils.[109]

We have seen that covered stents may also have good specific indications at other levels: supra-aortic vessels, renal and abdominal arteries, and hemodialysis fistula. More specific devices should be developed to enlarge their indications.

The indications for covered stents are still debated; however, the following indications are not debatable:

- aneurysms;
- arteriovenous fistulae (Fig. 13.23);
- arterial traumas;
- arterial rupture (Fig. 13.24).

Covered stents should be available in all catheterization laboratories in order to quickly treat arterial ruptures that may occur during an angioplasty procedure and thus avoid surgical repair.

Certain indications are more questionable, such as long occlusions or stenoses, long dissections, and ulcerated lesions.

Results obtained with covered stents seem encouraging and the use of new prostheses, with lower thrombotic risks, should allow the treatment of long lesions with success rates and results that are at least as good as those obtained with surgery.

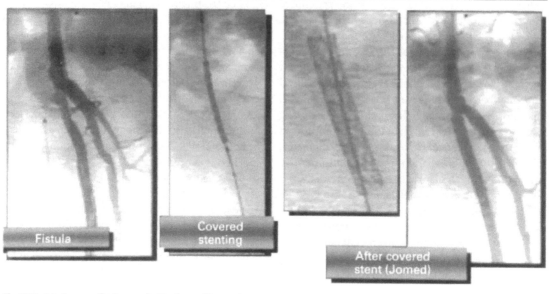

Fig. 13.23 Arteriovenous fistula treated with a Jostent™ covered stent.

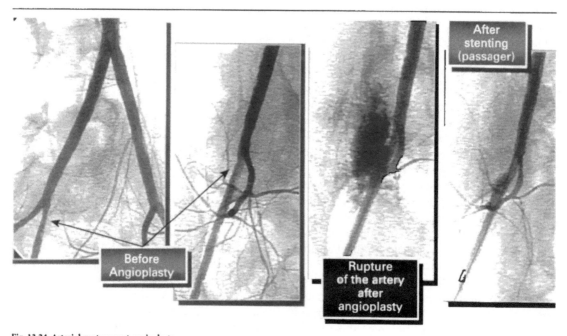

Fig. 13.24 Arterial rupture post-angioplasty.

Treatment with a Passager™ stent.

Results obtained with the Hemobahn™ and the new aSpire™ stent seem promising. New antiplatelet agents and new coated stents will probably improve long-term patencies.

CONCLUSION

Covered endoprostheses allow the operator to perform true internal bypass using the percutaneous access. The indications for their use should broaden and they could become an alternative to surgery. Improvements should come about, particularly with respect to thrombogenicity and the method of implantation. Randomized studies versus surgery and other types of stent are necessary in order to confirm the advantages of these new prostheses and their place as compared to non-covered prostheses.

REFERENCES

1. Johnson KW. Femoral and popliteal arteries: reanalysis of results of balloon angioplasty. Radiology 1992;183:767–71.
2. Capek P, McLean GK, Berkowitz HD. Femoropopliteal angioplasty. Factors influencing long-term success. Circulation 1991;83(suppl I):170–80.
3. Moore WS. Therapeutic options for femoropopliteal occlusive disease. Circulation 1991;83(suppl I):191–3.
4. Dotter CT. Transluminally placed coil-spring endarterial tube grafts: long-term patency in canine popliteal artery. Invest Radiol 1969;4:329–32.
5. Richter GM, Roeren TH, Loeldge G, et al. Superior clinical results of iliac stent placement versus percutaneous transluminal angioplasty: four-year success rates of a randomized study [abstract]. Radiology 1991;181(suppl):161.
6. Henry M, Amor M, Ethevenot G, et al. Palmaz-Schatz stent in the treatment of peripheral vascular diseases: two year follow up. A single center experience [abstract]. Circulation 1992;86:4.
7. Henry M, Amor M, Ethevenot G, et al. Le stent de Palmaz dans le traitement des artériopathies périphériques [in French]. Techno Cœur 1993;117–30.
8. Schatz RA. A view of vascular stents. Circulation 1989;79:445–57.
9. Palmaz JC. Intravascular stents: tissue–stent interactions and design considerations. AJR Am J Roentgenol 1993;160:613–18.
10. Parsson H, Cwikiel W, Johansson K, et al. Deposition of platelets and neutrophils in porcine iliac arteries after angioplasty and Wallstent placement compared with angioplasty alone. Cardiovasc Intervent Radiol 1994;17:190–6.
11. Hallisey MJ, Parker BC, von Breda A. Current status and extended applications of intravascular stents. Curr Opin Radiol 1992;4:7–12.
12. Palmaz JC, Garcia OJ, Schatz RA, et al. Placement of balloon-expandable intraluminal stents in iliac arteries: first 171 procedures. Radiology 1990;174:969–75.
13. Raillat C, Rousseau H, Joffre F, et al. Treatment of iliac artery stenoses with the Wallstent endoprosthesis. AJR Am J Roentgenol 1990;154:613–16.
14. Zollikofer CL, Antonuci F, Pfyffer M, et al. Arterial stent placement with the use of the Wallstent: midterm results of clinical experience. Radiology 1991;179:449–56.
15. Hausegger KA, Lammer J, Hagen B, et al. Iliac artery stenting. Clinical experience with the Palmaz stent, Wallstent and Strecker stent. Acta Radiol 1992;33:292–6.
16. White GH, Liew SCC, Waugh RC, et al. Early outcome and intermediate follow-up of vascular stents in the femoral and popliteal arteries without long-term anticoagulation. J Vasc Surg 1995;21:270–81.
17. Bray AE, Liu WG, Lewis WA, et al. Use of the Strecker stent in the femoropopliteal arteries. J Endovasc Surg 1995;2:150–60.
18. Bergeron P, Pinot JJ, Poyen V, et al. Long-term results with the Palmaz stent in the superficial femoral artery. J Endovasc Surg 1995;2:161–7.
19. Henry M, Amor M, Cragg A, et al. Occlusive and aneurysmal peripheral arterial disease: assessment of a stent-graft system. Radiology 1996;201:717–24.
20. Henry M, Amor M, Henry I, et al. Application of a new covered endoprosthesis in the treatment of occlusive and aneurysmal peripheral arterial diseases [in French]. Arch Mal Cœur Vaiss 1997;90:953–60.
21. Strecker EP, Hagen B, Liermann D, et al. Iliac and femoropopliteal vascular occlusive disease treated with flexible tantalum stents. Cardiovasc Intervent Radiol 1993;16:158–64.
22. Vorwerk D, Guenther RW, Schurmann K, et al. Primary stent placement for chronic iliac artery occlusions: follow-up results in 103 patients. Radiology 1995;194:745–9.
23. Vorwerk D, Guenther RW, Schurmann K, Wendt G. Aortic and iliac stenoses: follow-up results of stent placement after insufficient balloon angioplasty in 118 cases. Radiology 1996;198:45–8.
24. Palmaz JC, Laborde JC, Riviera FJ, et al. Stenting of the iliac arteries with the Palmaz stent: experience from a multicenter trial. Cardiovasc Intervent Radiol 1992;15:291–7.
25. Henry M, Amor M, Ethevenot G, et al. Palmaz stent placement in iliac and femoropopliteal arteries: primary and secondary patency in 310 patients with 2–4 year follow-up. Radiology 1995;197:167–74.
26. Henry M, Amor M, Ethevenot G, et al. Percutaneous endoluminal treatment of iliac occlusions: long-term follow-up in 105 patients. J Endovasc Surg 1998;5:228–35.
27. Bosch JL, Hunink MG. Meta-analysis of the results of percutaneous transluminal angioplasty and stent placement for aortoiliac occlusive disease. Radiology 1997;204:87–96.
28. Tetteroo E, van der Graaf Y, Bosch JL, et al. Randomized comparison of primary stent placement vs primary angioplasty followed by selective stent placement in patients with iliac-artery occlusive disease. Dutch Iliac Stent Study Group. Lancet 1998;351:1153–9.
29. Dake MD, Semba CP, Kee ST, et al. Early results of Hemobahn for the treatment of peripheral arterial disease. In: Ninth International Course Book of Peripheral Vascular Intervention. Endovascular Therapy Course; 1998, May 5–8; Paris, France. Toulouse: Europa Organization, 1998: 259–60.
30. Ohki T, Veith FJ. Endovascular grafts for the treatment of arterial lesions. In: Ninth International Course Book of Peripheral Vascular Intervention. Endovascular Therapy Course; 1998 May 5–8; Paris, France. Toulouse: Europa Organization, 1998: 269–82.
31. Sapoval MR, Long AL, Raynaud AC, et al. Femoropopliteal stent placement: long-term results. Radiology 1992;184:833–9.

32. Rousseau HP, Raillat CR, Joffre F, et al. Treatment of femoropopliteal stenoses by means of self-expandable endoprostheses: midterm results. Radiology 1989;172:961–4.

33. Lierman D, Strecker EP, Peters J. The Strecker stent: indications and results in iliac and femoropopliteal arteries. Cardiovasc Intervent Radiol 1992;15:298–305.

34. Damajaru S, Cuasay L, Le D, et al. Predictors of primary patency failure in Wallstent self-expanding endovascular prostheses for iliofemoral occlusive disease. Tex Heart Inst J 1997;24:173–8.

35. Gray BH, Sullivan TM, Childs MB, et al. High incidence of restenosis-reocclusion of stents in the percutaneous treatment of long segment superficial femoral artery disease after suboptimal angioplasty. J Vasc Surg 1997;25:74–83.

36. Cikrit DF, Dalsing MC. Lower extremity arterial endovascular stenting. Surg Clin North Am 1998;78:617–29.

37. Criado FJ. Endovascular treatment of occlusive lesions in the femoropopliteal territory. In: Criado FJ, ed. Endovascular Intervention: Basic Concepts and Techniques. Armonk, NY: Futura Publishing, 1999: 105–14.

38. Céjna M, Schoder M, Lammer J. PTA vs stent in femoropopliteal obstruction [in German]. Radiologe 1999;39:144–50.

39. Vroegindeweij D, Vos LD, Tielbeek AV, et al. Balloon angioplasty combined with primary stenting vs balloon angioplasty alone in femoropopliteal obstructions: a comparative randomized study. Cardiovasc Intervent Radiol 1997;20:420–5.

40. Zdanowski A, Albrechtsson U, Lundin A. Percutaneous transluminal angioplasty with or without stenting for femoropopliteal occlusions? A randomized controlled study. Int Angiol 1999;18:251–5.

41. TASC Document. J Vasc Surg 2000;31:S1–296.

42. Henry M, Henry I, Klonaris C, Hugel M. Clinical experience with the Optimed sinus stent in the peripheral arteries. J Endovasc Ther 2003;10:772–9.

43. Hayerizadeth BF, Zeller T, Krankenberg H, et al. Superficial femoral artery stenting using nitinol stents. A German multicenter experience in the Paris Course on Revascularization. Paris, May 2002.

44. Cragg AH, Lund G, Rysavy JA, et al. Nonsurgical placement of arterial endoprostheses: a new technique using nitinol wire. Radiology 1983;147:261–83.

45. Cragg AH, Lund G, Rysavy JA, et al. Percutaneous arterial grafting. Radiology 1984;150:45–9.

46. Cragg AH, De Jong SC, Barnhart WH, et al. Nitinol intravascular stent: results of pre-clinical evaluation. Radiology 1993;189:775–8.

47. Cragg AH, Dake MD. Percutaneous femoropopliteal graft placement. J Vasc Intervent Radiol 1993;4:445–63.

48. Parodi JC. Endovascular repair of abdominal aortic aneurysms and other arterial lesions. J Vasc Surg 1995;189:549–57.

49. Diethrich EB, Papazoglou CO, Lundquist P, et al. Early experience with aneurysm exclusion devices and endoluminal bypass prostheses. J Intervent Cardiol 1994;7:108–9.

50. Diethrich EB, Papazoglou CO, Rodriguez-Lopez J, et al. Endoluminal grafts for percutaneous aneurysm exclusion and intraluminal bypass. Circulation 1994;90:I206.

51. Papazoglou C, Lopez-Galarza L, Rodriguez-Lopez J, et al. Endoluminal grafting: the Arizona Heart Institute experience. J Endovasc Surg 1995;2:89–90.

52. Diethrich EB, Papazoglou CO. Endoluminal grafting for aneurysmal and occlusive disease in the superficial femoral artery: early experience. J Endovasc Surg 1995;2:225–39.

53. Papazoglou C, Diethrich EB, Lopez-Galarza L, et al. Percutaneous endoluminal grafting for iliofemoral aneurysmal and occlusive disease [abstract]. J Vasc Intervent Radiol 1995;6:40.

54. Marin ML, Veith FJ, Cynamon J, et al. Transfemoral endovascular stented graft treatment of aortoiliac and femoropopliteal occlusive disease for limb salvage. Am J Surg 1994;168:156–62.

55. Bergeron P. Stenting and endoluminal grafting of femoral and popliteal arteries [abstract]. J Endovasc Surg 1995;2:197–8.

56. Bray A. Superficial femoral endarterectomy with intra-arterial PTFE grafting. J Endovasc Surg 1995;2:297–301.

57. Sanchez LA, Marin ML, Veith FJ, et al. Placement of endovascular stented grafts via remote access sites: a new approach to the treatment of failed aortoiliofemoral reconstructions. Am Vasc Surg 1995;9:1–8.

58. Henry M, Amor M, Ethevenot G, et al. Initial experience with the Cragg Endopro System 1 for intraluminal treatment of peripheral vascular disease. J Endovasc Surg 1994;1:31–43.

59. Henry M, Amor M, Cragg A, et al. Occlusive and aneurysmal peripheral arterial disease: assessment of a stent-graft system. Radiology 1996;201:717–24.

60. Henry M, Amor M, Henry I, et al. Application d'une nouvelle endoprothèse couverte au traitement des artériopathies périphériques occlusives et anévrismales [in French]. Arch Mal Cœur 1997;90:953–60.

61. Scheinert D, Ragg JC, Vogt A, et al. The value of a fabric coated self expanding stent in iliac arterial occlusions or aneurysms. The primary and long-term results. Rofo Fortschr Geb Roentgenstr Nerren Bildgeb Verfahr 1998;169:302–9.

62. Link J, Muller-Hulsbeck S, Hackethal S, et al. Midterm follow up after Cragg stent placement in iliac arteries. Rofo Fortschr Geb Roentgenstr Nerren Bildgeb Verfarh 1997;167:412–7.

63. Dorffner R, Thurnher S, Puig S, et al. Treatment of arterial aneurysms of the pelvic leg vessels using dacron covered nitinol stents. Rofo Fortschr Geb Roentgenstr Nerren Bildgeb Verfahr 1998;168:275–80.

64. Formichi M, Raybaud G, Benichou H, et al. Rupture of the external iliac artery during balloon angioplasty: endovascular treatment using a covered stent. J Endovasc Surg 1998;5:37–41.

65. Beregi JP, Prat A, Willoteaux S, et al. Covered stents in the treatment of peripheral arterial aneurysms: procedural results and mid-term follow up. Cardiovasc Intervent Radiol 1999;22:13–19.

66. Scheinert D, Schroder M, Steinkamp H, et al. Treatment of iliac artery aneurysms by percutaneous implantation of stent grafts. Circulation 2000;102:253–8.

67. Cormier F, Alayoubi A, Laridon D, et al. Endovascular treatment of iliac aneurysms with covered stents. Ann Vasc Surg 2000;14:561–6.

68. Scheinert D, Ludwig J, Steinkamp HJ, et al. Treatment of catheter induced iliac artery injuries with self expanding endografts. J Endovasc Ther 2000;7:213–20.

69. Muller-Hulsbeck S, Schwarzenberg H, Hutzelmann A, et al. Intravascular ultrasound evaluation of peripheral arterial stent grafts. Invest Radiol 2000;35:97–104.

70. Donayre CE, Scoccianti M. Applications in peripheral vascular surgery: traumatic arteriovenous fistulae and pseudoaneurysms. In: Chuter TAM, Donayre CE, White R eds. Endoluminal Vascular Prostheses. Boston: Little, Brown, 1995: 217–55.

71. Dereume JP, Ferreira J, El Douaihy M, et al. Clinical experience with an integrated self-expandable stented graft (Corvita) for the treatment of various arterial lesions. In: Veith FJ, ed. Current Critical Problems in Vascular Surgery, Vol. 6. St. Louis: Quality Medical Publishing, 1995.

72. Dereume JP. Clinical experience with a self-expending endoluminal vascular prosthesis. Presented at Symposium of Vascular Surgery. September 1–2, 1995; Berlin, Germany.

73. Dake MD, Semba CP, Kee ST, et al. Hemobahn: results of a multicenter feasibility study. Presented at International Symposium on Vascular Diagnosis and Intervention. January 11–15, 1998; Miami, FL.

74. Lammer J, Dake MD, Bleyn J, et al. Peripheral arterial obstruction, prospective study of treatment with a transluminally placed self expanding stent graft. Interventional Trial Study Groups. Radiology 2000;217:95–104.

75. Bauermeister G. Endovascular stent grafting in the treatment of superficial femoral artery occlusive disease. J Endovasc Ther 2001;8:315–20.

76. Bleyn J. Superficial femoral artery stenting with Hemobahm. International Stenting Congress XV. February 2002; Scottsdale, AZ.

77. Steinkamp HJ, Werk M, Seibold S, et al. Treatment of arterial traumas by the Wallgraft endoprosthesis. Rofo Fortschr Geb Roentgenstr Nerren Bildgeb Verfahr 2001;173:97–102.

78. Kumins NH, Owens EL, Ogilvie SB, et al. Early experience using the Wallgraft in the management of distal microembolism from common iliac artery pathology. Ann Vasc Surg 2002;16:181–6.

79. Liistro F, Stankovic G, Dimario C, et al. Covered stent to exclude intravascular thrombus. J Endovasc Ther 2002;9:246–9.

80. Martin JD, Schubart P, Moll F, et al. A prospective evaluation of the Aspire covered stent and controlled expansion delivery system for the treatment of peripheral arterial occlusive disease: preliminary results. International Congress XV on Endovascular Interventions. February 2002; Scottsdale, AZ.

81. Inglese L, Calabrese E. Extracranial carotid aneurysm: interventional treatment. In: Henry M et al, eds. Angioplasty and stenting of the carotid and supra-aortic trunks. London: Martin Dunitz, 2004.

82. Mukherjee D, Roffi M, Yadav JS. Endovascular treatment of carotid artery aneurysms with stent grafts. J Endovasc Cardiol 2002;14:269–72.

83. Sangiorgi G, Arbustini E, Lanzarini P, et al. Non biodegradable expanded polytetrafluoroethylene-covered stent implantation in porcine peripheral arteries: histologic evaluation of vascular wall response compared with uncoated stents. Cardiovasc Intervent Radiol 2001;24(4):260–70.

84. Simionato F, Righi C, Melissano G, et al. Stent-graft treatment of a common carotid artery pseudoaneurysm. J Endovasc Ther 2000;7:136–40.

85. Scavee V, De Wispelaere JF, Mormont E, et al. Pseudoaneurysm of the internal carotid artery: treatment with a covered stent. Cardiovasc Intervent Radiol 2001;24:283–5.

86. Park JH, Chung JW, Joh JH, et al. Aortic and arterial aneurysms in Behçet disease: management with stent-grafts: initial experience. Radiology 2001;220(3):745–50.

87. Battaglia L, Bartolucci R, Minacci S, et al. Stent graft repair for rupture of the subclavian artery secondary to infection of a subclavian-to-carotid bypass graft. Ann Vasc Surg 2001;15(4):474–6.

88. Parodu JC, Ferreira LM, Bergan J. Endovascular stent-graft treatment of traumatic arterial lesions. Ann Vasc Surg 1999;13(2):121–9.

89. Geremia G, Bakon M, Brennecke L, et al. Experimental arteriovenous fistulae: treatment with silicone-covered metallic stents. Am J Neuroradiol 1997;18(2):271–7.

90. Eggebrecht H, Bruch C, Haude M, et al. Transluminal exclusion of a subclavian artery aneurysm with stent graft implantation. Z Kardiol 2000;89:761–5.

91. Hernandez JA, Pershad A, Laufer N, et al. Subclavian artery pseudoaneurysm: successful exclusion with a covered self expanding stent. J Invas Cardiol 2002;14:278–9.

92. Stecco K, Meier A, Seiver A, et al. Endovascular stent graft placement for treatment of traumatic penetrating subclavian artery injury. J Trauma 2000;48:948–50.

93. Chiaradio JC, Guzman L, Padilla L, et al. Intravascular graft stent treatment of a ruptured fusiform dissecting aneurysm of the intracranial vertebral artery: technical case report. Neurosurgery 2002;50:213–16.

94. Sapoval MR, Turmel Rodrigues LA, Raynaud AC, et al. Cragg covered stent in hemodialysis access: initial and mid-term results. J Vasc Intern Radiol 1997;7:334–5.

95. Becker GJ. Stent placement for peripheral arterial disease of the lower extremities. J Vasc Interv Radiol 1996;7:180–90.

96. Jeans WD, Armstrong S, Cole SE, et al. Fate of patients undergoing transluminal angioplasty for lower-limb ischemia. Radiology 1990;177:559–64.

97. Murray RR, Hewes RC, White RL, et al. Long-segment femoropopliteal diseases: is angioplasty a boon or a bust? Radiology 1987;162:473–6.

98. Clark T, Groffsky JL, Soulen MC. Determinants of long term patency following femoropopliteal angioplasty: results of the STAR registry. J Vasc Interv Radiol 2001;12:923–33.

99. Dutzel D, Bromet D, Kavinsky C, et al. Superficial femoral artery percutaneous intervention: outcomes in contemporary practice. Am J Cardiol 2002;90(suppl. 6A):63H.

100. Rutherford RB, Durham J. Percutaneous balloon angioplasty for arteriosclerosis obliterans: long term results. In: Yao JST, Pearce WH, eds. Techniques in Vascular Surgery. Philadelphia: WB Saunders, 1992: 329–45.

101. Henry M, Klonaris C, Amor M, et al. State of the art: which stent for which lesion in peripheral intervention? Tex Heart Inst J 2000;27:119–26.

102. Hunink MGM, Wong JB, Donaldson MC, et al. Revascularization for femoropopliteal disease: a decision and cost effectiveness analysis. JAMA 1995;274:165–71.

103. Krepel VM, Van Andel GJ, Van Erp WF, et al. Percutaneous dilatations of femoral artery: initial and long term results. Radiology 1985;158:325–8.

104. Capek P, MacLean GK, Berkowitz HD. Femoropopliteal angioplasty: factors influencing long term success. Circulation 1991;83(suppl. I):170–80.

105. Johnston KW. Femoral and popliteal arteries: reanalysis of results of balloon angioplasty. Radiology 1992;183:767–71.

106. Vogelzang R. Long term results of angioplasty. J Vasc Intern Radiol 1996;7:179–80.

107. Gallino A, Mahler F, Probst P, et al. Percutaneous transluminal angioplasty of the arteries of the lower limb: a 5 year follow-up. Circulation 1984;70(4):619–23.

108. Bergeron P, Pinot JJ, Poyen V, et al. Long term results with the Palmaz stent in the superficial femoral artery. J Endovasc Surg 1995;2:161–7.

109. Hayoz D, DoDai DO, Mahler F, et al. Acute inflammatory reaction associated with endoluminal bypass grafts. J Endovasc Surg 1997;4:354–60.

14. Drug-Eluting Stents

Philip A Morales and Richard R Heuser

INTRODUCTION

Stents have significantly changed the field of interventional therapy. They are becoming more widely used in everyday clinical practice. While endovascular stent-grafts in the aortoiliac vessels help maintain immediate and long-term patency rates that are comparable to that of surgery,[1-3] the same cannot be said for femoropopliteal vessels. Stents in femoropopliteal vessels do not significantly improve the long-term patency rates when compared to angioplasty alone.[4-6] The usual indications for stenting in the femoropopliteal vessels are therefore left for suboptimal balloon angioplasty results with residual stenosis or flow-limiting dissections. The long-term success of stenting is, however, hampered by in-stent restenosis. This is becoming a major clinical problem, as the increasing use of stents will only increase the incidence of in-stent restenosis. In addition, the treatment of in-stent restenosis can be, despite progresses in radiation therapy, technically challenging and costly.

In-stent restenosis is marked by exaggerated and uncontrolled neointimal hyperplasia,[7,8] and is considered to be a component of the general vascular response to injury. Catheter-induced injury consists of denuding of the intima and stretching of the media and adventitia. The wound-healing reaction starts with an inflammatory phase, characterized by platelets, growth factor and smooth muscle cell activation. Next, the granulation phase is characterized by smooth muscle cell and fibroblast migration and proliferation into the injured area. Finally, the remodeling phase is characterized by maturation of the neointima, proteoglycan and collagen synthesis, which replaces early fibronectin as major components of the extracellular matrix.

In-stent restenosis is associated with diabetes mellitus,[9] vessel size,[10] lesion length, extent of disease, number of stents, and minimal stent diameter

or area. Over the years, treating restenosis was focused on optimizing stent characteristics and placement technique. Systemic pharmacologic therapy has not been successful in totally eliminating restenosis.[11] One explanation for the repeated failure of clinical drug studies could be that these agents, when given systemically, cannot reach sufficient levels in the injured (treated) arteries. Local drug delivery can offer advantages not readily available through systemic drug delivery. The active drug, coated on a stent, can be applied to the vessel at the precise site and at the time of vessel injury (i.e. angioplasty and/or stenting). Higher tissue concentration of the drug is possible through local drug delivery. There would be reduced risk of remote systemic toxicity given the minimal systemic release of the drug.

POTENTIAL CANDIDATES FOR LOCAL DRUG DELIVERY

Ideally, the potential candidate or drug should effectively inhibit the multiple components of the complex restenosis process. Several pharmacologic agents with antiproliferative properties have failed to inhibit restenosis after intervention.[12] Table 14.1 lists the potential agents for local drug delivery. Even though there are a wide variety of potential agents, some have not shown convincing preclinical results that may lead to further testing in clinical trials. The potential agents that are being tested in randomized clinical trials are actinomycin, rapamycin, and paclitaxel. While the majority of drug-eluting stent trials deal with the treatment of coronary artery disease, one trial named SIROCCO (SIROlimus Coated Cordis SMART™ Nitinol Self-expandable Stent for the Treatment of Obstructive Superficial Femoral Artery Disease) deals with the treatment of superficial femoral arteries.

Table 14.1 List of potential candidates for local drug delivery

Antineoplastic
Paclitaxel (Taxol™)
Taxol derivative (QP-2)
Actinomycin D
Vincristine
Methotrexate
Angiopectin
Mitomycin
BCP 678
Antisense *c-muy*
Abbott ABT 578

Migration inhibitor/ECM modulators
Halofuginone
Propyl hydroxylase inhibitor
C-proteinase inhibitor
Metalloproteinase inhibitors
Batimastat

Antithrombus
Hirudin and Iloprost
Heparin
Abciximab

Immunosuppressants
Sirolimus (rapamycin)
Tacrolimus (FK506)
Tranilast
Dexamethasone
Methylprednisolone
Interferon gamma 1b
Leflunomide
Cyclosporin

Enhance healing/promote endothelial function
Vascular endothelial growth factor
17-β-estradiol
Tkase inhibition
BCP 671
HMG CoA reductase inhibitor

ACTINOMYCIN D (COSMEGEN™)

Actinomycin D is an antibiotic produced by various species of *Streptomyces* and is used for its antiproliferative properties in the treatment of various malignant neoplasms (e.g. Wilm's tumor, rhabdomyosarcomas, carcinoma of testis and uterus). It inhibits the proliferation of cells by forming a stable complex with double-strand DNA and inhibiting DNA-primed RNA synthesis.

There is no current published research documenting the use of actinomycin D for the treatment of coronary artery disease and restenosis. In 2001, a phase I randomized clinical trial named ACTION (ACTinomycin eluting stent Improves Outcomes by reducing Neointimal hyperplasia) was started to evaluate the safety and performance of the multilink tetra-D stent system. The enrollment is 360 patients randomized to receive an actinomycin D coated stent (high dose 10 mcg/cm²; low dose 2.5 mcg/cm²) or a non-coated stent for treatment of de novo lesions in native coronary arteries with a vessel caliber of 3.0–4.0 mm. Six-month angiographic follow-up was completed in 2002 and a 12-month clinical follow-up was completed subsequently.

RAPAMYCIN (SIROLIMUS, RAPAMUNE™)

Rapamycin has its roots in Easter Island where an actinomycete, *Streptomyces hygroscopicus*, was found to produce a macrolide antibiotic with potent antifungal, immunosuppressive, and antimitotic properties. Since 1999, rapamycin has been used as an antirejection drug in organ transplant recipients, particularly renal transplant recipients. It is a naturally occurring macrocyclic lactone that inhibits cytokine-mediated and growth-factor-mediated proliferation of lymphocytes and smooth muscle cells. Rapamycin blocks G1 to S cell cycle progression by interacting with a specific target protein (mTOR – mammalian Target of Rapamycin) and inhibits its activation. The inhibition of mTOR suppresses cytokine-driven T-cell proliferation. Rapamycin also prevents proliferation and migration of smooth muscle cells. Pre-clinical efficacy studies demonstrated a 35–50% reduction in in-stent neointimal hyperplasia for the rapamycin-coated stents as compared with bare metal stents at 28 days in the porcine and rabbit model.[13]

PACLITAXEL (TAXOL™)

Paclitaxel was originally isolated from the bark of the Pacific Yew tree. It is an antineoplastic agent that is currently used to treat several types of cancer, most commonly breast and ovarian cancer. It is a diterpenoid with a characteristic taxane skeleton of 20 carbon atoms and has a molecular weight of 853.9 Daltons. Its pharmacologic action is through formation of numerous decentralized and unorganized microtubules. This enhances the assembly of extraordinarily stable microtubules, interrupting proliferation, migration and signal transduction. Unlike other antiproliferative agents of the colchicine type which inhibit microtubule assembly, paclitaxel shifts the microtubule equilibrium towards microtubule assembly. It is highly lipophilic, which promotes a rapid cellular uptake, and has a long-lasting effect in the cell due to the structural alteration of the cytoskeleton.

Preliminary studies have shown that paclitaxel may prevent or attenuate restenosis.[14,15] In a rat balloon injury model, intraperitoneal administration of paclitaxel reduced neointimal area. Paclitaxel-eluting stents have been studied using different types of stent and different animal models.[16,17] These studies reveal a significant, dose-dependent inhibition of neointimal hyperplasia. Furthermore, the tissue response in paclitaxel-treated vessels includes incomplete healing, few smooth muscle cells, late persistence of macrophages, and dense fibrin with little collagen as well as signs of positive remodeling of the stented segment.

Some of the current clinical trials using paclitaxel-eluting stents include the ASPECT (Asian Paclitaxel Eluting stent Clinical Trial), ELUTES (European evaLUation of pacliTaxel Eluting Stent) and TAXUS I–IV (paclitaxel-eluting NIR™ stent trial).[18] These current trials are mainly in the treatment of coronary artery disease. There are no current trials that deal with the treatment of peripheral vessels, particularly superficial femoral arteries.

CLINICAL TRIALS USING
DRUG-ELUTING STENTS

RAVEL

The RAVEL (RAndomized, double-blind study with the sirolimus-eluting BX VElocity™ balloon expandable stent in the treatment of patients with de novo native coronary artery Lesions) trial is a multicenter prospective trial comparing a bare metal stent to a drug-coated stent.[19] In this trial, 238 patients were randomized to a single rapamycin-coated stent (140 mcg/cm^2) versus a bare metal BX Velocity™ stent. At 6-month follow-up, the degree of neointimal proliferation, manifested as the mean late lumen loss, was significantly lower in the sirolimus-stent group compared to the bare-stent group. The restenosis rate of the sirolimus-stent group was zero. There were no episodes of stent thrombosis. For the follow-up period of up to 1 year, the overall rate of major cardiac events was 5.8% in the sirolimus-stent group compared to 28.8% in the bare-stent group. Interestingly, the restenosis rate in the bare-stent group was 26.6%.

SIRIUS

The SIRIUS (a multicenter, randomized, double-blind study of the SIRolImUS-coated BX Velocity™ balloon expandable stent in the treatment of patients with de novo coronary artery lesions) trial is a prospective clinical trial being conducted in the United States. In this trial, 1100 patients with de novo coronary artery lesion were randomized to treatment with either a rapamycin-coated stent or a bare metal BX velocity stent. The primary endpoint of the SIRIUS trial is target vessel failure at 9 months. Secondary endpoints are core laboratory analysis of angiographic and intravascular ultrasound data to determine treatment effects on neointimal hyperplasia and in-stent restenosis.

SIROCCO

The SIROCCO (SIROlimus Coated Cordis SMART™ nitinol self-expandable stent for the treatment of Obstructive superficial femoral artery disease) trial is a multicenter, double-blind, randomized, prospective feasibility trial. Thirty-six patients with obstructive superficial femoral artery disease were randomized to either a sirolimus-coated stent or a bare metal SMART™ stent. At 6-

month follow-up, the restenosis rate of the treated group was zero and there was no target lesion revascularization.

TAXUS I–IV[19]

The TAXUS I trial is a 61 patient, randomized, double-blind, multicenter feasibility trial to evaluate the safety of a slow-release paclitaxel-coated (1.0 mcg/mm^2) NIR™ coronary stent. Six-month angiographic and intravascular ultrasound (IVUS) follow-up demonstrated a 50% reduction in late loss index for the paclitaxel-coated stent group compared to the bare-stent group. The TAXUS II trial is a 532 patient, double-blind, randomized, multicenter study that will evaluate the safety and performance of a slow and moderate-release paclitaxel-coated stent in de novo lesions. The TAXUS III-ISR trial is a feasibility study that will evaluate the safety of the paclitaxel-coated stent in the treatment of in-stent restenosis. The TAXUS IV trial is a 1600 patient pivotal, randomized, double-blind trial designed to study the safety and efficacy of moderate-release paclitaxel-coated stents in de novo and in-stent restenosis lesions.

CONCLUSION

Restenosis continues to be the 'Achilles heel' of percutaneous interventions. Drug-eluting stents represent a new and exciting approach to reduce the incidence of restenosis. It is a simple modification of a technology that still has not proven its efficacy in treating superficial femoral arteries. Planned and ongoing clinical trials will help determine their full potential, especially in the treatment of long lesions, small distal vessels, chronic total occlusions, and multilevel disease in the peripheral vessels. Future directions of drug-eluting stents include further study with the different classes of drug that are potential agents for the inhibition of restenosis to the combination of biodegradability with drug delivery, or local gene therapy (e.g. local expression of proliferation regulatory genes; trans-

fer of cytotoxic genes, vascular endothelial growth factor).

REFERENCES

1. Henry M, Amor M, Ethevenot G, et al. Percutaneous endoluminal treatment of iliac occlusions: long-term follow-up in 105 patients. J Endovasc Surg 1998;5:228–35.
2. Vorwerk D, Gunther RW, Schurmann K, et al. Primary stent placement for chronic iliac artery occlusions: follow-up results in 103. Radiology 1995;194:745–9.
3. Sullivan TM, Childs MB, Bacharach JM, et al. Percutaneous transluminal angioplasty and primary stenting of the iliac arteries in 288 patients. J Vasc Surg 1997;25:829–39.
4. Do-dai-Do, Triller J, Walpoth BH, et al. A comparison study of self-expandable stents vs. balloon angioplasty alone in femoropopliteal artery occlusions. Cardiovasc Intervent Radiol 1992;15:306–12.
5. Rosenfield K, Schainfeld R, Pieczek A, et al. Restenosis of endovascular stents from stent compression. J Am Coll Cardiol 1997;29:328–38.
6. Strecker EP, Hagen B, Liermann D, et al. Iliac and femoropopliteal occlusive disease treated with flexible tantalum stents. Cardiovasc Intervent Radiol 1993;16:158–64.
7. Kearny M, Pieczek A, Haley L, et al. Histopathology of in-stent restenosis in patients with peripheral artery disease. Circulation 1997;95:1998–2002.
8. Komatsu R, Ueda M, Naruko, T, et al. Neointimal tissue response at sites of coronary stenting in humans: macroscopic, histological, and immunohistochemical analyses. Circulation 1998;98:224–33.
9. Sobel BE. Acceleration of restenosis by diabetes: pathogenetic implications. Circulation 2001;103:1185–7.
10. Mintz GS, Popma JJ, Pichard AD, et al. Intravascular ultrasound predictors of restenosis after percutaneous transcatheter coronary revascularization. J Am Coll Cardiol 1996;27:1678–87.
11. Lefkovits J, Topol EJ. Pharmacological approaches for the prevention of restenosis after percutaneous coronary intervention. Prog Cardiovasc Dis 1997;40:141–58.
12. de Feyter PJ, Vos J, Rensing BJ. Anti-restenosis trials. Curr Interv Cardiol Rep 2000;2:326–31.
13. Suzuki T, Kopia G, Hayashi S-I, et al. Stent-based delivery of sirolimus reduces neointimal formation in a porcine coronary model. Circulation 2001;104:1188–93.
14. Sollott SJ, Cheng L, Pauly RR, et al. Taxol inhibits neointimal smooth muscle cell accumulation after angioplasty in the rat. J Clin Invest 1995;95:1869–76.
15. Axel DT, Kunert W, Goggelmann C, et al. Paclitaxel inhibits arterial smooth muscle cell proliferation and migration in vitro and in vivo using local drug delivery. Circulation 1997;96:636–45.
16. Farb A, Heller PF, Shroff S, et al. Pathological analysis of delivery of paclitaxel via a polymer-coated stent. Circulation 2001;104:473–9.
17. Heldman AW, Cheng L, Jenkins GM, et al. Paclitaxel stent coating inhibits neointimal hyperplasia at 4 weeks in a porcine model of coronary restenosis. Circulation 2001;103:2289–95.
18. Hiatt BL, Ikeno F, Yeung AC. Drug-eluting stents for the prevention of restenosis: in quest for the Holy Grail. Catheter Cardiovasc Interv 2002;55:409–17.
19. Morice MC, Serruys PW, Sousa JE, et al. A randomized comparison of a sirolimus-eluting stent with a standard stent for coronary revascularization. N Engl J Med 2002;346:1773–80.

15. Peripheral Vascular Brachytherapy

Ron Waksman

Ron Waksman

INTRODUCTION

With the growing popularity of peripheral vascular medicine, identifying a reliable treatment to the plaguing recurrence of restenosis will increase and augment the benefits of vascular intervention. Investigators have shown that the endovascular delivery of radiation therapy is one such treatment. Combating restenosis in the peripheral vascular system is contingent upon understanding the processes, mechanisms, and potential targets affected by using brachytherapy. The successful outcome of clinical trials in the coronary arteries facilitated recognition of vascular brachytherapy to become the standard of care for the treatment of in-stent restenosis. Expansion of the indications to de novo lesions identified not only the potential but also the limitations of the technology (late thrombosis and edge effect). Simultaneously investigators embarked on a series of studies utilizing vascular brachytherapy as adjunct therapy for intervention in peripheral arteries. The outcome of these trials will determine the future role of vascular brachytherapy as a tool for prevention of restenosis in the peripheral vascular system.

As the manifestation of coronary atherosclerosis and peripheral artery disease is primarily evident in older patient populations, and with the generation of baby boomers nearing their 60s, the full impact of peripheral and coronary atherosclerosis in the United States is upon us. Whereas coronary vascular procedures increase at a rate of 8% per year, there is greater growth in the frequency of peripheral procedures, estimated at 19% per year. Despite new advances such as stents, atherectomy devices, thrombectomy and endoluminal grafts, the restenosis rate after peripheral artery intervention continues to plague and compromise the overall success of these procedures. However, the main limitation of intervention in peripheral arteries remains restenosis and the need for repeat revascularization.

Vascular brachytherapy is a promising technology with the potential to reduce restenosis rates. To evaluate the effectiveness and safety of this technology, nearly 5000 patients have been enrolled in clinical trials. Five-year follow-up of clinical and angiographic data collection on patients treated with intracoronary radiation for the prevention of restenosis has recently been released. These studies demonstrate different levels of efficacy and raise further questions regarding proper dosimetry, the incidence of edge effect, the late thrombosis phenomenon, and late restenosis. While the majority of vascular brachytherapy trials have focused on the use of radiation therapy for the prevention of coronary in-stent restenosis, more data are still needed to determine the effectiveness of beta and gamma sources, and the use of centering delivery systems.

Currently, the clinical experience with vascular brachytherapy for the peripheral system is limited and planned trials are designed to evaluate the restenosis rates of several vascular sites with the use of endovascular radiation therapy following vascular intervention (i.e. balloon angioplasty, stent placement, atherectomy, or laser ablative techniques). Target sites for such preventive therapy have been identified as superficial femoral artery (SFA) lesions, renal artery stenosis, patients who are undergoing hemodialysis with arteriovenous (AV) graft stenosis, a subclavian or brachiocephalic vein, and following transjugular intrahepatic portosystemic shunt (TIPS) procedures for patients with portal hypertension.

MECHANISMS OF RESTENOSIS

The use of percutaneous transluminal angioplasty (PTA) has considerably improved the revascularization rates of many patients. Unfortunately, the long-term efficacy of PTA is limited by its 6–12 month high rate of restenosis.[1] Restenosis following PTA occurs in response to the healing process associated with overinflation of the balloon during angioplasty and subsequent overstretching of the vessel. The main mechanisms of restenosis are acute recoil, intimal hyperplasia, and late vascular constriction (negative remodeling).[2-5]

In the peripheral system, restenosis following PTA is mainly seen in small and medium peripheral arteries, such as the superficial femoropopliteal arteries and renal arteries. Although not as common, and found to have less of an effect on patency, lower rates of restenosis have also been reported in larger arteries, such as the aortoiliac and carotid arteries following intervention.[6-12] Other sites affected by restenosis include bypass graft anastomosis, AV dialysis grafts and following the placement of transjugular intrahepatic portosystemic shunts (TIPS).[13] Factors which affect long-term vessel patency following PTA include the length of the lesion, the degree of stenosis, the plaque burden, vessel size, and proximal and distal flow. For peripheral short focal lesions, short-term (6-month) patency rates as high as 75% have been reported. In contrast, more complex and longer areas of stenosis, those with poor distal runoff and those performed for limb salvage, may have a 6-month patency as low as 25%, and a 5-year patency of only 16%.[14]

Many attempts have been made to reduce restenosis by adding adjunct pharmacologic therapy to PTA, or by the use of mechanical devices, including atherectomy, laser angioplasty, and intravascular stenting. It appears that instrumentation of these vessels by balloon or other devices is responsible for inducing restenosis, as none of these alternative approaches significantly retards the neointimal hyperplasia or improves and preserves long-term vascular patency.[15-18] Indeed, the hyperplastic response post-revascularization remains an outstanding issue for all vascular interventional modalities.

Intraluminal delivery of radiation following vascular intervention is viewed as a viable solution to inhibit restenosis.[19-29] Exposing the vessels to low-dose radiation following angioplasty modifies wound healing by inhibiting the excessive neointima formation. Intravascular radiation in the peripheral system, however, requires special considerations when selecting the isotope and the delivery system to deliver the radiation to the target site.

RADIATION PHYSICS AND DOSIMETRIC CONSIDERATIONS

Different isotopes on various platforms and systems have been developed for the use of endovascular brachytherapy. The main platforms for radiation delivery are catheter-based systems and radioactive stents. Catheter-based systems contain a solid form such as line source wires, radioactive seeds or radioactive balloons, or non-solid sources such as radioactive gas and liquid-filled balloons.

There are several different gamma and beta isotopes available, and selecting the most appropriate one depends on the anatomy of the vessel, the properties of the treated lesion, and the proper identification of the target tissue that needs treatment. Anatomically important parameters which also need consideration include the diameter and the curvature of the vessel, the eccentricity of the plaque, the lesion length, the composition of the plaque, the amount of calcium, and the presence or absence of a stent in the treated segment. These factors influence which source to use, as different sources have varying properties which warrant using one over another.

Requirements for choosing the ideal radiation system for vascular brachytherapy should include dose distribution of a few millimeters from the source with a minimal dose gradient, low dose levels to surrounding tissues, and a dwell time less than 15 minutes. Other considerations for source selection include source energy, half-life for multiple applications, available activity, penetration, dose distribution, radiation exposure to both patient and operator, shielding requirement, availability, and cost.

In order to determine an accurate dosimetry, it is essential to identify the target tissue, the right dose, and the treatment margins. It has been argued that the adventitia is the target, but when considering the success of previous trials, it is difficult to deny the fact that the high dose exposure to the vessel wall and residual plaque may be essential to obtain efficacy.[30,31] The doses prescribed today in clinical studies are empirical; they are based on doses used in animal studies and the limited experience gained from treating other benign diseases. Since a wide range of doses demonstrated effectiveness in preclinical studies, a therapeutic window must exist that allows some flexibility in selecting the isotope for this application.

UNDERSTANDING GAMMA RADIATION

Gamma rays are photons originating from the center of the nucleus and differ from x-rays, which originate from the orbital outside of the nucleus. Gamma rays have deep penetrating energies from 20 keV to 20 MeV which require an excess of shielding, as compared to beta and x-ray emitters. The only gamma ray isotope currently in use is Iridium-192 (Ir-192). There are isotopes that emit both gamma and x-rays, such as Iodine-125 (I-125) and Palladium-103 (Pd-103). These isotopes have lower energies, however, and require higher activity levels in order to deliver a prescribed dose in the acceptable dwell time (<15 minutes). Using these isotopes for vascular brachytherapy is difficult, as they are either not available in high activity levels or too expensive for this application. The dosimetry of Ir-192 is well understood and is associated with an acceptable dose gradient, as Ir-192 has a lesser fall-off in dose than beta emitters. Iridium-192 is available in activities of up to 10 Ci, but due to high penetration, patients need to be transferred to the radiation oncology shielded room, as the average shielding of a catheterization laboratory will not be enough to handle more than 500 mCi source in activity. Focal stenosis in smaller diameter arteries can be treated with lower activities of Ir-192 in the catheterization laboratory and will require an average of 20 minutes of dwell time for doses above 15 Gy when prescribed at 2 mm radial distance from the source.

UNDERSTANDING BETA RADIATION

Beta rays are high-energy electrons emitted by nuclei and contain too many or too few neutrons. These negatively charged particles have a wide variety of energies, including transition energies, particularly between parent–daughter cells, and a diverse range of half-lives from several minutes (Cu-62) up to 30 years (^{90}Sr/Y). Beta emitters are associated with a higher gradient to the near wall, as they lose their energy rapidly to surrounding tissue and their range is within 1 cm of tissue. Vascular brachytherapy using beta emitters appears promising, as safety levels are high when radiation exposure to non-targeted areas is low. In order to use beta emitters for peripheral application they must be in proximity with the vessel wall and should be used with as high an activity level as possible.

RADIATION SYSTEMS FOR THE PERIPHERAL VASCULAR SYSTEM

Several radiation systems for peripheral endovascular brachytherapy have been suggested and are currently under development, as described below.

EXTERNAL RADIATION

External beam radiation is a viable option for the treatment of peripheral vessels. It allows a homogenous dose distribution with the possibility of fractionation. To date an attempt to treat SFA lesions and AV dialysis grafts with external radiation has been reported to be without success in reducing the restenosis rate. Using stereotactic techniques to localize the radiation to the target area may improve the results of this approach.

RADIOACTIVE STENTS

Radioactive stents are an attractive device since they require minimum shielding and are easy to use. The dosimetry of radioactive stents is even more complicated and depends on the geometry of the stent which varies across stent designs. Current tested radioactive stents lack dose homogeneity across the entire length of the stent. This could affect the biological response to radiation, especially at the stent edges. The lack of even-dose distribution may also result in an improper delivery to specific injury sites, causing additional growth. This problem, known as edge effect, and identified as the major limitation of radioactive stents in coronary trials, may result from a stimulatory response from the vessel. Low activity radioactive stents may be associated with an ineffective low dose rate. While radioactive stents with high activities may deliver toxic doses to the stented area that delay re-endothelialization, higher radiation doses might promote stent thrombosis and tissue necrosis to the area surrounding the stent. New studies are underway which will evaluate whether higher activities will minimize the edge effect phenomenon. Other approaches to improving the results with radioactive stents include changes to the geometry of the stent, and altering the isotope or the activity level at the stent's edges. A new approach with the use of radioactive nitinol self-expanding stents utilizing gamma emitters is currently under investigation as a potential therapy for primary SFA lesions.

CATHETER-BASED SYSTEMS

Several catheter-based systems are available for the peripheral vascular system. However, the only system used in clinical trials is the MicroSelectron™ HDR (Nucletron-Oldelft, The Netherlands) (Fig. 15.1). The system uses a high dose rate afterloader that consists of a computerized system which delivers a 3 mm stepping 10 Ci in activity of Ir-192 source into a centered closed end lumen segmented balloon radiation catheter. There are many advantages to using a remote afterloading system for vascular brachytherapy, namely that the remote afterloading system drives the radiation source quickly to the treatment site, avoiding radiation exposure to non-treated arteries. In addition, radiation exposure to clinical personnel is eliminated by remotely programming the automatic advancement of the radiation source from a shielded safe to the treatment site. The radiation dose can be con-

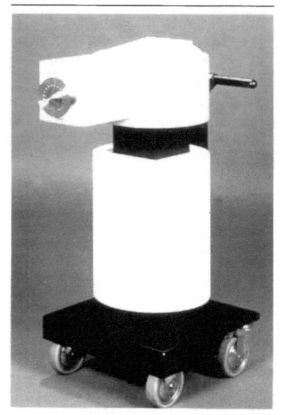

Fig. 15.1 MicroSelectron HDR™ afterloader.

trolled and shaped using the computerized afterloader device to accurately adjust the source position and treatment time. By using an afterloader, it continually monitors the radiation dose and automatically retracts the source into the shielded safe after treatment. Treatment time is automatically adapted for the radioactive decay of the source, and the afterloader can handle a very high activity source (10 Ci) which results in shorter dwell times.

The peripheral brachytherapy centering catheter (PARIS™ catheter) (Guidant, Santa Clara, CA) is currently being used in the multicenter Peripheral Artery Radiation Investigational Study (PARIS) (Fig. 15.2). This catheter is a double-lumen catheter with multiple centering balloons near its distal tip. One lumen is for inflation of the centering balloon and the second lumen is for the guidewire and for

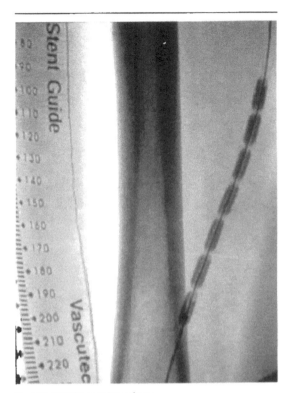

Fig. 15.2 PARIS™ centering catheter.

the closed end lumen sheath which, once the catheter is in position, is introduced following removal of the guidewire. The inflated balloons engage the walls of the vessel and allow centering. The shaft diameter is a 7F closed end lumen catheter and comes with balloons from 4 to 8 mm in diameter and from 10 to 20 cm in length, enabling the catheter to be in the center of the lumen of large peripheral vessels during inflation. Other catheter designs, such as the helical balloon, will overcome the centering problem and provide flow and perfusion during centering.

Another catheter-based system which is available for use in the catheterization laboratory includes the use of an Ir-192 radioactive wire which is delivered manually into a closed end lumen catheter. The activity of the source is limited to 500 mCi and the system is only practical to use for short lesions in small vessels (diameter <4.0 mm)

that require a dwell time of 20 minutes. Similar to this gamma system, the eventual use of a catheter-based system using high activity beta sources may also be an option for intermediate-sized vessels.

HOT BALLOONS

The angioplasty balloon is another platform which can be used to deliver radiation for the peripheral system. These balloons can be filled with either a liquid isotope such as Re-188 or Re-186, or radioactive Xenon-133 gas. The advantage of using these systems is the uniform dosimetry and proximity of the beta emitter to the vessel wall. Special care, however, is required when using the liquid-filled balloon to prevent spilling of the isotope outside of the balloon. The radioactive balloon catheter (Radiance, Irvine, CA) is particularly attractive for peripheral applications since it is associated with apposition of a solid beta P-32 source attached to the inner balloon surface. With inflation of the balloon, the source is attached to the lumen surface. The system is limited to lesions <33 mm in length with one step but can accommodate longer lesions with manual stepping. To date, there are no clinical data to support the use of this technology in peripheral arteries.

An alternative and attractive approach would be the use of low x-ray energy delivered intraluminally via a catheter. The emitter would be between 5 and 7 mm in length and between 1.25 and 2.0 mm in diameter. It could be administered distal to the lesion and pulled back to cover the entire lesion length. If effective, it would alleviate the need for the use of radioisotopes in the catheterization laboratory. Miniaturizing the emitter is a technical challenge and there are as yet no preclinical data to support this theory.

A modification of the Beta-Cath system to accommodate the beta systems with the ^{90}Sr/Y emitter to be used in the peripheral system, now called the Corona™ system (Fig. 15.3), is a balloon filled with CO_2 which allows centering and prevents dose attenuation. A clinical study in SFA for in-stent restenosis lesions entitled MOBILE was initiated.

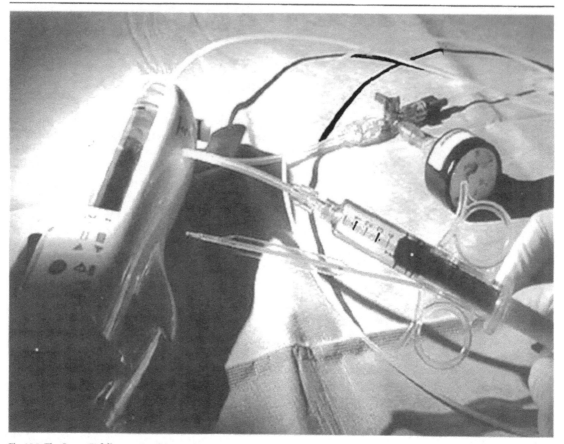

Fig. 15.3 The Corona™ delivery system (Novoste, Norcross, GA).

CLINICAL TRIALS

The first application of vascular brachytherapy for the prevention of restenosis was performed in the peripheral arteries and was initiated by Liermann and Schopohl (Frankfurt, Germany). Known as the Frankfurt Experience, the first pilot study of endovascular radiation was conducted in 30 patients with in-stent restenosis in their superficial femoral arteries.[32] The patients underwent atherectomy and PTA followed by endovascular radiation using the MicroSelectron™ HDR afterloader and a non-centering catheter. The gamma source Ir-192 was used to deliver a dose of 12 Gy, 3 mm into the vessel wall. The actual dose, however, varied from 8 to 28 Gy.

No adverse effects from the radiation treatment were reported up to 7 years follow-up. The 5-year patency rate of the target vessel was 82% with only 3/28 (11%) stenosis within the treated segment reported. Late total occlusion developed in 2/28 patients (7%) after 16 and 37 months respectively.

THE EMORY EXPERIENCE

A subsequent pilot study was conducted at Emory University in 1994, which studied the effects of endovascular radiation in the SFAs of four patients following PTA and stenting. Of the four patients, one with a Palmaz™ stent needed subsequent surgery 1-year post-radiation therapy because of a crushed stent. The histology of the irradiated stent segment in this patient demonstrated minimal intimal hyperplasia surrounding the stent struts, thus indicating the inhibitory effect of radiation therapy in stented SFAs.

THE VIENNA EXPERIENCE

The effectiveness of the MicroSelectron™ HDR system was tested in a randomized placebo-controlled trial in Vienna: 113 patients (63 men, 50 women; mean age 71 years) with de novo or recurrent femoropopliteal lesions were included in this randomized trial comparing the restenosis rate after PTA plus endovascular brachytherapy (BT) (57 patients, PTA+BT group) versus PTA (56 patients, PTA group) without stent implantation. The mean treated length was 16.7 cm (PTA+BT group) versus 14.8 cm (PTA group). In patients randomized to PTA+BT, a dose of 12 Gy was applied by an Ir-192 source 3 mm from the source axis. Follow-up examinations included measurement of the ankle–brachial index (ABI), color-flow duplex sonography, and angiography. The primary end point of the study was patency after 6 months. The overall recurrence rate after 6 months was 15 (28.3%) of 53 in the PTA+BT group versus 29 (53.7%) of 54 in the PTA group (χ^2 test, $p <0.05$). The cumulative patency rates at 12 months of follow-up were 63.6% in the PTA+BT group and 35.3% in the PTA group (log-rank test, $p <0.005$).[33] The group from Vienna continued to investigate a series of patients with higher dose 18 Gy to improve the outcome of the radiation group. In another series of studies the effectiveness of radiation as adjunct therapy with primary stenting of the SFA was evaluated in 33 patients. In this series, the recurrence rate at 6 months was 30% (10/33) but this was attributed to a high rate of late thrombosis. When thrombolytic patients were excluded, the in-stent restenosis rate fell to only 12%. Late thrombosis was reduced significantly once prolonged antiplatelet therapy was administered as shown in Vienna 5 in which 90 patients are randomized to stent plus radiation versus stent alone for the treatment of SFA lesions.

THE PARIS TRIAL

The PARIS Radiation Investigational Study is the first US Food and Drug Administration (FDA)-approved multicenter, randomized, double-blind control study involving 300 patients following PTA to SFA stenosis using a gamma radiation Ir-192 source. Utilizing the MicroSelectron™ HDR afterloader, the treatment dose is 14 Gy delivered via a centered segmented end lumen balloon catheter. The primary objectives of this study are to determine angiographic evidence of patency and a reduction of >30% of the treated lesion's restenosis rate at 6 months. A secondary endpoint is to determine the clinical patency at 6 and 12 months by treadmill exercise and by the ABI. The clinical endpoints are improvements in treadmill exercise time of >90 seconds, improvement of ABI of 0.10 compared to pre-PTA values, and an absence of repeat interventions to the treated vessel. This study was designed based on recently published recommendations and general principles of the evaluation of new interventional devices and technologies [34]. The data from this study should ultimately determine whether endovascular radiation therapy has a role in the prevention of restenosis in patients following PTA for SFA lesions.

In the feasibility phase of PARIS, 40 patients with claudication were enrolled. The mean lesion length was 9.9 ± 3.0 cm with a mean reference vessel diameter of 5.4 ± 0.5 mm. Following successful PTA, a segmented balloon-centering catheter was positioned to cover the PTA site.[34] The patients were transported to the radiation oncology suite and treated with radiation using a high dose rate MicroSelectron™ HDR afterloader. The isotope used for this study was Ir-192 (maximum of 10 Ci in activity) and the prescribed dose was 14 Gy to 2 mm into the vessel wall. ABI and maximum walking time were evaluated with a repeat angiogram at 6 months. Radiation was delivered successfully in all but two patients due to technical difficulties. There were no procedural, in-hospital, or 30-day complications in any of the treated patients. Maximum walking time on treadmill was increased from 3.56 ± 2.7 minutes at baseline to 4.53 ± 2.7 minutes at 3 months ($p = 0.01$) and ABI was also improved from 0.7 + 0.2 to 1.0 + 0.2. Among the first 20 patients that returned for 5-month angiographic follow-up, there was only one patient who required revascularization of the treated site. There has been no evidence of arterial aneurysms or perforations. The 6-month angiographic follow-up was completed on 30 patients; 13.3% of them had evidence of clinical restenosis. The feasibility study of PARIS demonstrated that the delivery of a high dose rate gamma radiation via a centering catheter is feasible and safe following PTA to SFA lesions. A list of SFA radiation trials is shown in Table 15.1.

ARTERIOVENOUS DIALYSIS STUDIES

A pilot study was initiated at Emory in 1994 to determine whether intravascular low dose radiation retards neointimal hyperplasia in patients who had failed PTA at the distal venous anastomosis of AV dialysis grafts.[35]

Patients who failed prior PTAs to their AV graft and had <50% luminal stenosis were enrolled in the study and underwent balloon dilation at the narrowed segment. Following PTA, a sheath was placed across the lesion and a closed end lumen 5F non-centered radiation delivery catheter was positioned at the angioplasty site. The catheter position was verified by radiopaque marker bands on a dummy source wire that was placed into the catheter. The sheath and the catheter were fixed to the skin and the patients were transported to the radiation oncology suite. The patients were treated with a high activity Ir-192 source delivered to the treatment site by a MicroSelectron™ HDR afterloader. The treatment dose was 14 Gy delivered to a depth of 2 mm into the arterial wall. After the radiation treatment, the sheath and the catheter were retrieved and the patients were sent home on the same day. Bimonthly clinical follow-up including color-flow Doppler evaluation was performed and the majority of the patients underwent angiographic follow-up at 6 months. Eleven patients with 18 lesions were treated. A 40% patency rate at 44 weeks was reported.

Although the procedure was successful in all patients, the long-term results of this study were similar to the practice reported so far by stand-alone PTA without radiation. In summary, this study demonstrated only the feasibility and safety of intravascular radiation therapy post-PTA using the MicroSelectron™ HDR afterloader for patients with AV dialysis graft stenosis.

This feasibility study had several limitations:

- the study population was small and heterogeneous;
- many patients had several PTA failures prior to the procedure;
- there was heterogenicity on the type of the treated grafted shunts.

Several patients in this study had thrombotic events within 3 months following the procedure and underwent thrombectomy or lytic therapy.

Table 15.1 Superficial Femoral Artery Radiation Trials

Study	No. of Patients	Randomized	Centering Catheter	Dose	@ mm	Patency (%)
Frankfurt	30	–	–	12 Gy	3	82
Vienna 1	10	–	No	12 Gy	3	60
Vienna 2	113	Yes	No	12 Gy	r+0	72
Vienna 3	134	Yes	Yes	18 Gy	r+2	77
Vienna 4	33	No	Yes	14 Gy	r+2	79
Vienna 5	98	Yes	Yes	14 Gy	r+2	88*
Swiss 4-arm study	346	Yes	Yes	12 Gy	r+2	72
Paris Pilot	40	No	Yes	14 Gy	r+2	88
PARIS Randomised	203	Yes	Yes	14 Gy	r+2	–

*Excluding the thrombosis cases.

Although the prescribed dose was 14 Gy, the actual calculated dose given to the patients ranged between 7 and 90 Gy. This occurred because a centering catheter was not utilized in a large conduit. The effectiveness of intravascular radiation therapy in AV dialysis grafts, however, is unclear. Utilizing a centered catheter to deliver radiation to large vessels will be essential to control the uniformity of the dose given to the vessel wall in such large conduits. Larger randomized studies are required to determine the value of this new technology for patients with AV dialysis graft failure.

Nori et al reported that a pilot study utilizing external radiation for AV dialysis in 10 patients failed to keep any of these grafts patent at 18 months follow-up. In this study dialysis patients with stenosis at the AV graft were subjected to balloon angioplasty and external radiation doses of 12 and 18 Gy in a fractionated method (two fractions for each dose. At 6 months the TLR (target lesion-revascularization) was 40% but at 18 months all grafts were failed and required intervention.

Cohen et al reported on the efficacy of low dose external beam irradiation in 31 patients with 41 lesions in their dialysis shunts. The patients were randomized to PTA or stent placement alone followed by external radiation, prescribed at 14 Gy in two 7 Gy fractions. The restenosis rate at 6 months was 45% in the irradiated and 67% in the control group. New studies for this application are currently underway using low dose external radiation to reduce restenosis of vascular access for AV grafts of hemodialysis patients. Other studies using a centering device to deliver an accurate homogenous dose of radiation following PTA are currently under design.

Recently a new study was initiated at SCRIPPS, utilizing endovascular radiation therapy for the prevention of restenosis following transjugular intrahepatic portosystemic shunts (TIPS) for patients with portal hypertension. Overall, the restenosis rate due to intimal hyperplasia of TIPS at 6 months has been reported to be as high as 70%. Complete thrombosis as early as 2 weeks after the procedure has also been reported.[36] However, in the long term, brachytherapy may be the best means of preventing occlusion for these patients.

Other potential targets for vascular brachytherapy include renal arteries and subclavian vein stenosis.

LIMITATIONS TO BRACHYTHERAPY

Although clinical trials using vascular brachytherapy for both coronary and peripheral applications have demonstrated positive results in reducing restenosis rates, these trials have also identified two major serious complications related to the technology: late thrombosis and edge stenosis effects seen at the edges of radiation treatment segments. Late thrombosis is probably due to the delay in healing associated with radiation. It has been estimated that late thrombosis can be remedied through the prolonged administration of antiplatelet therapy following intervention.

Identified as a major limitation to radioactive stents and explained above, the edge effect phenomenon is not exclusive to stented lesions; edge effect has also been known to occur with catheter-based systems utilizing both beta and gamma emitters, especially when the treated area is not covered with wide enough margins. The main explanation for the incidence of edge effect is a combination of low dose at the edges of the radiation source and an injury created by the device for intervention which is not covered by the radiation source. It is hypothesized that wider radiation margins of radiation treatment to the intervening segment may eliminate or significantly reduce the edge effect seen so far in all radiation trials.

CONCLUSION

Despite new technologies and devices, restenosis remains the major limitation of intervention in the peripheral vascular system. The results from preliminary studies demonstrate that radiation has the potential to alter the rate of restenosis following intervention. With the further progression of these studies and their promising results, the use of vascular brachytherapy will dramatically change the practice of peripheral intervention, resulting in an improved long-term patency for our patients.

REFERENCES

1. Tripuraneni P. Catheter-based radiotherapy for peripheral vascular restenosis. Vascular Radiotherapy Monitor 1999;1(3):70–7.

2. Haude M, Erbel R, Issa H, Meyer J. Quantitative analysis of elastic recoil after balloon angioplasty and after intracoronary implantation of balloon-expandable Palmaz–Schatz stents. J Am Coll Cardiol 1993;21:26–34.

3. Consigny PM, Bilder GE. Expression and release of smooth muscle cell mitogens in arterial wall after balloon angioplasty. J Vasc Med Biol 1993;4:1–8.

4. Mintz GS, Popma JJ, Pichard AD, et al. Arterial remodeling after coronary angioplasty. A serial intravascular ultrasound study. Circulation 1996;94:35–43.

5. Isner JM. Vascular remodeling. Honey, I think I shrunk the artery. Circulation 1994;89:2937–41.

6. Murray RR Jr, Hewes RC, White RI Jr, et al. Long-segment femoro-popliteal stenoses: is angioplasty a boon or a bust? Radiology 1987;162:473–6.

7. Johnston KW. Femoral and popliteal arteries: re-analyses of results of balloon angioplasty. Radiology 1992;183:767–71.

8. Vroegindeweij D, Kemper FJ, Teilbeek AV, Buth J, Landman G. Recurrence of stenosis following balloon angioplasty and Simpson atherectomy of the femoropopliteal segment. A randomized comparative 1 year follow-up study using color flow duplex. Eur J Vasc Surg 1992;6:164–71.

9. Rees CR, Palmaz JC, Becker GJ, et al. Palmaz stent in atherosclerotic stenosis involving the ostia of the renal arteries: preliminary report of a multicenter study. Radiology 1991;181:507–14.

10. Hunink MFM, Magruder CD, Meyerovitz MF, et al. Risks and benefits for femoropopliteal percutaneous balloon angioplasty. J Vasc Surg 1993;17:183–94.

11. White GF, Liew SC, Waugh RC, et al. Early outcome of intermediate follow-up of vascular stents in the femoral and popliteal arteries without long term anticoagulation. J Vasc Surg 1995;21:279–81.

12. Kotb MM, Kadir S, Bennett JD, Beam CA. Aortoiliac angioplasty: is there a need for other types of percutaneous intervention? J Vasc Interv Radiol 1992;3:67–71.

13. Dolmatch BL, Gray RJ, Horton KM, Rundback JH, Kline ME. Treatment of anastomotic bypass graft stenosis with directional atherectomy: short-term and intermediate-term results. J Vasc Interv Radiol 1995;6:105–13.

14. Johnston KW. Femoral and popliteal arteries: reanalysis of results of angioplasty. Radiology 1987;162:473–6.

15. Robinson KA. Arterial biologic response to ionizing radiation. In: Waksman R, Bonan R, eds. Vascular Brachytherapy: State of the Art. London: Remedica Publishing, 1999: 15–24.

16. Hillegass WB, Ohman EM, Califf RM. Restenosis: the clinical issues. In: Topol EJ, ed. Textbook of Interventional Cardiology, 2nd edn, Vol. 1. Philadelphia: WB Saunders, 1994: 415–35.

17. Pickering JG, Weir L, Jekanowski J, et al. Proliferative activity in peripheral and coronary atherosclerotic plaques among patients undergoing percutaneous revascularization. J Clin Invest 1993;91:1469–80.

18. Strandness DE, Barnes RW, Katzen B, Ring EJ. Indiscriminate use of laser angioplasty. Radiology 1989;172:945–6.

19. Waksman R, Robinson KA, Crocker IR, et al. Long term efficacy and safety of endovascular low dose irradiation in a swine model of restenosis after angioplasty. Circulation 1995;91:1533–9.

20. Weidermann JG, Marboe C, Amols H, Schwartz A, Weinberger J. Intracoronary irradiation markedly reduces restenosis after balloon angioplasty in a porcine model. J Am Coll Cardiol 1994;23:1491–8.

21. Weidermann JG, Marboe C, Amols H, Schwartz A, Weinberger J. Intracoronary irradiation markedly reduces neointimal proliferation after balloon angioplasty in swine: persistent benefit at 6-month follow-up. J Am Coll Cardiol 1995;25:1456–61.

22. Mazur W, Ali MN, Dabhagi SF, Criscard C, et al. High dose rate intracoronary radiation suppresses neointimal proliferation in the stented and balloon model of porcine restenosis. Int J Radiat Oncol Biol Phys 1996;36:777–88.

23. Borok TL, Bray M, Sinclair I, et al. Role of ionizing irradiation for keloids. Int J Radiat Oncol Biol Phys 1988;15:865–70.

24. Van den Brenk HAS, Minty CCJ. Radiation in the management of keloids and hypertrophic scar. Br J Surg 1959/1960;47:595–607.

25. Nickson JJ, Lawrence W, Rachwalsky I, Tyree E. Roentgen rays and wound healing. II. Fractionated irradiation; an experimental study. Surgery 1953;34:859–62.

26. Insalsingh CHA. An experience in treating 501 patients with keloids. Johns Hopkins Med J 1974;134:284–90.

27. Grillo HC, Potsaid MS. Studies in wound healing. Ann Surg 1961;154:741.

28. MacLennon I, Keys HM, Evarts CM, Rubgin P. Usefulness of post-operative hip irradiation in the prevention of heterotrophic bone formation in a high risk group of patients. Int J Radiat Oncol Biol Phys 1984;10:49–53.

29. Van den Brenk HAS. Results of prophylactic post-operative irradiation in 1300 cases of pterygium. AJR Am J Roentgenol 1968;103:723.

30. Mintz GS, Pichard AD, Kent KM, et al. Endovascular stents reduce restenosis by eliminating geometric arterial remodeling: a serial intravascular ultrasound study. J Am Coll Cardiol 1995;35A:701–5.

31. Waksman R, Rodriquez JC, Robinson KA, et al. Effect of intravascular irradiation on cell proliferation, apoptosis and vascular remodeling after balloon overstretch injury of porcine coronary arteries. Circulation 1996;96:1944–52.

32. Liermann DD, Bottcher HD, Kollath J, et al. Prophylactic endovascular radiotherapy to prevent intimal hyperplasia after stent implantation in femoropopliteal arteries. Cardiovasc Intervent Radiol 1994;17:12–16.

33. Minar E, Pokrajac B, Maca T, et al. Endovascular brachytherapy for prophylaxis of restenosis after femoropopliteal angioplasty: results of a prospective randomized study. Circulation 2000;102:2694–9.

34. Waksman R, Laird JR, Jurkovitz CT, et al. Intravascular radiation therapy after balloon angioplasty of narrowed femoropopliteal arteries to prevent restenosis: results of the PARIS feasibility clinical trial. J Vasc Interv Radiol 2001;12:915–21.

35. Waksman R, Crocker IA, Kikeri D, et al. Long term results of endovascular radiation therapy for prevention of restenosis in the peripheral vascular system. Circulation 1996;94(8)I-300:1745.

36. Nori D, Parikh, S et al. External beam radiotherapy to prevent post-angioplasty restenosis of compromised arteriovenous dialysis accesses: A Phase I Study. Int J Radiat Oncol Biol Phys 1998;42(Suppl 1):347.

37. Cohen GS, Freeman H, Ringold MA. External beam irradiation as an adjunctive treatment in failing dialysis shunts. JVIR 2000;11:321–326.

38. Raat H, Stockx L, Ranschaert E, et al. Percutaneous hydrodynamic thrombectomy of acute thrombosis in Transjugular Intrahepatic Portosystemic Shunt (TIPS): a feasibility study in five patients. Cardiovasc Interv Radiol 1997;20:180–3.

16. Chronic Total Occlusions: New Therapeutic Approaches

Raghunandan Kamineni and Richard R Heuser

INTRODUCTION

Peripheral vascular disease (PVD) is an often unrecognized or untreated component of systemic atherosclerotic disease. The prevalence of PVD in the general population ranges from 1 to 6% with a significant increase in the prevalence in patients with established coronary artery disease.[1] More than 50% of all lesions of peripheral arterial obstructive disease are localized in the femoropopliteal segment. Lesions in this vascular segment are rarely focal stenosis and are frequently total occlusions. Moreover, these femoropopliteal occlusions are long and are often seen with multi-level atherosclerotic disease. Screening for PVD is an important step in the evaluation of patients with established or suspected coronary artery disease. Ankle–brachial index (ABI) and segmental blood pressure measurements with pulse volume recordings (PVR) are the standard non-invasive screening tools.[2] Although these tests can objectively determine the severity of limb ischemia (ABI) and localize the level of arterial disease (PVR), they cannot distinguish a simple stenosis from a chronic occlusion. Despite magnetic resonance angiography (MRA) or ultrafast computed tomography (CT) angiography increasing the sensitivity of diagnosing PVD (particularly total occlusions), invasive angiography is still considered the gold standard in establishing the diagnosis and extent of PVD (i.e. stenosis vs occlusions).

SURGICAL VERSUS PERCUTANEOUS INTERVENTIONS

The first application of percutaneous transluminal angioplasty was reported by Dotter[3] in the femoropopliteal circulation and further developed by Gruntzig with the addition of balloon dilation. Percutaneous endovascular treatment of vascular disease has since evolved rapidly during the past four decades. With the increasing use of peripheral stents or endovascular grafts in clinical practice, guidelines have been formed to help direct physicians determine the appropriate choice of therapy (i.e. percutaneous vs surgical intervention). For example, recent guidelines for interventions of the distal abdominal aorta and lower extremity vessels classified the severity of peripheral vascular disease into four categories:[1]

- Category 1 lesions: suitable for percutaneous intervention alone;
- Category 2 lesions: suitable for percutaneous intervention in conjunction with surgical intervention;
- Category 3 lesions: can be treated by percutaneous intervention but may have a lower rate of initial technical success and long-term benefit compared with surgical intervention;
- Category 4 lesions: more suitable for surgical intervention with a limited role for percutaneous intervention.

However, these guidelines are not strict. Endovascular techniques and materials are rapidly advancing and the boundaries between these predefined categories are becoming blurred. Many patients that were formerly referred for surgery (e.g. aortoiliac occlusions, long superficial femoral occlusions, infrapopliteal occlusions) are now being treated with percutaneous interventions. This chapter discusses the currently available therapeutic approaches for treatment of chronic total occlusions in the peripheral arteries.

RATIONALE FOR TREATMENT

Revascularization of chronic total occlusions in the peripheral arteries has long been a subject of debate.[4] The rationale for percutaneous treatment of peripheral arterial chronic total occlusions is to improve the lifestyle-limiting claudication and decrease the need for vascular bypass surgery. A further incentive of such treatment is the reduced likelihood of developing critical limb ischemia and the threat of amputation. Also, by decreasing the need for vascular bypass surgery, saphenous veins can be spared for future use (i.e. coronary artery bypass surgery). However, it should be borne in mind that there are limited data substantiating the benefit of such treatment.[5] A relevant disadvantage of percutaneous transluminal angioplasty and stenting is a high incidence of restenosis and reocclusions of approximately 50% in peripheral arteries.[6,7]

CONVENTIONAL MEANS OF TREATMENT

Acute or subacute total occlusions are usually treated with conventional methods of angioplasty and/or stenting with adjunctive thrombolysis or fibrinolysis. However, such conventional methods are usually not successful in treating chronic total occlusions. The major limitation of conventional recanalization techniques is the inability to cross total occlusions with a length of more than 5 cm in up to 50% of the cases. Hydrophilic wires (e.g. Terumo) have considerable success in crossing chronic total occlusion but run the risk of distal perforation. A variety of new techniques designed to treat chronic total occlusion have been developed and are described in the subsequent sections.

PIER – PERCUTANEOUS INTENTIONAL EXTRALUMINAL (SUBINTIMAL) RECANALIZATION

Bolia et al[8] first described this alternative technique to conventional PTA in 1990 before the introduction of stents. Although this technique has gained limited recognition it is a relatively simple technique and is worth describing.

TECHNIQUE

An antegrade puncture of the common femoral artery is performed. The guidewire and the guiding catheter are then advanced through the femoral artery and positioned in the stump, just cranial to the occluded superficial femoral artery (SFA). A 5F rigid catheter with a slightly angled tip is the best catheter for this technique. The catheter is slowly pushed forward with slight rotation. After initial resistance the catheter will suddenly jump forward a few millimeters, indicating that the catheter tip has now entered the extraluminal space from subintimal dissection. Alternatively, a curved tip guidewire can be used to enter the extraluminal space. Once the catheter is in the extraluminal space, a standard 0.035 inch angled guidewire (e.g. Terumo) is pushed down until it forms into a large loop configuration. With this loop the extraluminal space is explored distally. The wire loop can be supported by the catheter, but the loop must always be ahead to make the subintimal dissection. By pushing the loop and the catheter towards the distal patent part of the vessel, a suddenly decreased resistance can be felt with the wire seeming to move down freely, suggesting that the wire has now entered the lumen of the vessel. The catheter is brought down and the wire is removed. The intraluminal position of the catheter should be checked by contrast injection. Care should be taken to prevent damage to the first major collateral artery by avoiding a too distal re-entry site. After re-entry into the true patent distal lumen is confirmed with contrast injection, heparin can be administered. The new false lumen is now dilated in a standard fashion with appropriately sized balloon catheters, eventually with prolonged dilation times up to 3 minutes to improve the initial results. PIER can also be safely and effectively performed via the retrograde popliteal approach when the standard PIER is unsuccessful or contraindicated.[9] Cumulative patency rates of 66% at 6 months, 62% at 1 year and 59% at 18 months with PIER technique have been reported.[9]

NEW DEVICES

LASER ANGIOPLASTY

The idea of using laser energy to vaporize atherosclerotic material obstructing the vessel lumen was introduced in the early 1980s.[10] Early results were fraught with disastrous complications such as perforations and the enthusiasm for laser angioplasty quickly waned. The initial systems used continuous wave laser irradiation, a powerful but inadequate energy source that could cause considerable transversal temperature rise leading to unavoidable thermal damage of adjacent tissue structures.[11] Over the years, various types of laser angioplasty catheter have been developed. Some of these laser catheters have proved ineffective (i.e. the argon laser, metal tips, or sapphire laser) or, quite simply, never made it into clinical practice (i.e. 'smart laser', angioscopically guided laser).[10] Nowadays, with improvements in catheter design and the use of the saline infusion technique, there has been a renewed interest in laser angioplasty.

Currently, excimer laser angioplasty is considered a valuable alternative or adjunct to conventional means for chronic occlusion angioplasty. In contrast to the vaporization caused by the continuous wave lasers, the excimer laser is a pulsed system which induces photoablation during an athermic process.[12] Photoablation (optical breakdown) is simply the disruption of chemical bonds at very high-energy densities with short interaction times. The system uses xenon chloride 308 nm as the source of energy. At this wavelength, the ablation of the irradiated tissue is no longer a photochemical disruption of chemical bonds, but a localized, very fast microexplosion provoked by an extremely high temperature rise of the irradiated volume with energy densities of about 3–6 J/cm^2. As a result of the excimer laser beam's small penetration depth and extremely short pulse duration, the thermal damage to the adjacent tissues is minimal even when high energy densities are used.[12]

TECHNIQUE

The contralateral access with subsequent crossover recanalization of the occlusion can be considered the standard approach for recanalization of long SFA occlusions. After achieving a retrograde femoral artery access, a hydrophilic guidewire (Terumo 0.035 inch, stiff type, angled tip; Terumo, Tokyo, Japan) is advanced to the origin of the occlusion. Then, the multifiber excimer laser catheter (7F or 8F) is placed at the origin of the occlusion and the activated catheter is advanced the first few millimeters into the occlusion without wire guidance. Further recanalization of the occluded vessel segment is done by slowly advancing the activated laser catheter stepwise for a short (<5 mm) distance without wire guidance, followed by further crossing with the guidewire in a step-by-step fashion. The advancement of the activated laser catheter should not exceed 1 mm/s.

To enter the patent distal segment of the occluded artery it is recommended that the last 2 cm of the occlusion be crossed with the guidewire alone. Care should be taken to avoid dissections distal to the original occlusion. Fluoroscopic 'road mapping' can be used throughout to verify the alignment of guidewires and catheters to the vessel lumen. Also, the vessel should be thoroughly flushed with saline before lasering to remove any contrast medium as the interaction of laser energy with the contrast medium can produce shock waves, which may result in disruption of the vessel wall.

After the initial laser passage, the 0.035 inch hydrophilic guidewire is exchanged for a 0.018 inch guidewire to allow distal saline flushing for a subsequent second or third passage of the obstructed area. Finally the recanalization procedure is completed by balloon dilation in a standard fashion with appropriately sized balloon catheters. During intervention all patients should receive 5000–10,000 international units of unfractionated heparin. Anticoagulation may be continued for 24 hours with a target activated partial thromboplastin time of 60–80 seconds. Also, all patients should be given aspirin.

OUTCOME RESULTS

Scheinert et al[13] published results from a large series of patients that underwent excimer laser assisted revascularization of chronic SFA occlusions. With a total number of 318 patients (411 limbs or lesions, mean occlusion length 19.4 ± 6.0 cm) being treated with excimer laser assisted angioplasty, the primary success rate for revascularization was 83.2% (342/411 cases). A secondary attempt was performed in 44 cases, including using the retrograde popliteal approach in 39 cases. The total technical success rate was 90.5% (372/411 cases). Relevant interventional complications were acute reocclusion (1.0%), perforation (2.2%), and embolization/distal thrombosis (3.9%). Restenosis was detected in more than 50% of the cases; however, using secondary interventions, the majority of the reobstructions were treatable on an outpatient basis. As a result, the clinical benefit was maintained in 75.1% of the patients after 1 year.

Similarly, Steinkamp et al[14] reported results of laser angioplasty of short occlusions of the SFA (total number of patients 312, mean occlusion length 7.5 cm). The success rate for recanalization of the SFA was 91.7% (286/312 cases). In 26 patients recanalization was not possible. The major causes of failure were obstructing calcifications and aberrant anatomy of the SFA. The primary, primary assisted and secondary patency rates at 36 months were 49.2%, 76.5% and 86.3% respectively.

LUMEND FRONTRUNNER CTO™ CATHETER

The LuMend Frontrunner CTO™ catheter (LuMend, Redwood, CA) is a bioptome-like device specifically designed to cross chronic total occlusions in the coronaries and has recently been approved for clinical use in coronary arteries only. It consists of a 3.0 or 4.0 mm metallic blunt distal tip, a 4F shaft (135 cm long), and a hand-held distal tip control device at the proximal end of the catheter. The distal tip of the catheter can be opened and closed, much like the tip of the bioptomes used for percutaneous endomyocardial biopsies. The catheter makes blunt microdissec-tions, separating atherosclerotic plaques and creates a passage through the occlusion enabling the guidewire to be placed distally. Whitlow et al[15] reported the largest series of patients so far (n = 100) with coronary chronic total occlusions who underwent treatment using the Frontrunner™ catheter. These patients had earlier failed the use of conventional means in crossing total occlusions. The chronic total occlusion was successfully crossed in 79% of the patients. Roukoz et al[16] reported their experience with the Frontrunner™ catheter used to treat 16 chronic SFA occlusions with an average occlusion length of 11 cm; 15/16 (94%) lesions were crossed successfully and there were no perforations. One patient had a short subintimal dissection that resolved after stenting. Mean fluoroscopic time to cross the total occlusion was 4.2 minutes.

These early reports suggest that the device appears to be a safe and effective tool to treat chronic total occlusions and may one day be approved for use in treating chronic occlusion in peripheral arteries.

MOLLRING CUTTER™

This is a remote endarterectomy device designed to transect the distal end of an atheromatous core in chronic occlusions. The MollRing Cutter™ (Vascular Architects, San José, CA) consist of stainless steel double ring cutters and a hypotube with angled interior blades. The ring diameters come in many sizes, from 5 mm (for femoral arteries) to 10 mm (for iliac arteries). A detailed description of the device and the technique for using it can be seen in a review by Teijink et al.[17]

SAFE-CROSS™ TO RF GUIDEWIRE SYSTEM

This 'forward-looking' fiberoptic guidewire system, recently approved by the US Food and Drug Administration (FDA) for use in both coronary and peripheral arterial occlusions, is based on the principle of low-coherence interferometry.[18] In general, a light source is divided into two beams: a reference arm and a sample arm. The light in the reference arm is reflected at a determinable path length and, for measurement purposes, the path length can be changed. Light in the sample arm is also reflected or scattered by the material present in the sample. The reflections and the backscattered light are combined at the coupler and if the path lengths of the two arms are within the coherence length of the light, the beams will recorrelate or interfere with one another. The detector measures the interference intensity. Since the reference arm length is known and adjustable, the intensity profile of scattered light from a sample arm can be determined as a function of the reference arm path length. The resolution of the system is largely dependent on the coherence length of the light. Since the coherence length is inversely proportional to the bandwidth, a broadband source is desirable. Resolution of approximately 10 μm can be obtained with commercially available sources and components.[19]

OCR SYSTEM

The optical coherence reflectometry (OCR) system consists of an optical interferometer, a demodulation-computer unit and monitor, fiberoptic cables, and a light source (Fig. 16.1). The Safe-Cross™ TO RF guidewire system (Intraluminal Therapeutics, Carlsbad, CA) consists of an OCR system, optical guidewire, and catheter (Fig. 16.2). The optical interferometer operates in an A-scan mode to detect the distance to the normal arterial wall interface through plaque or thrombus. No real imaging is attempted with the optical guidewire; rather, the optical fiber in the guidewire illuminates the tissue in front of the distal tip of the guidewire and collects the backscattered light, hence the derived nomenclature of optical coherence reflectometry.[20]

The backscattered light is analyzed through the low-coherence interferometer, producing a signal tracing that is displayed and updated every half-

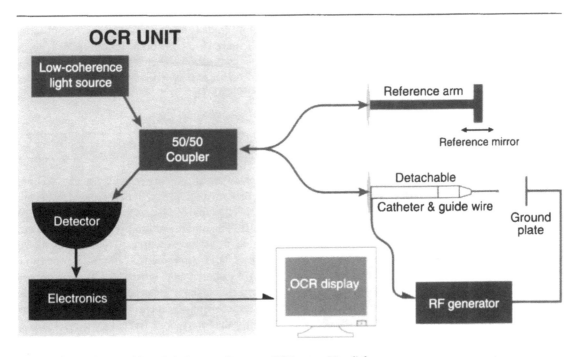

Fig. 16.1 Schematic diagram of the optical coherence reflectometry (OCR) system. RF, radiofrequency.

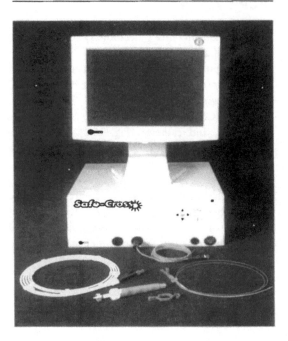

Fig. 16.2 The console and guidewire control system.

second on an OCR monitor. The signal tracing is monitored through a series of algorithms to determine if the normal arterial wall interface is within the field of view. If the normal arterial wall is detected, a visual indication of a red bar across the top portion of the signal tracing is displayed to the operator and the relative distance to the arterial wall is shown. If the normal arterial wall is not in the field of view, a green bar is displayed, indicating the guidewire can be advanced. This simple method allows the interventionist to navigate safely through the total occlusion within the vessel.

The Safe-Cross™ TO RF guidewire is equipped with radiofrequency (RF) energy that is delivered at the tip of the wire to facilitate crossing occlusions. The RF energy ablates through the atherosclerotic plaques. As an added safety feature, the RF energy cannot be applied and becomes automatically disabled when the guidewire identifies an arterial wall. Early experience with the guidewire was successful with chronic coronary as well as peripheral arterial occlusions.[21]

RESULTS

GRIP TRIAL

The Guided Radio Frequency in Peripheral Total Occlusions (GRIP) Registry study was designed to evaluate the safety and effectiveness of the Safe-Cross™ TO RF guidewire system to traverse total occlusions in the peripheral arteries of the lower extremities (Figs 16.3–16.5). Thirteen investigational sites enrolled a total of 72 consecutive patients (75 lesions) with total occlusion in the native peripheral arteries of the lower extremities (Wholey MH reported preliminary results of this study in *Endovascular Today*). Mean age was 66.1 ± 11.5 years, and 68% of the patients were male. The key inclusion criteria were that the total occlusion be in a native lower extremity and that the total occlusion could not be crossed with conventional guidewires after a minimum of 10 minutes of guidewire manipulation. Device success rate (defined as the achievement of distal lumen position with no occurrence of vessel perforation), dissection (grade C or greater), or distal embolization was achieved in 74.7% of the lesions treated. For 56 lesions that were recanalized, the mean pre-procedural ABI was 0.59; the post-procedural ABI was 0.86 ($p < 0.001$).

CONCLUSION

With the advancements in endovascular technology, balloon angioplasty/stenting is rapidly becoming the therapy of choice for peripheral vascular disease. The initial and long-term results are comparable to surgical outcomes. Technologies such as excimer laser angioplasty, LuMend Frontrunner CTO™ catheter, and 'fiberoptic' guidewires with optical coherence reflectometry now make it possible to successfully treat chronic occlusions percutaneously that were once treated by surgical means only. Despite these advances, chronic total occlusions of the peripheral vessels remain a therapeutic challenge. Small reports of treating peripheral

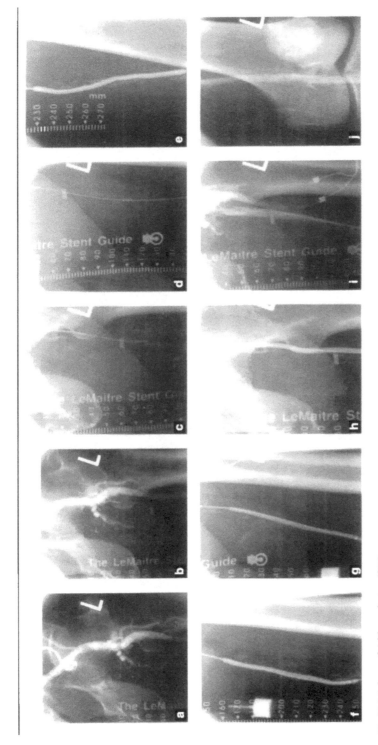

Fig. 16.3 Left superficial femoral artery (SFA).

(a) Left SFA occlusion near the femoral bifurcation. (b) Safe-Cross™ guidewire tip across the initial part of the left SFA occlusion. (c) Safe-Cross™ guidewire tip further advanced distally in the left SFA occlusion. (d) Further advancement of the Safe-Cross™ guidewire in the distal SFA. (e–h) Successive balloon angioplasties along the length of the SFA (from distal SFA to SFA origin). (i) Post-angioplasty angiogram confirming a patent left SFA. (j) Post-angioplasty angiogram confirming a patent left popliteal artery.

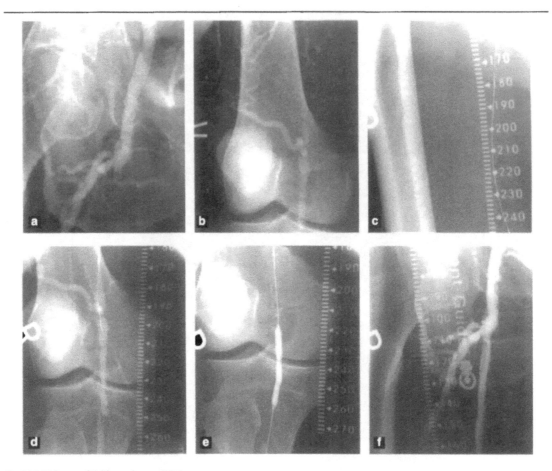

Fig. 16.4 Right superficial femoral artery (SFA).

(a) Right SFA occlusion at the femoral bifurcation. (b) Distal end of the right SFA occlusion with right popliteal artery filling in via collateral vessels. (c) Safe-Cross™ guidewire tip across the right SFA occlusion and positioned in the distal right SFA. (d) Safe-Cross™ guidewire tip completely across the right SFA occlusion and positioned in the right popliteal artery. (e) Balloon angioplasty of the distal portion of the right total occlusion. (f) Post-angioplasty angiogram confirming a patent right SFA.

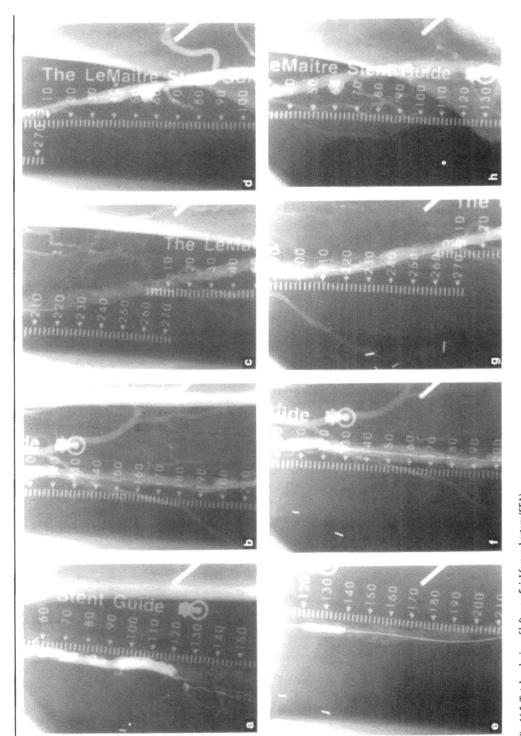

Fig. 16.5 Total occlusion of left superficial femoral artery (SFA).

(a) Total occlusion at mid-level of left SFA (ruler marker 122). (b) Safe-Cross™ guidewire tip across the total occlusion (positioned between ruler markers 200 and 210). (c) Safe-Cross™ guidewire tip (ruler marker 220) advanced further into the left SFA occlusion. (d) Angiogram through the glide catheter confirming the catheter's intraluminal position in the left popliteal artery. Safe-Cross™ guidewire was removed for angiogram. (e) Balloon angioplasty at the original site of the left SFA occlusion. (f) Post-angioplasty angiogram confirming a patent mid-level left SFA. (g,h) Post-angioplasty angiograms confirming a patent left distal SFA and popliteal artery.

chronic occlusions with 'drug-eluting stents' are promising in reducing the rate of restenosis.[22] With the continued enthusiasm to develop new endovascular technologies, it may eventually be possible to treat almost all chronic occlusions in the peripheral arteries non-surgically.

REFERENCES

1. Pentecost MJ, Criqui MH, Dorros G, et al. Guidelines for peripheral percutaneous transluminal angioplasty of the abdominal aorta and lower extremity vessels. A statement for health professionals from a special writing group of the Councils on Cardiovascular Radiology, Arteriosclerosis, Cardio-Thoracic and Vascular Surgery, Clinical Cardiology, and Epidemiology and Prevention, the American Heart Association. Circulation 1994;89:511–31.

2. Hirsch AT, Criqui MH, Treat-Jacobson D, et al. Peripheral arterial disease detection, awareness, and treatment in primary care. JAMA 2001;286:1317–24.

3. Dotter CT, Judkins MP. Transluminal treatment of arteriosclerotic obstruction. Description of a new technique and a preliminary report of its application. Circulation 1964;30:654–70.

4. Puma JA, Sketch MH Jr, Tcheng JE, et al. Percutaneous revascularization of chronic coronary occlusions: an overview. J Am Coll Cardiol 1995;26:1–11.

5. Roukoz B, Haider AW, Surabhi S, et al. Initial experience with the LuMend Frontrunner Catheter for treatment of chronic superficial femoral artery occlusions. Abstracts of the 15th annual symposium: Transcatheter Cardiovascular Therapeutics. September 15–17, 2003. Washington, DC, USA. Am J Cardiol 2003;92:1L–252L.

6. Hewes RC, White RI Jr, Murray RR, et al. Long-term results of superficial femoral artery angioplasty. AJR Am J Roentgenol 1986;146:1025–9.

7. Colapinto RF, Harries-Jones EP, Johnston KW. Percutaneous transluminal angioplasty of peripheral vascular disease: a two-year experience. Cardiovasc Intervent Radiol 1980;3:213–8.

8. Bolia A, Miles KA, Brennan J, Bell PR. Percutaneous transluminal angioplasty of occlusions of the femoral and popliteal arteries by subintimal dissection. Cardiovasc Intervent Radiol 1990;13:357–63.

9. Yilmaz S, Sindel T, Ceken K, Alimoglu E, Luleci E. Subintimal recanalization of long superficial femoral artery occlusions through the retrograde popliteal approach. Cardiovasc Intervent Radiol 2001;24:154–60.

10. Meier B. Coronary angioplasty in chronic total occlusion. Rev Port Cardiol 1999;18 Suppl 1:I55–60.

11. Dorschel K, Biamino G, Brodzinski T, Axel T, Muller G. Comparison of the feasibility of laser angioplasty using heater probes, sapphire tips, and bare fibers. Eur Heart J 1988;9(suppl.):331.

12. Grundfest WS, Litvack F, Forrester JS, et al. Laser ablation of human atherosclerotic plaque without adjacent tissue injury. J Am Coll Cardiol 1985;5:929–33.

13. Scheinert D, Laird JR Jr, Schroder M, et al. Excimer laser-assisted recanalization of long, chronic superficial femoral artery occlusions. J Endovasc Ther 2001;8:156–66.

14. Steinkamp HJ, Wissgott C, Rademaker J, et al. Short (1–10 cm) superficial femoral artery occlusions: results of treatment with Excimer laser angioplasty. Cardiovasc Intervent Radiol 2002;25:388–96.

15. Whitlow PL, Selmon M, O'Neill W. Treatment of uncrossable chronic total occlusions with the Frontrunner: multicenter experience. J Am Coll Cardiol 2002;39:1A–578A.

16. Roukoz B, Haider AW, Surabhi S, et al. Initial experience with the LuMend Frontrunner Catheter for treatment of chronic superficial femoral artery occlusions. Am J Cardiol 2003;92:158L.

17. Teijink JA, van den Berg JC, Moll FL. A minimally invasive technique in occlusive disease of the superficial femoral artery: remote endarterectomy using the MollRing Cutter. Ann Vasc Surg 2001;15:594–8.

18. Zou XY, Wang LJ, Mandel L. Induced coherence and indistinguishability in optical interference. Phys Rev Lett 1991;67:318–21.

19. Newton S. Optical coherence and quantum optics. Photonic Spectra 1991:118–26.

20. Neet JM, Winston TR, Hedrick AD. Navigating a guidewire through total occlusions: clinical experience. In: Anderson RR, Bartels KE, Bass LS, et al, eds. Lasers in Surgery: Advanced Characterization Therapeutics, and Systems X. Pro SPIE 2000;3907:536–43.

21. Morales PA, Heuser RR. Chronic total occlusions: experience with fiber-optic guidance technology – optical coherence reflectometry. J Interv Cardiol 2001;14:611–6.

22. Duda SH, Pusich B, Richter G, et al. Sirolimus-eluting stents for the treatment of obstructive superficial femoral artery disease: six-month results. Circulation 2002;106:1505–9.

17. Complications of peripheral interventions

Raghunandan Kamineni, Lisa Kelly and Richard R Heuser

INTRODUCTION

Percutaneous vascular interventions (coronary or peripheral) are inherently associated with certain complications. As technology is improving and new procedures and devices are being introduced to the interventional field, operators will face both a positive and a negative impact on the complications associated with peripheral interventional procedures.

As peripheral interventional procedures are almost always performed by the femoral approach, femoral access site (groin) complications represent the most common localized complications. A second group of complications are directly related to the angioplasty site. These complications can result in adverse outcomes, exposing patients to significant discomfort, additional risk, longer hospital stay, and consumption of additional institutional resources. It is very important for interventionists to have a thorough understanding of complications associated with peripheral interventional procedures. They should also understand the steps that should be taken to minimize the consequences when a complication occurs. In this chapter we describe the complications associated with peripheral interventional procedures as well as the methods to handle the complications.

Groin complications can be classified as follows:

- Local bleeding and hematoma
- Pseudoaneurysm
- Retroperitoneal hemorrhage
- Arteriovenous fistula
- Groin infection
- Thrombotic occlusion
- Arterial laceration and perforation
- Arterial dissection
- Femoral neuropathy.

LOCAL BLEEDING AND HEMATOMA

Local bleeding and formation of hematoma represent the most common access site complications (up to 50% of the bleeding complications) encountered after the catheterization procedure. As a precise and uniform definition of bleeding in clinical trials is lacking, the true incidence of this complication is not known. The reported incidence of hematomas from observational studies and randomized trials varies widely – from 0.5 to 7%.[1-5] Several contributing factors have been identified as increasing the risk of access site bleeding (Table 17.1).

Table 17.1 Factors Predisposing to Vascular Access Site Bleeding Complications

Anatomic factors
Elderly patient
Obese patient
Female patient
Calcified vessels

Procedural factors
Through-and-through puncture
High puncture (above inguinal ligament)
Low puncture (profunda or superficial femoral artery)
Multiple punctures
Large sheath size
Prolonged procedure time
Prolonged indwelling sheath time

Hemodynamic factors
Severe hypertension

Hematologic factors
Multiple platelet antagonists (aspirin, clopidogrel, glycoprotein IIb/IIIa antagonists)
Antithrombotic agents (warfarin)
Thrombolytic agents (tPA, TNKase)
Underlying coagulopathy or thrombocytopenia

Human factors
Inexperience
Inability to gain 'control' of site upon sheath removal
Short duration of pressure applied to obtain hemostasis

Groin bleeding can be insidious, especially in obese patients, leading to a significant blood loss before it is recognized. Fortunately, in most cases bleeding is trivial and responds to local compression with no antecedent complications. Persistent bleeding, if not attended to promptly, can result in an enlarging mass surrounding the puncture site, the cardinal sign of hematoma (space-occupying collection of blood). In some instances, groin hematomas can cause femoral nerve compression leading to quadriceps weakness that may take weeks to months to resolve. If the ongoing bleeding stops with manual compression, the hematoma will gradually resolve in 1–2 weeks as the blood is reabsorbed from the soft tissues. If a through-and-through puncture is made in the femoral artery above the inguinal ligament the hematoma may extend into the retroperitoneal space. This bleeding is not evident from surface inspection and should be suspected if the patient develops unexplained hypotension, tachycardia, fall in hematocrit, or ipsilateral flank pain following a femoral catheterization procedure.

Groin bleeding from femoral artery cannulation is usually treated with direct manual compression of the bleeding site. Mechanical clamp or pneumatic compression when used to control bleeding should be applied very cautiously without prolonged (>3 minutes) occlusion of distal flow, and with continuous monitoring until control is obtained. Mechanical devices should be avoided in patients with severe peripheral vascular disease, or prior aortofemoral or femoropopliteal bypass surgery due to the higher risk of development of femoral thrombosis. Large hematomas may require transfusion but surgical repair is generally not required. In patients with a large hematoma resulting in hypotension, stabilization of hemodynamics with rapid volume replacement (crystalloid or blood) is critical. In hypertensive patients, blood pressure should be lowered with nitrates or vasodilators. If the bleeding cannot be controlled, urgent surgical exploration with repair of the vascular access site may be required. Uncontrollable free bleeding around the sheath suggests laceration of the femoral artery. This problem can usually be managed by replacement of the sheath with the next-larger-diameter sheath. Bleeding can be restricted with manual compression around the sheath until the procedure is completed. If heparin is used during the procedure it should be reversed and the sheath should be removed; prolonged compression (30–60 minutes) of the access site (either manually or with a compression device) should then be applied.

Bleeding complications can be minimized by meticulous attention to the access site, recognition of predisposing factors (see Table 17.1), avoidance of post-procedural heparin, and prompt removal of vascular sheaths (activated clotting time (ACT) <160 seconds). Adequate time should be allowed to compress the access site and achieve complete hemostasis after removal of the sheath.

PSEUDOANEURYSM

A pseudoaneurysm is an encapsulated hematoma that communicates with the artery due to dissolution of clot plugging the arterial puncture site. Pseudoaneurysm usually results from inadequate compression and incomplete hemostasis following sheath removal. The factors associated with increased risk of pseudoaneurysm formation are shown in Table 17.2. Distinguishing a pseudoaneurysm from an expanding hematoma is frequently difficult. Generally the pseudoaneurysm is identified as a tender, pulsatile mass with audible

---

Table 17.2 Factors Associated with Increased Risk of Pseudoaneurysm Formation

- Low vascular access in the superficial femoral or profunda artery (i.e. puncture below the bifurcation of the common femoral)
- Severe peripheral vascular disease
- Large sheaths
- Prolonged sheath time
- Prolonged anticoagulation
- Impaired platelet function
- Premature ambulation

bruit over the mass. Any patient with a large or painful hematoma or when a hematoma is associated with femoral nerve palsy should be evaluated for pseudoaneurysm. Duplex ultrasound scanning confirms the diagnosis of pseudoaneurysm.

Treatment of a pseudoaneurysm depends on the size, expansion and the need for anticoagulation. Pseudoaneurysms <3 cm usually do not need surgical repair. A follow-up ultrasound in 1–2 weeks after the initial diagnosis is useful to reassess the expansion of the pseudoaneurysm. By this time spontaneous thrombosis occurs in most cases, requiring no further treatment. Large pseudoaneurysms (>3 cm) are less likely to undergo spontaneous thrombosis and may pose the risk of enlargement and rupture. Techniques used to close pseudoaneurysms include ultrasound-guided compression,[6] surgical repair, insertion of coils,[7] ultrasound-guided direct thrombin injection,[8,9] fluoroscopically guided direct thrombin injection,[10] and covered stents.[11,12] Kang et al[8] reported that 75% of pseudoaneurysms thrombosed within 15 seconds of using direct thrombin injection.

Of the above-described techniques, ultrasound-guided compression has become the initial therapy in patients with suitable anatomy. Pseudoaneurysm with a long and thin neck has a success rate of 92–98% when further anticoagulation is not needed. Those needing anticoagulation have success rates of 54–86%.[13–16] Surgical repair is considered for failed ultrasound compression or when the femoral nerve is involved.[17]

The key to avoiding pseudoaneurysm formation is:

1. accurate puncture of the common femoral artery;
2. fluoroscopic localization of the skin nick to overlie the inferior border of the femoral head;
3. use of small sheaths whenever possible and prompt sheath removal after the ACT falls to subtherapeutic level (<175 seconds);
4. avoidance of post-procedural anticoagulation;
5. treatment of hypertension at the time of sheath removal and adequate groin compression with achievement of complete hemostasis.

RETROPERITONEAL HEMORRHAGE

Femoral puncture above the inguinal ligament may result in bleeding that tracks posteriorly into the retroperitoneal space. The reported incidence of retroperitoneal hematoma is <1% after interventional procedures.[3,5] Retroperitoneal bleeding is not evident from the surface, especially in obese patients. Frequently the diagnosis is suspected from a fall in hematocrit levels, unexplained hypotension and tachycardia, vague abdominal pain, ipsilateral flank pain[18,19] and abdominal distention. Retroperitoneal hematoma that is adjacent to the psoas muscle may lead to hip pain and inability to flex the hip. Large retroperitoneal hematoma can mimic acute appendicitis with right lower quadrant pain and fever.[20] Severe retroperitoneal hemorrhage can also cause hemodynamic collapse, shock, liver/renal failure, and disseminated intravascular coagulation.

CT scanning or ultrasound of the abdomen and pelvis can confirm the diagnosis of retroperitoneal hematoma. Treatment is usually expectant with attention to hemodynamic status. Rapid replacement of volume with crystalloid or blood is important. Vital signs should be closely monitored. Heparin should be reversed with protamine. Vascular sheaths should be promptly removed and adequate time should be allowed to compress the access site. If the above measures fail, urgent surgical exploration is warranted.

Careful localization of the femoral artery entry site, accurate single anterior wall puncture, avoidance of excessive anticoagulation, and careful manipulation of the guidewire help to prevent retroperitoneal hemorrhage. The inguinal crease is an unreliable marker for deep vascular anatomy, especially in obese patients,[21] and fluoroscopic localization of the medial third of the femoral head can be a useful guide for a femoral artery access site.

ARTERIOVENOUS FISTULA

Puncturing the femoral artery and the overlying femoral vein can result in arteriovenous (AV) fistula after sheath removal (Fig. 17.1). Also, ongoing

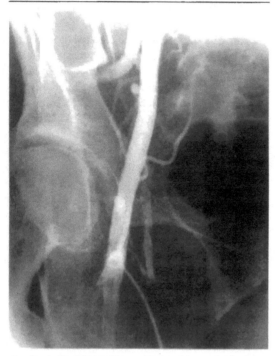

Fig. 17.1 Angiographic appearance of an arteriovenous fistula with simultaneous filling of the right superficial femoral artery (left) and vein (right).

bleeding from the femoral puncture site may decompress into the adjacent venous puncture site to form an AV fistula. The factors that increase the risk of AV fistula formation are:

- multiple punctures to obtain vascular access;
- low puncture (superficial femoral or profunda, transecting a small venous branch);
- high puncture (common femoral artery and lateral femoral circumflex vein);
- impaired clotting.

AV fistulae are not evident immediately and may take days to develop after the femoral catheterization procedure.[22] Clinical signs associated with AV fistulae are to-and-fro continuous bruit over the puncture site, and a swollen, tender extremity due to venous dilation. Small AV fistulae with low-volume AV flow by Duplex scan can be managed conservatively, since many of these close spontaneously.[3] Some authors suggest prompt surgical repair of large AV fistulae due to the fear of the patient developing high-output heart failure if left untreated. However, two recently reported reviews of a large group of patients with persisting femoral AV fistula, followed prospectively over a period of 2–3 years, showed no increased incidence of cardiac volume overload or limb damage.[23,24] Surgical repair, if considered, involves excision or division of the fistula, or synthetic grafting of the involved vessels. Experience with non-surgical techniques such as ultrasound-guided compression[13] and endovascular stent grafting is limited.[11,12]

GROIN INFECTION

Groin infections after catheterization procedure are rare. Cleveland and Gelfand[25] observed only three infectious complications in 4669 patients who underwent catheterization procedure. Smith et al[26] reported only five infectious complications in 2003 patients at the vascular access site. Thus, the overall reported incidence of groin infection following catheterization is 0.25%. Gram-positive organisms, especially staphylococcus species, are the predominant cause of groin abscesses and endarteritis associated with femoral arterial cannulation.[25,27,28] Risk factors for the development of groin infections after catheterization procedure are the presence of hematoma or foreign material within the lumen of the artery.[29,30] Groin infections are more frequently associated with the use of vascular closure devices compared to manual compression.[31] The braided polyester suture used in the Perclose™ device may act as a nidus for infection.

Groin infections manifest with access site erythema, painful induration, or exudative drainage. Systemic involvement can cause fever and/or rigors. A local reaction such as phlebitis at the access site responds to hot soaks and elevation of the affected limb. Cellulitis or exudative drainage requires antibiotics. Large abscesses may require surgical drainage in addition to parenteral antibiotic therapy.

THROMBOTIC OCCLUSION

Local thrombosis of the femoral artery access site is a rare complication except in patients with a small common femoral artery lumen in whom a large diameter catheter or sheath has been placed. The reported incidence of femoral artery thrombosis after interventional procedures is <1%. Femoral artery thrombosis, especially in the presence of pre-existing peripheral vascular disease, can lead to subsequent complications such as limb ischemia (21%), leg amputation (11%) and death (2%).[32] Risk factors associated with thrombotic occlusion of the access site include peripheral vascular disease, advanced age, hypercoagulable state, cardiomyopathy, small-caliber vessels, female gender, and small body habitus. Vessel spasm and dissection often contribute to arterial thrombosis.

Femoral artery occlusion manifests with sudden onset of limb pain, pallor, cyanosis, absence of distal pulse and a cool extremity. Physical examination looking for the above signs and duplex scanning may be used to diagnose femoral artery thrombosis. Arteriography may be needed for confirmation of the diagnosis and to guide therapy.

If the vascular sheath itself is causing obstruction to antegrade flow, removal of the sheath resolves the limb ischemia. Persistent limb ischemia with diminished or absent pulses despite removal of the vascular sheath suggests femoral artery thrombosis or dissection at the puncture site. This requires urgent surgical consultation and treatment with heparinization and urgent thrombectomy to prevent late complications such as muscle necrosis and limb amputation. Various types of thrombectomy – such as Fogarty catheter thrombectomy, percutaneous rheolytic thrombectomy (Possis AngioJet™) – have been used to treat femoral artery thrombosis. If thrombectomy fails, surgical thromboendarterectomy or bypass grafting may be considered.

Using small sheaths in high-risk patients with peripheral vascular disease, small vessels, or hypercoagulable states can reduce femoral artery thrombosis. Regular flushing and avoiding delays in vascular sheath removal are essential. If an indwelling sheath is necessary, infusion of pressurized heparinized saline through the sheath will help prevent local thrombosis.

ARTERIAL LACERATION AND PERFORATION

Advancement of guidewires, catheters or other devices can result in arterial tear or perforation. Also, deep skin nicks in patients with a superficially lying femoral vessel can cause significant arterial laceration. Arterial perforation can occur at the access site or at a site remote from the puncture site.

Uncontrollable bleeding around the vascular sheath suggests arterial laceration. Perforation is suspected when the patient complains of acute pain during guidewire or catheter manipulation. Continuous bleeding results in hypotension. Catheter or guidewire withdrawal can cause more discomfort as extravasation increases when the defect gets exposed. Bleeding from guidewire perforation can be slow, small and less obvious. Contrast injection may confirm extravasation of blood, but small perforations may be missed. Digital subtraction angiography is a more sensitive tool to diagnose arterial perforations. Free bleeding around the vascular sheath usually responds to replacement with a next-larger-diameter sheath. However, if the bleeding persists, manual compression around the sheath during the procedure is indicated.

Most guidewire-induced arterial perforations are benign and resolve spontaneously without significant blood loss. If the bleeding is ongoing, anticoagulation should be reversed immediately. Lost blood volume should be replaced with crystalloid or blood. Depending on its location and extent, the perforation can be treated with prolonged balloon inflation, stent grafting, therapeutic coil embolization or surgical repair.

Arterial perforation can be avoided with careful and gentle advancement of guidewires, catheters or other interventional devices. The tip of the guidewire should always be observed under fluoroscopy during catheter advancement. If resistance is met during guidewire advancement the guidewire should be withdrawn and redirected: never force a guidewire or catheter to advance when resistance is encountered. Hydrophilic wires provide poor tactile feedback and should be used very cautiously under fluoroscopic guidance.

ARTERIAL DISSECTION

Access site arterial dissection occurs during retrograde advancement of guidewires, especially hydrophilic guidewires or catheters (Fig. 17.2). The reported incidence of such dissection with interventional procedures is 0.01–0.4%.[33-37] However, the true frequency is probably higher, as most minor dissections may go unnoticed. Patients with peripheral vascular disease are more likely to develop dissection during interventional procedures.

Serious consequences from iatrogenic access site arterial dissection with interventional procedures are rare. However, unrecognized local dissection at the access site may sometimes lead to development of late thrombosis or pseudoaneurysm formation. As most access site vascular dissections are retrograde from the advancement of guidewires or catheters, antegrade flow will usually 'tack down'

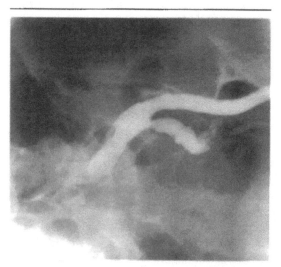

Fig. 17.2 Angiographic appearance of a non-flow limiting arterial wall dissection of the left iliac artery caused by a guidewire.

the flap without the need for further therapy. Dissections associated with thrombosis and/or distal flow impairment need immediate surgical or percutaneous treatment with stenting.

The principles described to prevent arterial perforation also apply to arterial dissection. Use of non-hydrophilic, soft-tip or J-tip guidewires will reduce the likelihood of dissection. Dilators and vascular sheaths should always be advanced over a leading guidewire to keep them off the arterial wall.

FEMORAL NEUROPATHY

Femoral neuropathy usually develops from inadvertent direct injury to the femoral nerve with the needle in an attempt to gain vascular access or due to impingement of the nerve with a large groin hematoma or pseudoaneurysm from femoral artery puncture. Also, transient femoral neuropathy can be seen with the use of large amounts of topical lidocaine (lignocaine) at the access site.

Femoral neuropathy manifests as sensory and/or motor impairment in the distribution of the femoral nerve. Patients may be unable to ambulate or bear weight due to quadriceps weakness. Femoral neuropathy due to topical lidocaine (lignocaine) resolves in several hours as the effect of lidocaine (lignocaine) wears off. However, neuropathy occurring due to large groin hematoma may take weeks or even months to resolve. Femoral neuropathy due to pseudoaneurysm improves following treatment of the pseudoaneurysm.

VASCULAR CLOSURE DEVICES

Vascular closure devices (VCDs) are gradually becoming an important tool in the management of patients following diagnostic and interventional catheterization procedures. Vascular closure devices were introduced in 1990s to increase patient comfort and convenience with early mobilization and discharge from the hospital, and to decrease complication rates associated with vascular access. Although achieving these objectives, VCDs are still associated with complications such as hematoma, retroperitoneal bleeding, pseudoaneurysm, late bleeding, groin infection, acute femoral artery closure and rarely death. As with all new devices, the complications are more frequent during the operator's learning phase.[38] The early use of these devices generated reports from the surgical literature on complications that were considered different[39,40] and more devastating[41,42] than the usual complications experienced from manual compression. More recent studies have shown a decrease in complication rates in both control and device-treated patients.[43,44]

Factors associated with an increased rate of vascular complications are outlined in Table 17.3. These factors, when present, may preclude the use of closure devices. In addition, the following factors should be considered when using VCDs:

- Vascular closure devices should not be used to treat patients with suspected double-wall punctures, as punctures of the posterior wall are not closed with these devices.
- The risk of bleeding at the puncture site should be carefully weighed against the benefits of using a vascular hemostasis device when treating patients with bleeding disorders.
- The groin puncture site should be carefully monitored to minimize the occurrence of complications with vascular hemostasis devices.

ANGIOPLASTY SITE

A second group of complications are related directly to the angioplasty site as well as distal to this site. These complications include acute vessel thrombosis, vessel dissection (Fig. 17.3), perforation (Fig. 17.4), and distal embolization. With improving technology (development of low-profile non-compliant balloons, miniaturization of the balloon catheters, introduction of vascular stents) such complications have decreased in frequency. In the pre-stent era, for most complications such as dissections and perforations, surgery was the only option. Now these complications are easily treated with vascular stents or covered stents and are usually not reported.

Table 17.3 Factors Associated with Increased Rate of Vascular Complications

- Severely calcified femoral artery
- Small-caliber femoral artery
- Low punctures (below the common femoral artery bifurcation)
- Inguinal scarring
- Significant peripheral vascular disease
- Age >70 years
- Activated clotting time >300 seconds

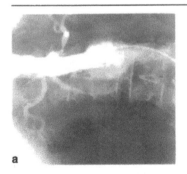 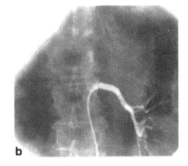 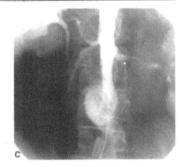

a b c

Fig. 17.3 Renal artery dissection during angioplasty and stent placement.

(a) Severe ostial stenosis of the left renal artery. (b) Angiogram following stent placement in the left renal artery. (c) Angiogram revealing dissection at the left renal artery.

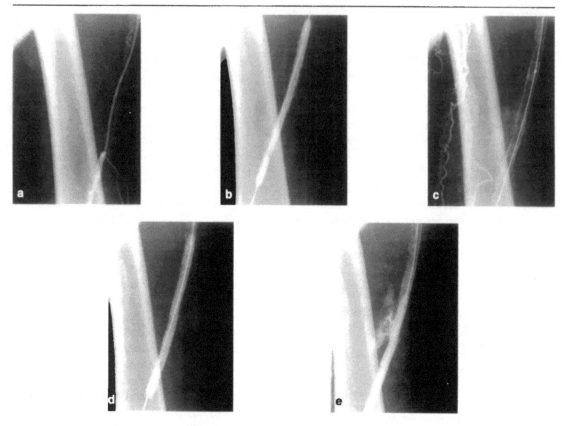

Fig. 17.4 Superficial femoral artery (SFA) perforation during angioplasty.

(a) Total occlusion of the left SFA. (b) Balloon angioplasty of the left SFA. (c) Serial stent placements to a long segment of the left SFA. (d) Post-stent balloon angioplasty. (e) Angiogram revealing perforation after post-stent balloon angioplasty.

ABRUPT CLOSURE/THROMBOSIS

Abrupt closure or acute thrombosis occurred in 2–4% of cases with balloon angioplasty in the pre-stent era.[45-47] Multivessel disease and complex lesions were predictors of acute occlusion during or after the procedure. Angiographic characteristics associated with abrupt closure with balloon angioplasty included long lesions, dissection, use of oversized balloons relative to the reference segment, residual stenosis >50%, intraluminal thrombus, and multivessel disease.

Abrupt closure is commonly caused by dissection from balloon angioplasty with superimposed thrombosis. Clinical features associated with increased risk of abrupt closure include diabetes mellitus, inadequate antiplatelet therapy, female gender, and extreme age. Stenting has essentially decreased abrupt closure at the end of a procedure to <1%. Also, use of peri-procedural aspirin has been shown to reduce abrupt closure during intervention. Use of heparin with ACT >300 seconds in the absence of glycoprotein IIb/IIIa antagonists is recommended.

ACUTE/SUBACUTE STENT THROMBOSIS

With the introduction of stents to treat peripheral vascular disease came the complication of acute and subacute stent thrombosis.[48] Stent thrombosis occurred at an unacceptably higher rate in the earlier days of coronary stenting. Fortunately, the frequency of acute/subacute stent thrombosis has decreased due to several reasons including high-pressure balloon deployment, and antiplatelet treatment for several weeks after stent placement. Dual antiplatelet therapy (aspirin and clopidogrel) has been shown to significantly reduce the incidence of subacute stent thrombosis with coronary stenting.[49] Given that the vascular biological response to stent placements may be somewhat similar in the coronary circulation compared to that in the peripheral circulation, many interventionists will use the same if not similar antiplatelet regimen following peripheral vascular stenting.

SYSTEMIC

CONTRAST-INDUCED COMPLICATIONS

The adverse effects of contrast media can be divided in two categories: anaphylactoid and toxic.

- Anaphylactoid reactions include urticaria, angioedema, bronchospasm, and circulatory shock.
- Toxic effects include nausea, a hot flushing sensation, vascular congestion, metallic taste, and arrhythmias – particularly bradycardia and asystole.

The use of newer low-osmolar non-ionic contrast media has decreased the incidence of some adverse effects, especially arrhythmias.[50]

Contrast-induced nephropathy (CIN) is generally defined as a greater than 0.5 mg/dl increase in serum creatinine within 48 hours of contrast exposure. The serum creatinine usually peaks within 4–5 days and in most cases returns to normal or near normal in 1–3 weeks. The incidence of CIN varies widely to as high as 70% in various populations undergoing catheterization,[51,52] reflecting the differences in the definition of nephropathy and the risk factors of the population undergoing the procedure.

The risk factors for developing CIN include pre-existing renal disease (serum creatinine >1.5 mg/dl), diabetes mellitus, multiple myeloma, congestive heart failure, volume of contrast administered, and repeat dye exposure within 24 hours. Of these risk factors, pre-existing renal disease and diabetes mellitus seem to have the highest risk for developing CIN.

The only effective strategy in preventing CIN is the use of aggressive hydration before and after the use of contrast, minimizing the use of contrast volume, and avoiding repeat exposure within 48–72 hours. Comparison of saline infusion alone with either mannitol or forced diuresis with furosemide (frusemide) has shown that saline infusion alone is superior in preventing CIN.[53] Other trials using dopamine, aminophylline, or atrial natriuretic peptide have not shown any consistent benefit.[54,55] Other agents such as fenoldepam mesylate (selective dopamine A1 receptor agonist), and N-acetyl-cysteine (Mucomyst) have shown some promise in the prevention of CIN.[52]

RADIATION INJURIES

During the last 15 years, x-ray technologies have substantially improved our ability to treat patients using fluoroscopically guided interventional techniques. Fluoroscopically guided diagnostic and interventional procedures can be associated with excessive radiation exposure causing radiation injuries. Current fluoroscopes are easily capable of producing dose rates in the range of 0.2–0.4 Gy (20–40 rads) per minute.[56] Patients undergoing multiple or prolonged procedures are at increased risk of injury from the cumulative effects of radiation on the skin.[57-59] Radiation-induced skin injuries consist of both acute and chronic changes. Signs of acute radiation injury become apparent within 10 weeks of exposure and range from erythema (6 Gy) and hyperpigmentation to desquamation (10–15 Gy) and ulceration (18–20 Gy).[60] Chronic manifestations such as dermal atrophy, telangiectases, ulceration, and fibrosis are seen as early as 10 weeks, but may take years to fully develop.[60]

Unfortunately, many physicians who use fluoroscopy have no training or credentials in the management of radiation or the biological effects associated with its use. In 1994, the US Food and Drug Administration (FDA) Advisory Committee warned that training of physicians for modern-day use of the fluoroscope was insufficient and needed to be expanded. The American College of Cardiology and the American Heart Association also stated the urgent need for such training.[61] The Laboratory Performance Standards Committee of the Society for Cardiac Angiography and Interventions has devised guidelines for catheterization personnel about appropriate radiation monitoring and protection.[62] In summary, radiation injuries are preventable and physicians who use fluoroscopic radiation should receive adequate training in radiation physics, radiation biology, and radiation safety.

CONCLUSION

Emphasis on improved management of access sites is essential to achieve better patient care and reduced health care costs. Although vascular closure devices decrease the discomfort of prolonged compression and allow early ambulation, clinical trials have failed to demonstrate any significant reduction in major vascular complications compared with manual compression. The technology and devices to treat peripheral vascular disease are constantly being improved and it is likely that in the future the improvement will further reduce the complications associated with these procedures. Until then, operators should be prepared to handle the complications associated with peripheral vascular interventional procedures.

REFERENCES

1. Muller DW, Shamir KJ, Ellis SG, Topol EJ. Peripheral vascular complications after conventional and complex percutaneous coronary interventional procedures. Am J Cardiol 1992;69:63–8.
2. Kalinowski EA, Trerotola SO. Postcatheterization retroperitoneal hematoma due to spontaneous lumbar arterial hemorrhage. Cardiovasc Intervent Radiol 1998;21:337–9.
3. Kent KC, Moscucci M, Mansour KA, et al. Retroperitoneal hematoma after cardiac catheterization: prevalence, risk factors, and optimal management. J Vasc Surg 1994;20:905–10; discussion 910–13.
4. Omoigui NA, Califf RM, Pieper K, et al. Peripheral vascular complications in the Coronary Angioplasty Versus Excisional Atherectomy Trial (CAVEAT-I). J Am Coll Cardiol 1995;26:922–30.
5. Grines CL GS, Bakalyar D, et al. Predictors of bleeding complications following coronary angioplasty [abstract]. Circulation 1991;84:II-591.
6. Agarwal R, Agarwal SK, Roubin GS, et al. Clinically guided closure of femoral arterial pseudoaneurysms complicating cardiac catheterization and coronary angioplasty. Cathet Cardiovasc Diagn 1993;30:96–100.
7. Pan M, Medina A, Suarez de Lezo J, et al. Obliteration of femoral pseudoaneurysm complicating coronary intervention by direct puncture and permanent or removable coil insertion. Am J Cardiol 1997;80:786–8.
8. Kang SS, Labropoulos N, Mansour MA, Baker WH. Percutaneous ultrasound guided thrombin injection: a new method for treating postcatheterization femoral pseudoaneurysms. J Vasc Surg 1998;27:1032–8.
9. Brophy DP, Sheiman RG, Amatulle P, Akbari CM. Iatrogenic femoral pseudoaneurysms: thrombin injection after failed US-guided compression. Radiology 2000;214:278–82.
10. Samal AK, White CJ, Collins TJ, Ramee SR, Jenkins JS. Treatment of femoral artery pseudoaneurysm with percutaneous thrombin injection. Catheter Cardiovasc Interv 2001;53:259–63.
11. Waigand J, Uhlich F, Gross CM, Thalhammer C, Dietz R. Percutaneous treatment of pseudoaneurysms and arteriovenous fistulas after invasive vascular procedures. Catheter Cardiovasc Interv 1999;47:157–64.
12. Thalhammer C, Kirchherr AS, Uhlich F, Waigand J, Gross CM. Postcatheterization pseudoaneurysms and arteriovenous fistulas: repair with percutaneous implantation of endovascular covered stents. Radiology 2000;214:127–31.
13. Schaub F, Theiss W, Heinz M, Zagel M, Schomig A. New aspects in ultrasound-guided compression repair of postcatheterization femoral artery injuries. Circulation 1994;90:1861–5.
14. Moote DJ, Hilborn MD, Harris KA, et al. Postarteriographic femoral pseudoaneurysms: treatment with ultrasound-guided compression. Ann Vasc Surg 1994;8:325–31.
15. Cox GS, Young JR, Gray BR, Grubb MW, Hertzer NR. Ultrasound-guided compression repair of postcatheterization pseudoaneurysms: results of treatment in one hundred cases. J Vasc Surg 1994;19:683–6.
16. Chatterjee T, Do DD, Kaufmann U, Mahler F, Meier B. Ultrasound-guided compression repair for treatment of femoral artery pseudoaneurysm: acute and follow-up results. Cathet Cardiovasc Diagn 1996;38:335–40.
17. Kazmers A, Meeker C, Nofz K, et al. Nonoperative therapy for postcatheterization femoral artery pseudoaneurysms. Am Surg 1997;63:199–204.
18. Shires T. Principles of Surgery. New York: McGraw Hill, 1984: 240–1.

19. Boylis SM LE, Gilas NW. Traumatic retroperitoneal hematoma. Am J Surg 1962;103:477.

20. Haviv YS, Nahir M, Pikarski A, Shiloni E, Safadi R. A late retroperitoneal hematoma mimicking acute appendicitis – an unusual complication of coronary angioplasty. Eur J Med Res 1996;1:591–2.

21. Grier D, Hartnell G. Percutaneous femoral artery puncture: practice and anatomy. Br J Radiol 1990;63:602–4.

22. Smith SM, Galland RB. Late presentation of femoral artery complications following percutaneous cannulation for cardiac angiography or angioplasty. J Cardiovasc Surg (Torino) 1992;33:437–9.

23. Perings SM, Kelm M, Jax T, Strauer BE. A prospective study on incidence and risk factors of arteriovenous fistulae following transfemoral cardiac catheterization. Int J Cardiol 2003;88:223–8.

24. Kelm M, Perings SM, Jax T, et al. Incidence and clinical outcome of iatrogenic femoral arteriovenous fistulas: implications for risk stratification and treatment. J Am Coll Cardiol 2002;40:291–7.

25. Cleveland KO, Gelfand MS. Invasive staphylococcal infections complicating percutaneous transluminal coronary angioplasty: three cases and review. Clin Infect Dis 1995;21:93–6.

26. Smith TP, Cruz CP, Moursi MM, Eidt JF. Infectious complications resulting from use of hemostatic puncture closure devices. Am J Surg 2001;182:658–62.

27. Maki DG, McCormick RD, Uman SJ, Wirtanen GW. Septic endarteritis due to intra-arterial catheters for cancer chemotherapy. I. Evaluation of an outbreak. II. Risk factors, clinical features and management, III. Guidelines for prevention. Cancer 1979;44:1228–40.

28. Brummitt CF, Kravitz GR, Granrud GA, Herzog CA. Femoral endarteritis due to *Staphylococcus aureus* complicating percutaneous transluminal coronary angioplasty. Am J Med 1989;86:822–4.

29. Frazee BW, Flaherty JP. Septic endarteritis of the femoral artery following angioplasty. Rev Infect Dis 1991;13:620–3.

30. Dougherty SH. Pathobiology of infection in prosthetic devices. Rev Infect Dis 1988;10:1102–17.

31. Carey D, Martin JR, Moore CA, Valentine MC, Nygaard TW. Complications of femoral artery closure devices. Catheter Cardiovasc Interv 2001;52:3–7; discussion 8.

32. Humphries AW. Evaluation of the Natural History and Result of Treatment involving the Lower Extremities. New York: McGraw-Hill, 1973.

33. Connors JP, Thanavaro S, Shaw RC, et al. Urgent myocardial revascularization for dissection of the left main coronary artery: a complication of coronary angiography. J Thorac Cardiovasc Surg 1982;84:349–52.

34. Bourassa MG, Noble J. Complication rate of coronary arteriography. A review of 5250 cases studied by a percutaneous femoral technique. Circulation 1976;53:106–14.

35. Guss SB, Zir LM, Garrison HB, et al. Coronary occlusion during coronary angiography. Circulation 1975;52:1063–8.

36. Feit A, Kahn R, Chowdhry I, et al. Coronary artery dissection secondary to coronary arteriography: case report and review. Cathet Cardiovasc Diagn 1984;10:177–81.

37. Morise AP, Hardin NJ, Bovill EG, Gundel WD. Coronary artery dissection secondary to coronary arteriography: presentation of three cases and review of the literature. Cathet Cardiovasc Diagn 1981;7:283–96.

38. Morice MC. Immediate post PTCA percutaneous suture of femoral arteries with the Perclose Device: results of high volume users. J Am Coll Cardiol 1998;31(suppl. A):1033–104.

39. Pipkin W, Brophy C, Nesbit R, Mondy Iii JS. Early experience with infectious complications of percutaneous femoral artery closure devices. J Vasc Surg 2000;32:205–8.

40. Nehler MR, Lawrence WA, Whitehill TA, et al. Iatrogenic vascular injuries from percutaneous vascular suturing devices. J Vasc Surg 2001;33:943–7.

41. Sprouse LR 2nd, Botta DM Jr, Hamilton IN Jr. The management of peripheral vascular complications associated with the use of percutaneous suture-mediated closure devices. J Vasc Surg 2001;33:688–93.

42. Eidt JF, Habibipour S, Saucedo JF, et al. Surgical complications from hemostatic puncture closure devices. Am J Surg 1999;178:511–6.

43. Baim DS, Knopf WD, Hinohara T, et al. Suture-mediated closure of the femoral access site after cardiac catheterization: results of the suture to ambulate and discharge (STAND I and STAND II) trials. Am J Cardiol 2000;85:864–9.

44. Sesana M, Vaghetti M, Albiero R, et al. Effectiveness and complications of vascular access closure devices after interventional procedures. J Invas Cardiol 2000;12:395–9.

45. Becker GJ, Katzen BT, Dake MD. Noncoronary angioplasty. Radiology 1989;170:921–40.

46. Gardiner GA Jr, Meyerovitz MF, Stokes KR, et al. Complications of transluminal angioplasty. Radiology 1986;159:201–8.

47. Pentecost MJ, Criqui MH, Dorros G, et al. Guidelines for peripheral percutaneous transluminal angioplasty of the abdominal aorta and lower extremity vessels. A statement for health professionals from a special writing group of the Councils on Cardiovascular Radiology, Arteriosclerosis, Cardio-Thoracic and Vascular Surgery, Clinical Cardiology, and Epidemiology and Prevention, the American Heart Association. Circulation 1994;89:511–31.

48. Sigwart U, Puel J, Mirkovitch V, Joffre F, Kappenberger L. Intravascular stents to prevent occlusion and restenosis after transluminal angioplasty. N Engl J Med 1987;316:701–6.

49. Berger PB, Bell MR, Hasdai D, et al. Safety and efficacy of ticlopidine for only 2 weeks after successful intracoronary stent placement. Circulation 1999;99:248–53.

50. Baim DS, Grossman W. Complications of cardiac catheterization. In: Cardiac Catheterization, Angiography, and Intervention. Baltimore: Williams and Wilkins, 1996: 17–38.

51. Porter GA. Contrast-associated nephropathy. Am J Cardiol 1989;64:22E–26E.

52. Lepor NE. Radiocontrast nephropathy: the dye is not cast. Rev Cardiovasc Med 2000;1:43–54.

53. Solomon R, Werner C, Mann D, D'Elia J, Silva P. Effects of saline, mannitol, and furosemide to prevent acute decreases in renal function induced by radiocontrast agents. N Engl J Med 1994;331:1416–20.

54. Gare M, Haviv YS, Ben-Yehuda A, et al. The renal effect of low-dose dopamine in high-risk patients undergoing coronary angiography. J Am Coll Cardiol 1999;34:1682–8.

55. Abizaid AS, Clark CE, Mintz GS, et al. Effects of dopamine and aminophylline on contrast-induced acute renal failure after coronary angioplasty in patients with preexisting renal insufficiency. Am J Cardiol 1999;83:260–3, A5.

56. den Boer A, de Feijter PJ, Serruys PW, Roelandt JR. Real-time quantification and display of skin radiation during coronary angiography and intervention. Circulation 2001;104:1779–84.

57. Koenig TR, Wolff D, Mettler FA, Wagner LK. Skin injuries from fluoroscopically guided procedures: part 1, characteristics of radiation injury. AJR Am J Roentgenol 2001;177:3–11.

58. Koenig TR, Mettler FA, Wagner LK. Skin injuries from fluoroscopically guided procedures: part 2, review of 73 cases and recommendations for minimizing dose delivered to patient. AJR Am J Roentgenol 2001;177:13–20.

59. Vano E, Goicolea J, Galvan C, et al. Skin radiation injuries in patients following repeated coronary angioplasty procedures. Br J Radiol 2001;74:1023–31.

60. Archambeau JO, Pezner R, Wasserman T. Pathophysiology of irradiated skin and breast. Int J Radiat Oncol Biol Phys 1995;31:1171–85.

61. Archer BR. High-dose fluoroscopy: the administrator's responsibilities. Radiol Manage 2002;24:26–32; quiz 33–5.

62. Balter S. Guidelines for personnel radiation monitoring in the cardiac catheterization laboratory. Laboratory Performance Standards Committee of the Society for Cardiac Angiography and Interventions. Cathet Cardiovasc Diagn 1993;30:277–9.

Index

Note to index: page locators in bold indicate tables

T - #0330 - 101024 - C0 - 246/189/12 [14] - CB - 9781841843469 - Gloss Lamination